**INTERDISCIPLINARY
INVESTIGATION OF THE BRAIN**

ADVANCES IN BEHAVIORAL BIOLOGY

Editorial Board:

Jan Bures   *Institute of Physiology, Prague, Czechoslovakia*

Irwin Kopin   *Laboratory of Clinical Science, National Institute of Mental Health, Bethesda, Maryland*

Bruce McEwen   *Department of Biology, Rockefeller University, New York, New York*

James McGaugh   *Department of Psychobiology, University of California, Irvine, California*

Karl Pribram   *Department of Psychology, Jordan Hall, Stanford University School of Medicine, Stanford, California*

Jay Rosenblatt   *Institute of Animal Behavior, Rutgers University, Newark, New Jersey*

Lawrence Weiskrantz   *Institute of Experimental Psychology, University of Oxford, Oxford, England*

Volume 1 • BRAIN CHEMISTRY AND MENTAL DISEASE
Edited by Beng T. Ho and William M. McIsaac • 1971

Volume 2 • NEUROBIOLOGY OF THE AMYGDALA
Edited by Basil E. Eleftheriou • 1972

Volume 3 • AGING AND THE BRAIN
Edited by Charles M. Gaitz • 1972

Volume 4 • THE CHEMISTRY OF MOOD, MOTIVATION, AND MEMORY
Edited by James L. McGaugh • 1972

Volume 5 • INTERDISCIPLINARY INVESTIGATION OF THE BRAIN
Edited by J. P. Nicholson • 1972

INTERDISCIPLINARY INVESTIGATION OF THE BRAIN

The Proceedings of a Symposium held at
Oxford, April 11th – 13th, 1972

**Edited by
J. P. Nicholson**

*Physics Department
Westminster Hospital
Page Street Wing
London SW1
ENGLAND*

Φ PLENUM PRESS · LONDON–NEW YORK · 1972

Library of Congress Catalog Card Number: 72-91037

ISBN 0-306-37905-8

©1972 by Plenum Publishing Company Ltd

Plenum Publishing Company Ltd
Davis House
8 Scrubs Lane
Harlesden
London NW10 6SE

Telephone 01-969 4727

U.S. Edition published by

Plenum Publishing Corporation
227 West 17th Street
New York, New York 10011

All Rights Reserved

No part of this book may be reproduced, stored in a
retrieval system, or transmitted, in any form or by
any means, electronic, mechanical, photocopying,
microfilming, recording or otherwise, without
written permission from the Publisher.

Set in cold type by Academic Industrial Epistemology,
London
Printed in Great Britain by J.W. Arrowsmith Ltd,
London and Bristol

PREFACE

This volume contains the Proceedings of a Conference on "Interdisciplinary Investigation of the Brain" held at Oxford, 11-13th, April 1972.

The Congress was organised by the UK Liaison Committee for Sciences Allied to Medicine and Biology (SAMB). This organisation was set up in 1965 to promote the interdisciplinary approach to medical and biological problems. The present Conference is the third to be held under the auspices of SAMB. It was planned to cover a wide range of interests by inviting workers from various disciplines to speak about their work in progress.

It is hoped that the present volume will be of interest and will vindicate this multidisciplinary approach.

SESSIONAL CHAIRMEN

R. Cooper
    Burden Neurological Centre, Stapleton, Bristol, England

E.S. Watkins
    Department of Neurosurgery, London Hospital, Whitechapel,
    London, E1, England

W.A. Cobb
    National Hospital for Nervous Diseases, Queens Square,
    London, WC1, England

J.P.M. Tizard
    Institute of Child Health, Hammersmith Hospital,
    London, W12, England

G.B. Arden
    Institute of Opthalmology, London, WC1, England

C.R. Evans
    Division of Computer Science, National Physical Laboratory,
    Teddington, Middlesex, England

CONTRIBUTORS

D. Albe-Fessard
    Laboratoire de Physiologie des Centres Nerveux, Paris, France

J. Andrew
    Middlesex Hospital, London, W1, England

M.A. Armstrong James
    London Hospital, Whitechapel, London, E1, England

B.G. Batchelor
    Electronics Department, University of Southampton,
    Southampton, England

C.D. Binnie,
    Department of Clinical Neurophysiology, St. Bartholomew's
    Hospital, London, EC1, England

M.V. Driver
    Maudsley Hospital, London, SE5, England

I.D. Eversden
   Atkinson Morley's Hospital, Wimbledon, London, SW20, England

P. Fenwick
   Institute of Psychiatry, De Crespigny Park, London, SE5, England

I.J. Good
   Department of Statistics, Virginia Polytechnic Institute, Blacksburg, Virginia, U.S.A.

J.A.B. Gray
   Medical Research Council, London, England

R.L. Gregory
   Department of Anatomy, University of Bristol, Bristol, England

M.L. Hyde
   Audiology Group, ISVR, University of Southampton, Southampton, England

D.S.L. Lloyd
   Department of Clinical Neurophysiology, St. Bartholomew's Hospital, London, EC1, England

D.G. McDowall
   Department of Anaesthetics, University of Leeds, Leeds, England

B.B. MacGillivray
   National Hospital, Queens Square London, WC1, England

D. Regan
   Department of Communications, University of Keele, Staffordshire, England

J.O. Rowan
   Institute of Neurological Sciences, Southern General Hospital, Glasgow, Scotland

N. de M. Rudolf
   Department of Clinical Neurophysiology, West London Hospital, Hammersmith, London, W6, England

J.C. Shaw
   MRC Clinical Psychiatry Unit, Graylingwell Hospital, Chichester, Sussex, England

I.A. Silver
   Department of Pathology, Medical School, Bristol, England

H. Spekreijse
   Laboratory for Medical Physics, Herengracht 196, Amsterdam, The Netherlands

H.G. Vaughan
   Albert Einstein College of Medicine, New York, U.S.A.

CONTENTS

Preface v

Contributors vii

Inaugural Address 1
   J.A.B. Gray

The Regulation of Cerebral Blood Flow and
Intracranial Pressure 9
   D.G. McDowall

Measurement of Cerebral Blood Flow with
Special Reference to the Use of Radioisotopes 15
   J.O. Rowan

The Measurement and Interpretation of
Cerebral Oxygen Tension 29
   I.A. Silver

Intracranial Pressure Measurements -
A Review of Available Methods 39
   I.D. Eversden

Micro-Electrode Recordings in the Human
Thalamus during Stereotaxic Surgery 53
   J. Andrew and N. de M. Rudolf

Integration Techniques for Localisation
during Stereotaxic Exploration of the
Thalamus and Basal Ganglia 73
   M.A. Armstrong-James

Upon the Possible Role and Origin of
Rhythmic Activities Observed in Parkinsonian
Patients' Thalamus 83
   D. Albe-Fessard

EEG Assessment in Clinical Medicine 97
   M.V. Driver

Clinical Electroencephalography and
Computing 109
   B.B. MacGillivray

Signal Analysis 119
   P. Fenwick

Topographic Analysis of the EEG 133
   J.C. Shaw

Electric Response Audiometry 147
   M.L. Hyde

Pattern Recognition in EEG 153
   B.G. Batchelor, C.D. Binnie
   and D.S.L. Lloyd

A Note on the Visual Neurosensorium 167
   H.G. Vaughan

Cortical Evoked Potentials 177
   D. Regan

System Analysis Approach to the
Problems of Vision 193
   H. Spekreijse

Food for Thought 213
   I.J. Good

A Look at Biological and Machine
Perception 229
   R.L. Gregory

INAUGURAL ADDRESS TO THE CONGRESS ON INTERDISCIPLINARY
INVESTIGATION OF THE BRAIN, OXFORD - APRIL 11-13th 1972

J.A.B. GRAY

Secretary of the Medical Research Council
20 Park Crescent, London W1N 4AL

Mr. Chairman, ladies and gentlemen. First I must thank you for inviting me to give the opening address to this meeting. This is a meeting which it gives me particular pleasure to address, first because it brings me back for a moment to problems of the nervous system, which was my own scientific interest until I moved to an administrative post. I am also pleased because in many fields a multidisciplinary approach can be of considerable value and importance and the Medical Research Council actively tries to foster teams to undertake multidisciplinary attacks on a variety of problems. I am glad of an opportunity to consider not only the advantages of interdisciplinary investigations of the brain, but also an opportunity to talk about some of the realities and practical difficulties that do arise in organizing multidisciplinary teams.

When giving this talk I intend first to look briefly at what the study of nervous systems involves. Then I will go on to say something about the nature and needs of a multidisciplinary approach and I hope I am not wrong in using this somewhat wider term than the term interdisciplinary used in your title. Finally, I want to turn to some of the factors which have to be taken into account in organizing multidisciplinary teams.

THE NERVOUS SYSTEM

The nervous system as an object of study has certain characteristics. It is, for a biological topic, relatively circumscribed but at the same time it is perhaps the most complex and difficult probelm which one can find. It is not surprising, therefore, that the reasons which make us study the nervous system are complex; furthermore the reasons which persuade the country to find the money for such studies are also complex. The most fundamental reason for research on the nervous system is in my view that the very machine we use to solve other problems must have a particular attraction as a problem in itself. Nevertheless many of us, and not least the public who fund research, have more practical ideas connected with improving our ability to deal with real life problems, for example disorders of health. The nature of the motive and objective can significantly alter the emphasis to be placed on particular lines of work at particular times and places but they do not in themselves alter the fundamental pattern of the problem. In any case, the really important practical point is that neither the formal logic of the problem nor the demand of practical needs can alter the fact that the most important pragmatic arbiter of what can be done and what is done is practicability.

Let me now look briefly at the structure of the fundamental problem: I deliberately use the singular. We are faced with understanding a mysterious black box, or rather I should say a set of black boxes, which are all fundamentally similar but exhibit a considerable range of differences. Basic to our studies must therefore be a knowledge of what they do and how they behave. Behavioural studies involve at least three major elements: the description of behaviour in the usual living environment; observing the behavioural responses to experimental situations; the study of abnormal behaviour. The overall problem requires them on a significant sample of our set of black boxes. The range of expertise required for such studies obviously includes every speciality in the behavioural sciences from psychiatry to invertebrate behaviour. The behavioural patterns must be explained in terms of the underlying mechanisms. Behaviour is a response to circumstances. Basically information is received, complex events take place in the nervous system and finally some external expression of a response takes place and can be observed. At the least we can be sure that these complex processes must depend on two factors; one must be structural features, macro or micro, which are genetically determined, the other is the information stored in the system as a result of previous experience. There are therefore a series of basic questions: what are the processes in operational terms; how is information coded in transmission, in analysis and in storage; what are the transformations between these; and how are the operations performed in terms of code signals. These questions are very complex, involving as they do the interactions of large numbers of units and so far, despite considerable increases in knowledge, we are still only scratching the surface. As a background to these problems we need knowledge of the function of individual units and in this area there has been very great progress in recent years and these advances have involved many disciplines, but particularly neurophysiology, neuropharmacology and electron microscopy.

Generally the keynote in any approach to the problems of the nervous system is to find some way of simplifying and reducing the complexity of the problems; hence the need to classify the characteristics of the elements of the nervous system in respect, for example, to their anatomical localization, to their morphology, to their behaviour, to the character of their transmitters and other features of such a kind. Hence the need to look for general principles, e.g. in the similar behaviour of units and their signal patterns, and in features in the coding of information, common to different parts of a nervous system or to different nervous systems. Ideas of localization and characterization have given rise to an important group of studies - studies of abnormalities or of changes in behaviour resulting from lesions or stimulations which can modify a part characterized in some way; these lesions may be brought about by disease or by experiment. For example, there can be interference related to anatomy, such as experimental coagulations or naturally-occurring tumours. There can be interference related to chemistry, for example through the administration of substances believed to have a particular effect in relation to a group of cells having a particular transmitter. And then there can be interference related to previous learning situations; these affect features of a nervous system characterized in yet another way. Alongside such investigations of the machinery which underlies behaviour there are important areas of study concerned with the supplies needed for building and running the machine and the manner in which they are used.

In what I have just said I have talked as if the problem could be treated solely as an intellectual exercise constrained by practicability. But, as we all know, many important questions arise (and some can even be answered) from practical need and empirical finding. For example many conditions of disorder have been studied to determine the characteristics of the disorder or the nature of the lesion to the nervous system. Empirical methods have been used to improve the treatment or care of patients and studies have been needed to understnad and improve the situation. Clearly such practical studies merge into and depend on work of the kind I have already mentioned.

There have been great advances in techniques in recent years but it is all too obvious that both conceptual methods and intrumentation for recording the required information still need to develop very much further. The need to develop conceptual methods relates to the complexity of the problem and the need for simplification. This implies the need to determine what are the most useful simplifications and these might perhaps eventually prove to be simplifications which are determined by the operational properties of the system rather than simplifications based on, for example, anatomy or transmitter characteristics. Such thinking is long term. More immediately there are other technical gaps.

One group of techniques in particular I would mention. Man is a particularly special animal in studies of the nervous system. Man is the only species that can be used for many behavioural investigations; it is only man that can describe certain kinds of response and it is only in man that one gets the behavioural disorders which are of such major social importance; it is to benefit man that the practical objectives of work on the nervous system are determined. However, man's brain is inaccessible and for this reason, despite major advances, our methods for looking at the physical and chemical activity of the human brain are inevitably very inadequate compared to those which can be used with experimental animals. This gap is very important. It is important because of the practical needs of man but it is also important because of its theoretical implications. Crudely, man is unique for behavioural studies but experimental study of the underlying machine must be carried out almost entirely on experimental animals; the links between the two may be crucial and the barrier around the human nervous system demands major advances in technique.

THE NEEDS FOR MULTIDISCIPLINARY WORK

The problem I have outlined involves many disciplines and these interact at many levels and in many ways. Within this pattern multidisciplinary teams or multidisciplinary studies can mean a number of different things. I would like to put these in three categories. First, there is the collaboration between individuals of different biological disciplines but each working on the nervous system: for example, psychiatrists, neuro-surgeons, neurophysiologists, neuropharmacologists, as well as others such as developmental biologists and biophysicists working on the nervous system. These are all people working in the neuro-sciences and for any particular problem several disciplines may be involved. For example, a project arising from the intrinsic logic of the problem, such as an investigation of memory, can involve behavioural, anatomical and physiological techniques in combination, while a practical question related to say biogenic amines can involve psychiatrists, biochemists and pharmacologists. Collaborations of this kind all involve collaborations between people whose basic interest is the study of the nervous system, but whose background training and knowledge of techniques is different. Close collaborations are usually fairly straightforward and of course there are quite a number of individuals who have developed a competence in more than one of the methods applicable to the study of the nervous system.

The second type of collaboration I would like to mention is that between people working in the neuro-sciences and people who can develop new methodology. There can be problems here. Such a collaboration needs to be between individuals who have at least a minimum level of a common language. A neurobiologist needs to be able to understand enough of the technical problems to make a contribution to the definition of what is needed and the individual responsible for the method, be he engineer, physicist or chemist, needs to have sufficient understanding and sympathy with the problem to be solved if anything more than a tidying up on existing techniques is to be achieved. While of course there are many successful, some very highly successful, collaborations of this kind, they can raise problems. How far can the engineer or physicist become a specialist in improving methods for investigating nervous systems? How much time can he spend without having to make it his whole career, and if he does make it his whole career, what are his career prospects? Has he cut himself off completely from the more orthodox steps in his profession, and if he stays in the neuro-sciences can he, with his background, have adequate opportunity to lead the team or must he usually be in a position of helping somebody else to solve that other person's problem. Posts can be and have been created but that does not answer all these questions.

Then there is the third group whom we must consider, that is, those who by their work on non-biological systems have learnt methods of handling complex processes and may be in a position to introduce new ideas into thinking about nervous systems. I am of course talking about mathematicians and physicists and engineers interested in such problems as communication or control systems.

Their rôle in the neuro-sciences is of course still controversial, though less so than it was; I am sure we must encourage people of this type. The problems are very difficult and there is probably a long way to go before any major success is achieved but there will be no major progress unless the ground is explored and smaller advances made. I think it is unlikely that a quick excursion into the neuro-sciences for any such people is likely to be productive. Those that get into this field need to be really original and need to be prepared and in a position to spend a great deal of time on the subject; they need to be throughout in close contact with neuro-biologists of all kinds so that they are in a position to get a deep understanding of nervous systems so that their thinking is clearly based on the realities of the biological evidence.

PRACTICAL ASPECTS

I would now like to turn to some of the practical problems that arise in organizing multidisciplinary teams. It is one thing to praise multidisciplinary studies - like being against sin, we're all for multidisciplinary studies. What is important is the solution of the practical questions: how should work in the neuro-sciences be organized and what is the place of multidisciplinary teams? What are the practical difficulties about organizing such teams? I would like to look briefly at these two questions.

In relation to the first question one must realize that a vast amount of work in the neuro-sciences is being done and can be done by individuals working within a single discipline, usually within a university or hospital department. This of course does not mean that many of these individuals do not from time to time undertake a collaborative project with a colleague from a neighbouring laboratory or department in a different discipline, but these arrangements can come and go as is appropriate and opportunity arises. It is good that much research does go on in this way - indeed, it is necessary that it should. It is through this kind of situation that the work in the neuro-sciences retains close contact with all the many other problems which have been and are being tackled through the methodology of the parent disciplines in fields other than the nervous system. But there is, I believe, more than this to the answer to the question of how the neuro-sciences should be organized. The work of individuals needs to be complemented by that of multidisciplinary teams working in defined areas or towards defined objectives. In my view such teams need to be placed in such a way that they not only carry out their own particular task but also act as a centre and catalyst for interdisciplinary collaboration between individuals working in discipline-based laboratories or departments.

The second question concerns the practical problems which arise in organizing successful teams. In my view there are three important conditions which must be met. First there must be a reasonably circumscribed common aim for the team within the vast field of the neuro-sciences. Second there needs to be a significant amount of genuine collaborative work between all the various individuals making up the team, and third the individuals need to be chosen and the team so placed that although part of a multidisciplinary team they do not become isolated from developments in their own discipline relevant to the neuro-sciences.

We must remember that the operative word for this element in multidisciplinary research is 'team'. This means that the continuance of the basic conditions and ultimate success depend on a willingness of all the staff to act as members of a team and for the more senior staff to provide continuously the leadership that is essential to make a team viable. Within the general framework I have indicated, teams can obviously be run successfully in different ways. For example there may be a specific objective and all work may be organized within a single collaborative plan or alternatively the area of operation may be less well defined and individuals may carry out separate programmes within this common area for part of their time while participating in various collaborative studies as well. However, whatever the pattern, there must be leadership and there must be a general willingness to put team work first. If on the contrary individuals work in multidisciplinary establishments and withdraw from working on common problems with those of other disciplines, they may become even more isolated than individualists in disciplinary departments for they will find themselves in a situation in which they have neither a problem nor a discipline in common with their colleagues. The members of a multidisciplinary team need to be of a somewhat gregarious character, they need not only to work with their fellows, but on behalf of the team manintain day to day contact with other areas of their own discipline. For the latter reason it is usually desirable to place teams within a university environment.

These concepts of multidisciplinary teamwork do have considerable implications for the individuals concerned and in particular for those at the age when they are establishing their individual reputations. A contribution, however important, to the output of a team sometimes does not have, or at least may not be thought to have, the same impact on a career as an individual contribution. On the other hand multidisciplinary teams cannot normally operate unless there are workers of some seniority capable of directing one or two juniors in each major discipline concerned. Furthermore as the work of a team develops the objectives will need to be adjusted and from time to time greater shifts of emphasis may be desirable. Such shifts and changes in a team's programme may not coincide with what would be the first choices of the individual members of the team. In short, teamwork demands give and take and understanding leadership if conflicting interests are to be reconciled. I have been talking about multidisciplinary teams in the neuro-sciences but these problems arise whenever circumstances force scientists into working in teams rather than as individuals. Experience has shown that when teams are really necessary, as for example in 'Big Science', attitudes adapt to the new situation. Multidisciplinary team work as a component of work on the nervous system is increasingly recognized as at least desirable and in some circumstances essential. In consequence attitudes are adapting to the realities of the situation.

CONCLUSION

The study of the nervous system is of immense complexity and the bases on which one can simplify, classify and manipulate the material derive from techniques which belong to a wide range of biological disciplines. The development of methodology is a special problem, and collaboration with engineers, physicists, chemists and others for this purpose is essential. It is also desirable to bring into the field of the neuro-sciences those experienced with the ways of handling problems having some similarities amongst man-made systems.

The multidisciplinary approach to the neuro-sciences can mean simply that individuals working in the environment of their own discipline actively collaborate from time to time with colleagues working in departments devoted to other disciplines. But the pattern of work in the neuro-sciences is not complete without multidisciplinary teams. If such teams are to provide a truly multidisciplinary approach, they must each have a purpose. This means the acceptance of common leadership in a common area of endeavour with at least a proportion of collaborative work. There are real difficulties in developing successful teams and it seems to me that there will need to be more widespread acceptance of the need to work in teams in the neuro-sciences and of the problems this creates than is perhaps at present the case.

THE REGULATION OF CEREBRAL BLOOD FLOW AND INTRACRANIAL PRESSURE

D.G. McDOWALL

Department of Anaesthesia, The University of Leeds

MAJOR ARTERIES TO THE BRAIN

The arterial input to the brain, in man, is entirely through the two internal carotids and two vertebral arteries; the latter joining together to form the basilar artery. Each internal carotid artery and the basilar artery delivers approximately one-third of the cerebral blood supply. These three input vessels link up at the base of the brain to form the Circle of Willis. From this arterial anastomosis the major medium-sized intracranial arteries arise. The advantage of this system is that variations in calibre of the vessels in the neck, due for example to movements of the neck, are compensated for by re-routing of blood through the Circle of Willis.

Under normal conditions the vascular resistance offered by these major vessels is small, so that the arterial pressure measured at the Circle of Willis is 80-95% of that in the femoral artery (Symon, 1967). These carotid and vertebral arteries are, however, richly supplied with sympathetic fibres, and are capable of active vasoconstriction. Clinically, this can sometimes be seen in response to the insertion of a needle into these vessels during carotid angiography. Atheromatous obstruction of these vessels also occurs, though Brice et al. (1964) have shown that the cross-sectional area has to be reduced below 5 sq. mm. before flow is affected. Many patients can withstand complete occlusion of one internal carotid artery without signs of cerebral ischaemia, so great is the reserve capacity of the other supply vessels to the Circle of Willis.

MAJOR VEINS FROM THE BRAIN

Blood from the brain mainly leaves via the two internal jugular veins. These veins lie in the loose tissue of the neck, and so venous pressure within them is virtually atmospheric. Just within the skull lie the jugular bulbs, and in these the venous pressure is above atmospheric due to the rigid outflow orifices.

CEREBROVASCULAR RESISTANCE

Cerebrovascular resistance is conventionally defined as mean aortic pressure minus jugular bulb pressure, divided by the cerebral blood flow. This calculated resistance therefore includes the resistance of the internal carotids and vertebral arteries which, as we have already seen, is normally low. It also includes the resistance of the medium-sized and small cerebral arteries, as well as that of the rather rigid intracranial venous sinuses.

An alternative method of calculating vascular resistance is to derive the perfusion pressure by subtracting mean intracranial CSF pressure from mean arterial blood pressure, and this yields values of cerebrovascular resistance which do not include the contribution to resistance made by the venous sinuses.

The sympathetic nerve fibres which travel with the internal carotid arteries and the vertebral arteries have been traced along the medium-sized and small cerebral arteries, but appear to stop short of the arterioles. It seems likely, therefore, that on the arterial side there are two components of vascular resistance: the large, medium and small arteries, which appear to be capable of neurogenically initiated responses, and the arterioles which are controlled by the local factors discussed below. Of these two components the arteriolar resistance is normally much the more important, but under pathological conditions - e.g. arterial spasm - the major part of total vascular resistance may be exerted proximal to the arterioles.

CONTROL OF ARTERIOLES

The cerebral arterioles to the factors listed in the Table below. This, however, is not intended as a complete list.

CO_2	High PCO_2 lowers resistance; lower PCO_2 increases resistance.
Blood-pressure	Autoregulation, i.e. resistance is adjusted so that flow remains constant over a range of cerebral perfusion pressures.
O_2	The brain is rather insensitive to changes in oxygen tension unless arterial PO_2 is reduced below 45 mm Hg, equivalent to a venous PO_2 of about 25 mm Hg.
Metabolic control	Arteriolar resistance adapts so that there is a balance between local blood supply and local metabolic needs.

All the points listed in the above Table are well-known, so I will enlarge on only a few aspects. Firstly, autoregulation is a very sensitive mechanism and is readily deranged with only minimal trauma or insult. Secondly, the metabolic flow control mechanism is extremely rapid in action. In a recent study of a new anaesthetic drug, cerebral flow fell within seconds of metabolic depression produced by the deepening of anaesthesia (Pickerodt et al: *Postgrad. Med. J.*, (in press)). Thirdly, it is remarkable that an organ which is so susceptible to oxygen deprivation should possess flow control mechanisms which appear to be much more sensitive to PCO_2 change than to PO_2 change.

The most popular hypothesis of cerebral arteriolar control at the moment is that this largely depends on the pH of the extracellular fluid of the arteriolar smooth muscle wall. It is stated that an acid shift in this extracellular fluid pH causes vasodilatation, and vice versa. Figure 1 illustrates this hypothesis and demonstrates that the CO_2 and O_2 responsiveness of the cerebral circulation can be explained in this manner. It also emphasizes, incidentally, that the pH of the arteriolar blood is not important to cerebral arteriolar tone, because the blood brain barrier limits the interchange of hydrogen and bicarbonate ions. In this way large gradients of hydrogen ion concentration can exist between blood and brain.

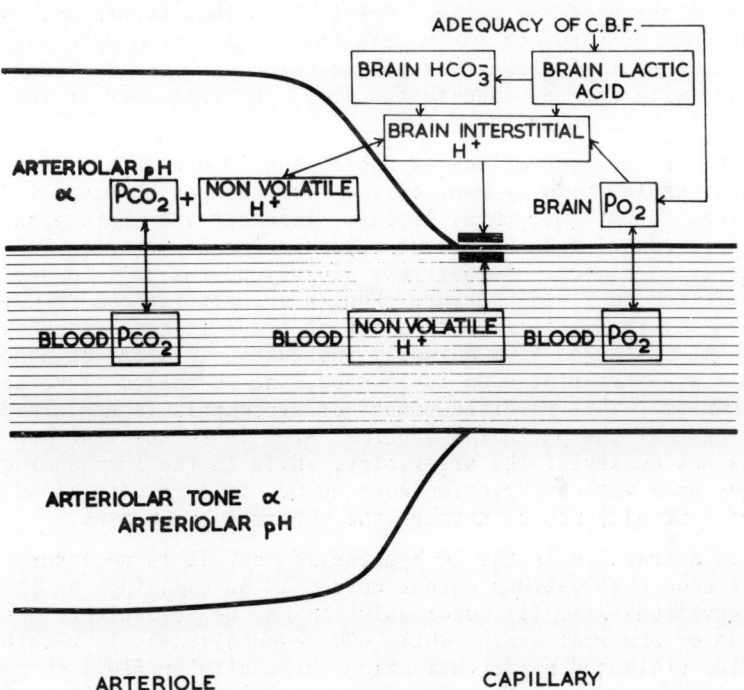

Figure 1 - The brain tissue pH hypothesis of cerebral blood flow regulation. From this figure it can be seen that changes in blood PCO_2 influence the interstitial pH of the arteriolar smooth muscle by diffusion through the vessel wall, while changes in blood H^+ ion concentration do not directly affect interstitial pH. Diminution in cerebral oxygen supply due to either hypoxic or ischaemic hypoxia affects interstitial pH through the formation of lactic acid as a consequence of increased anaerobic metabolism. (Reproduced from *General Anaesthesia*, (3rd edition., Vol. 1), (eds. Gray, T.C. and Nunn, J.F.), (Butterworths, London), (1971), p.276, by kind permission of the publishers).

Autoregulation to perfusion pressure change may also be mediated via tissue pH, but it has also been ascribed to the myogenic reactivity of the cerebral arterioles to the intravascular distending pressure.

The adaptation of flow to metabolic needs of the brain may be mediated by the pH mechanism, e.g. an increase in local metabolism will produce an increase in local PCO_2, and so a fall in extracellular fluid pH. The difficulty with this explanation has always been the problem of understanding how a down-stream change in tissue PCO_2 and pH signals to an up-stream vascular control site, i.e. the arteriole. A tentative explanation currently sustained is that vasomotion, i.e. the intermittent opening and closing of individual capillary beds, would allow such up-stream signalling during the no-flow phase of the cycle. Critical to this hypothesis is the frequency of vaso-motion in relation to the speed with which metabolic control of flow is exercised. From the observations cited above, with the new anaesthetic drug, the frequency of vaso-motion would need to be rapid.

One of the attractions of the tissue pH hypothesis is that it allows explanation of many of the flow changes observed in pathological situations; thus, tumours, infarcts and brain trauma commonly produce areas of tissue acidosis and low extracellular pH. Such areas commonly demonstrate 'luxury perfusion', loss of autoregulation to blood-pressure changes and alterations in CO_2 responsiveness; in relation to the last of these it has been shown that in some instances flow actually increases, in areas of abnormal brain when arterial PCO_2 is lowered, the so-called 'inverse steal' mechanism. This reversed effect of hypocapnia is explained by assuming that the pH in the abnormal area is so low that hypocapnia does not constrict the arterioles, while in the surrounding normal areas such vasoconstriction does occur; as a result, blood flow is preferentially routed through the abnormal brain area.

So attractive is the pH hypothesis that it is necessary to recall that some observations cannot currently be explained by it; these observations are: (i) autoregulation may be selectively lost in areas of abnormal brain, while CO_2 responsiveness is retained; (ii) during prolonged hyperventilation extracellular fluid pH returns to normal some hours before flow returns to normal; (iii) hyperbaric oxygen, even during controlled ventilation, causes cerebral vasoconstriction.

It is not possible to discuss intracranial pressure regulation in any detail. I will only make one point on this subject, and that is that when a space-occupying lesion enlarges within the skull intracranial pressure does not rise for a considerable period, because of compensatory mechanisms mainly involving the movement of cerebro-spinal fluid and venous blood volume out of the skull. However, during this phase of compensation the intracranial contents are becoming increasingly compressed, so that any sudden expansion of intracranial blood volume will produce an exaggerated increase in intracranial pressure, and may lead to the accentuation of intracranial pressure gradients; such sudden expansion in intracranial blood volume can be produced by certain anaesthetic drugs and by hypercapnia; great care is therefore necessary when a patient with an intracranial space-occupying lesion is given a cerebral vasodilating drug or a respiratory depressant drug (Fitch and McDowall, 1971).

REFERENCES

Brice, J.B., Dowsett, D.J. and Lowe, R.D. (1964). Haemodynamic effects of carotid artery stenosis, *Brit. Med. J.*, **2**, 1363.

Fitch, W. and McDowall, D.G. (1971). Effect of halothane on intracranial pressure gradients in the presence of space-occupying lesions, *Brit. J. Anaesth.*, **43**, 904.

Symon, L. (1967). A comparative study of middle cerebral pressure in dogs and macaques, *J. Physiol.*, **191**, 449-465.

MEASUREMENT OF CEREBRAL BLOOD FLOW
WITH SPECIAL REFERENCE TO THE USE OF RADIOISOTOPES

J.O. ROWAN

*Institute of Neurological Sciences
and Department of Clinical Physics and Bio-engineering, Glasgow*

It is not possible in this communication to cover all methods of cerebral blood flow measurement in detail. Since radioisotope methods are more widely used than any others, these will be outlined more fully, while some of the other methods will be described briefly together with their advantages and disadvantages.

RADIOISOTOPE METHODS

Both diffusible radioactive tracers, i.e. radioisotopes which diffuse physically between blood and tissue, and non-diffusible radioactive tracers, i.e. radioisotopes which remain in the blood stream during the time of the investigation have been used in the attempt to measure cerebral blood flow.

DIFFUSIBLE TRACERS

Which Radioisotope?

The tracer employed should be metabolically inert and should diffuse rapidly between blood and tissue. The radioisotopes which have been commonly used are:

(a) Krypton 85 - half-life 10.6 years - main emission - 670 keV gamma radiation (Lassen and Ingvar, 1961);

(b) Xenon 133 - half-life 5.27 days - main emission - 81 keV gamma-radiation (Harper et al., 1964).

The use of beta counting techniques is limited because the beta particles travel only a short distance in tissue before being absorbed, e.g. the maximum range of Krypton 85 beta particles in tissue is only 2.6 mm. Beta radiation is, therefore, only employed for measuring cerebral blood flow in the exposed superficial brain cortex. Furthermore, only 0.4% of the total Krypton 85 disintegrations result in the emission of 510 keV gamma radiation giving rise to low count rates and the need for considerable amounts of lead in collimation to define the field of view at this energy. As a consequence, Xenon 133 has been widely used in recent years. (For a general review, see Lassen and Ingvar (1972) and Rowan (1972)).

Method

Methods using diffusible tracers are based on the Fick principle, which states that the quantity of a substance, Q_t, taken up by an organ at a specific time, t, is the product of the blood flow, F, and the arterial venous difference for that substance at that time, $C_{at} - C_{vt}$, i.e.

$$Q_t = F(C_{at} - C_{vt}),$$

$$F = \frac{Q_t}{(C_{at} - C_{vt})}$$

The flow in a period, T, is found by integration, i.e.

$$F = \frac{\int_0^T Q_t dt}{\int_0^T (C_{at} - C_{vt}) dt}$$

If C_{Bt} is the concentration of the substance in brain tissue at time, t, and W_B is the weight of the brain tissue, then

$$Q_t = C_{Bt} W_B.$$

If equilibrium is reached within the time, T, the concentration of the substance in the brain tissue will be equal to the final venous concentration C_{vT} multiplied by a constant, λ, the partition coefficient expressing the ratio of the solubility of the substance in brain tissue and blood,

$$F = \frac{C_{vT} W_B \lambda}{\int_0^T (C_{at} - C_{vt}) dt},$$

that is,

$$\frac{F}{W_B} = \frac{C_{vT} \lambda}{\int_0^T (C_{at} - C_{vt}) dt}$$

It is usual to express the cerebral blood flow measurement in flow per 100 gm weight of tissue per minute.

The Kety Schmidt method, the first successful technique based on the Fick principle did not use a radioisotope tracer, but used stable nitrous oxide. With this method the patient inhaled nitrous oxide over a 10 minute period and samples of arterial and venous blood were taken serially and measured for nitrous oxide content. The use of a radioactive tracer with this method, overcomes the problems of estimating the amounts of nitrous oxide in the blood

MEASUREMENT OF CEREBRAL BLOOD FLOW

since the amount of radioactive tracer in the blood can be found by normal counting techniques.

However, the most frequently used technique employs intra-carotid artery injections of Xenon 133 and externally mounted radiation detectors to monitor the clearance of the tracer from brain tissue. With this technique the need for blood sampling is obviated and cerebral blood flow can be measured in defined regions of the brain as well as just in the brain as a whole.

When Xenon 133 dissolved in saline is injected as a bolus into the internal carotid artery, the tracer is carried to the cerebral tissue by arterial blood. Equilibration between blood and tissue takes place rapidly. Since the inert gas is highly soluble in air, about 95% of the tracer reaching the lungs is excreted and there is, therefore, no significant recirculation. On completion of the injection, the fresh arterial blood containing no radioisotope clears the tracer from the tissue and the rate of this clearance depends on the cerebral blood flow.

Detection and Data Processing

A number of collimated scintillation detectors are mounted around the patient's head. The size of the detectors and the degree of collimation are chosen to define the regions of the brain to be studied. The output pulses from each detector are fed to pulse height analysers and the selected pulses can be processed in the following ways:

(1) The pulses can be fed to a multi-track digital magnetic tape recorder with a monitoring head, such that any chosen channel can be monitored by a ratemeter and scaler to allow immediate data analysis. The ratemeter output can be recorded on a paper chart recorder to give the shape of the clearance curve, while a scaler can be used to display the total number of counts detected, i.e. the area under the clearance curve.

This is the simplest way of storing data, so that detailed analysis can be carried out on all channels at some later stage. However, the tape recording system imposes definite dead time limitations on the acceptable count rate and if these limits are exceeded, gross loss of counts will result.

(2) The pulses can be fed via a multiplexing system to a multi-channel analyser set to operate in 'multi-scaler mode' and the data can be stored in the instrument's ferrite core memory in the form of time histograms with selectable time intervals. Depending on the multiplexing system, this method may also be dead time limited.

(3) The pulses can be fed on-line to a laboratory digital computer, where again the data can be collected in the form of time histograms. In addition to the ferrite core memory, use can also be made of magnetic tape files. Analysis can be carried out using the computer and the results for every regional channel obtained in a very short time.

Sources of Error

The attempts to measure cerebral blood flow in smaller and smaller regions of the brain is often accompanied by the temptation to use systems which are unable to provide the necessary spatial resolution.

The regions of the brain defined by some systems have been assessed using point sources. The response of a scintillation detector to a point source of radiation depends on:

   (a) the inverse square of the distance of the source to the detector,
   (b) the area of the crystal exposed to radiation,
   (c) the attenuation produced by the intervening tissue.

When cerebral blood flow is being measured, the source is not a point and the result of this kind of assessment is misleading because due to the inverse square law effect, it tends to suggest that the effective volume from which gamma radiation is being detected is confined to a localised region close to the scintillation detector. However, if thin infinite uniform sources perpendicular to the axis of the detector are considered, then the detector response to such a source is independent of the source to detector distance. This is because the detector response to any point source within the extended source is inversely proportional to the square of the source to the detector distance, whereas the area of the extended source 'viewed' is directly proportional to the square of the source to detector distance and the two squared distance factors cancel. In the practical situation, however, the detector response will fall off with distance from the detector due to absorption in the intervening tissue, but this reduction in response is not as severe as that predicted by point source assessment. If a multidetector system has been designed using point source assessment, there will be considerable overlap in the adjacent detector fields of view and the idea of well defined regions of measurement using such a system is questionable.

This situation is aggravated even more due to Compton scatter within the tissue of the 81 keV gamma rays of Xenon 133. If large pulse height analyser window widths are employed, a significant percentage of the detected rays in fact, originate outwith the collimated detector field of view, again limiting the regionality of the measurement. With Xenon 133 as the tracer, the optimum setting of the lower threshold on the analyser is of the order of 75 keV eliminating all first order scatter greater than 60°. This, of course, reduces the counting sensitivity and, as the detector size is reduced more and more in the attempt to measure the cerebral blood flow from smaller regions of the brain, the effect on the counting sensitivity is considerable.

Furthermore, if the comparisons of cerebral blood flow measurements from different small regions of the brain are to be meaningful, then not only must all the nucleonic channels be set up accurately in the same way, but each detector gamma ray energy response must be the same.

The accuracy of cerebral blood flow measurements using the clearance technique also depends on the uniformity of partial pressure of Xenon within the tissue. This becomes a problem where the region under consideration is small and consists of inhomogeneous tissue. At microscopic levels, in a situation where flow is high, the

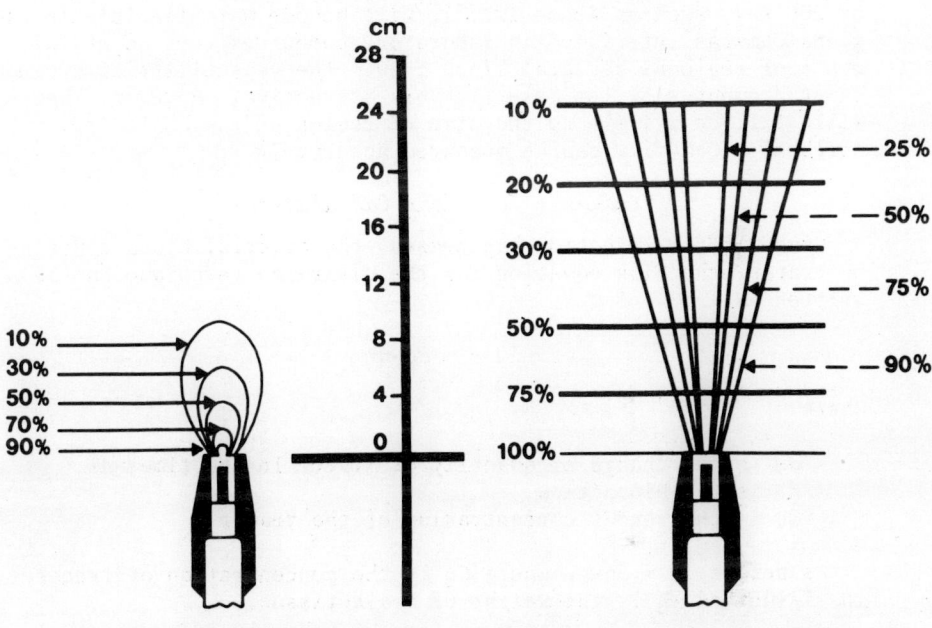

Figure 1 - Comparison of point source response and plane source response for a collimated scintillation detector. (From Gillespie, F.C. (1968). Some factors influencing the interpretation of regional blood flow measurement using inert gas clearance techniques, *Blood Flow Through Organs and Tissues*. Published by kind permission of E.& S. Livingstone).

Xenon partial pressure will decrease more rapidly than where flow is low and as a result, partial pressure gradients can be set up around different tissue boundaries. The inert gas will then diffuse from areas of high mean partial pressure to areas of low mean partial pressure altering the mean rate of clearance of both regions. The lower the mean flow in the whole region, the more significant this effect will be and this further imposes a lower limit on the size of the region from which meaningful cerebral blood flow measurements can be made, since if measurements are being made from a region of fast flow, and from an adjacent region of slow flow, diffusion of Xenon will take place between regions modifying the clearance curves obtained.

With present day detectors and using Xenon 133 as the radioactive tracer, it is indeed questionable if there are any advantages to be gained in attempting to measure cerebral blood flow from more than about eight different regions of the brain. With the introduction of cyclotron produced isotopes with energies in the region of 200 keV, such as Xenon 127, it will become more feasible to use gamma cameras interfaced to laboratory computers for the measurements of regional cerebral blood flow. The versatility of a gamma camera/computer system makes it very attractive. However, there will still be a limit to the size of region of the brain from which cerebral blood flow can be measured accurately.

Clearance Technique Calculations

Since, after injection has ceased, the arterial blood contains no tracer, the Fick equation for the clearance technique can be written as

$$dQ = - FC_V dt,$$

where

dQ is the change of quantity of tracer in the time, dt,
F is the blood flow,
C_V is the venous concentration of the tracer.

As before, $Q = C_B W_B$, where C_B is the concentration of tracer in tissue and W_B is the weight of brain tissue.

Therefore,

$$dC_B = - \frac{FC_V dt}{W_B},$$

$$C_V = \frac{C_B}{\lambda},$$

where λ is the partition coefficient, and hence

$$\frac{dC_B}{C_B} = - \frac{F dt}{W_B \lambda}.$$

The solution of this equation is

$$C_B = C_{B0} \exp(-Ft/W_B \lambda),$$

where C_{BO} is the concentration at time 0.

This is an equation of an exponential decay and when points are plotted on semi-log paper a straight line will result. After intra-carotid injection of Xenon 133, two exponential components can be extracted. These are understood to represent the distribution of flows in grey and white matter of the brain. The exponential stripping process can be carried out manually by plotting the clearance curve on semi-log paper and fitting a straight line to the latter part of the curve. This defines the slow component and the fast component can be obtained by subtraction from the initial part of the curve. Of course, this can be done more accurately and more quickly using a computer.

The slopes of the two components can be expressed as clearance half time, $T_{\frac{1}{2}}$, and from these $T_{\frac{1}{2}}$ values flow values can be calculated for grey and white matter from the following equations:

$$\text{Flow(grey matter)} = \frac{\lambda_g \cdot \ln(2 \times 100 \times 60)}{T_{\frac{1}{2}}(\text{fast component})} = \frac{3370}{T_{\frac{1}{2}}(\text{fast component})},$$

$$\text{Flow(white matter)} = \frac{\lambda_w \cdot \ln(2 \times 100 \times 60)}{T_{\frac{1}{2}}(\text{slow component})} = \frac{6237}{T_{\frac{1}{2}}(\text{slow component})},$$

where

$T_{\frac{1}{2}}$ is the half time in seconds,
λ_g is the partition coefficient for grey matter,
λ_w is the partition coefficient for white matter.

The mean cerebral blood flow through the whole region of the brain under investigation can be calculated from the peak count rate obtained and the area under the clearance curve using the formula

$$\text{Mean Flow}_{(m\ell/100g/min)} = \frac{(H_{max} - H_{10})\lambda_b \times 100 \times 60}{A_{10}},$$

where

H_{max} is the peak count rate of the clearance curve,
H_{10} is the count rate 10 minutes after injection,
A_{10} is the area under the clearance curve (i.e. the total number of counts recorded in 10 minutes),
λ_b is the partition coefficient for whole brain.

The relation was basically formulated by Zieler (1965), but it can also be proved using the more general occupancy principle enunciated by Orr and Gillespie (1968).

The use of 10 minute measurement period is a practical approximation. In cases of very slow flows, tracer clearance may have to be monitored for a longer period or when a computer is being used used, the slow component can be extrapolated to infinity assuming a mono-exponential clearance. The mean flow calculated using the 10 minute correction will, on average, over estimate the flow by about 15%.

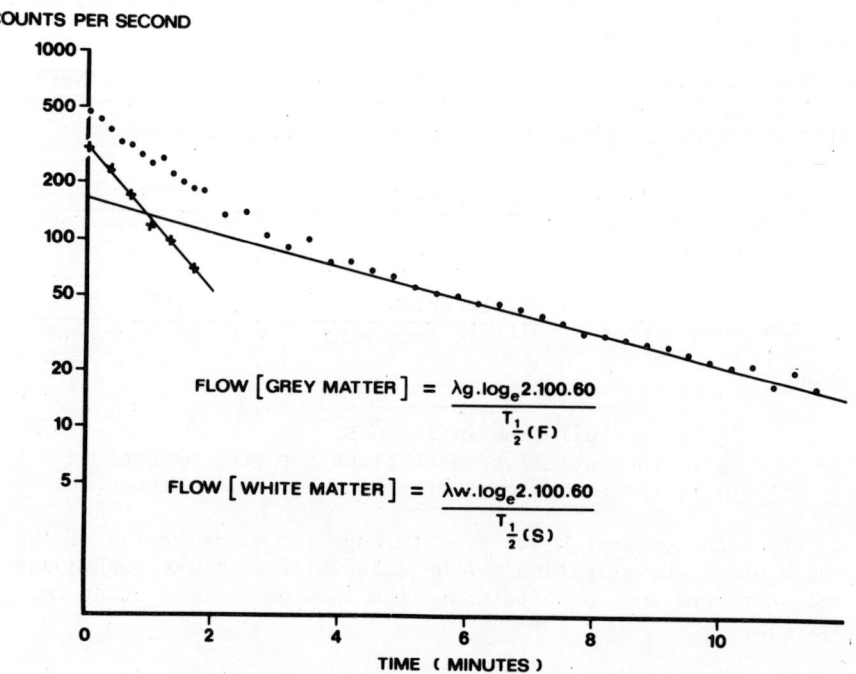

Figure 2 - Semi-log plot of biexponential Xenon 133 clearance curve.

Use has been made of the initial slope of the clearance curve over the first one to two minutes together with an empirical constant in order to make an early estimate of blood flow thus:

$$\text{Flow(initial)} = \frac{K}{T_{\frac{1}{2}}(\text{initial})},$$

where

K is an empirical constant,
$T_{\frac{1}{2}}(\text{initial})$ is the initial clearance half time.

With normal and slow flows this will give a value close to mean cerebral blood flow since the initial part of the clearance curve is constituted by both fast and slow components. With fast flows the initial slope estimate will be weighted towards grey matter flows.

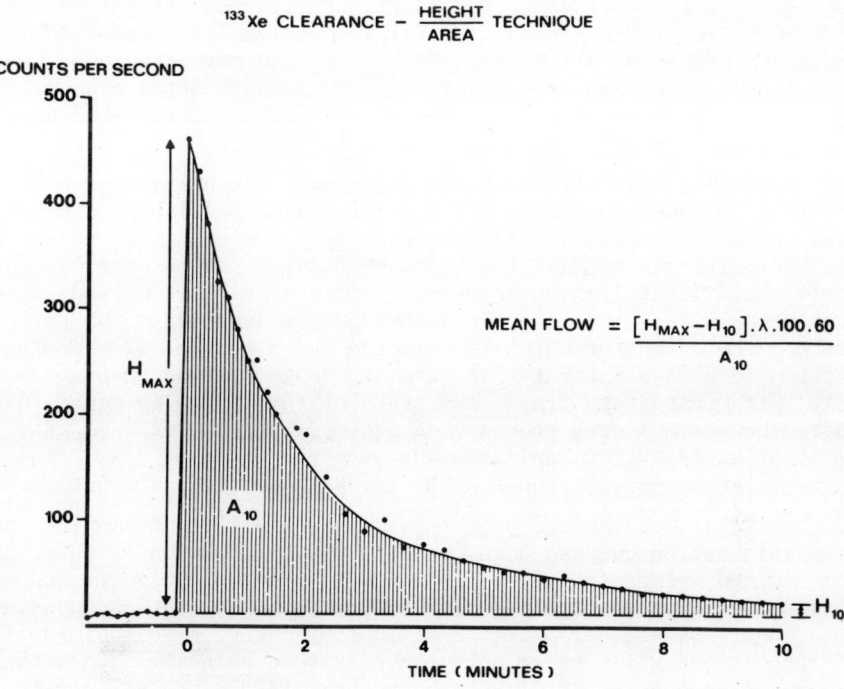

Figure 3 - Linear plot of Xenon 133 clearance curve.

Inhalation Technique

The most clinically attractive technique of measuring cerebral blood flow is the Xenon 133 inhalation technique introduced by Mallett and Veall in 1963 and also developed by Obrist. In this method Xenon 133 is inhaled by the patient for 1-5 minutes and the brain tissue clearance curve is monitored by externally mounted detectors. Since no arterial punctures or blood samples are necessary, this technique is completely atraumatic. However, there are two major disadvantages. During inhalation, all the body tissues take up Xenon and the consequent recirculation distorts the clearance curve appreciably. A correction is applied by measuring the Xenon activity in the expired air and this reflects the arterial concentration. The clearance curves are also distorted due to isotope in the extracranial tissues. It would appear that the real practical use of this technique will be to determine initial slope flows and fast componenet flows using computer analysis to carry out the exponential stripping procedure and apply the necessary corrections.

NON-DIFFUSIBLE TRACERS

There have been a number of attempts to find a less traumatic and simpler alternative to the inert gas clearance technique with its intra-carotid injections and fairly complex data processing. A method proposed by Oldendorf (1962), utilised the measurement of the circulation time of a non-diffusible isotope after a bolus injection. The method has been taken up by other workers and has been applied to patients with various intracranial disorders.

The method basically consists of injecting a bolus of a non-diffusible isotope intravenously (0.5 mCi iodine 131 labelled hippuran and 1 mCi Technetium 99m have been used) and monitoring the passage of radioactivity through the brain by means of an externally mounted collimated scintillation detector. After amplification and pulse height analysis, the detector output pulses are fed to the ratemeter, the output of which is filtered and electronically differentiated to give a recording of rate of change of count rate (activity) with respect to time. The peaks of this bi-polar curve indicate the maximum rate of entry of activity and the maximum rate of exit of activity into and from the detector field of view. The time interval between these peaks is the mode circulation time.

The relative simplicity of this method makes it attractive, but the information one can acquire about the circulation in this way is limited, since the method provides an index of velocity and not a measure of cerebral blood flow (Rowan et al., 1970). Fundamental theory shows that under conditions of changing radius, the flow through tubes will change more markedly than velocity. Investigations using baboons in Glasgow have shown that circulation time is not a reliable index of cerebral blood flow. Furthermore, in a series of 200 patients studied in the Institute of Neurological Sciences in Glasgow, many patients with gross intracranial pathology showed no abnormal circulation velocity, although the average mode circulation time for groups of patients with ischaemia, haematoma and subarachnoid haemorrhage was increased (Rowan et al., 1970). This is of limited value, however, since when faced with an individual patient, the clinician is very likely to be confronted with a mode circulation time result which will be within the expected range for normal patients. This is due to the rather wide range of mode circulation times found in normal subjects. The assumption that changes in flow will be refleceted in changes in velocity is valid in such restricted circumstances that it seems unwise to base clinical decisions on such measurements.

NON - RADIOISOTOPE METHODS

Skull Window Techniques

In the mid 19th century, studies on the cerebral circulation were carried out by exposing the pial vessels and observing them directly or through a window in the skull. Later, in 1930, Wolff and Lennox, using this technique, observed the vasodilatation effect of carbon dioxide. In recent years, Meyer has used this technique to investigate blood flow in leptomeningeal vessels following occlusion of the mid cerebral artery.

Hydrogen Clearance Technique

Hydrogen gas saturates blood rapidly allowing immediate analysis of partial pressure in blood using hydrogen electrodes. Hydrogen can be given either as a bolus injection into the carotid artery, or by allowing the patient to inhale a hydrogen gas mixture consisting of 2.5% hydrogen, 21% oxygen and 76.5% nitrogen from a face mask until venous equilibrium has been achieved. Due to the relative insolubility of hydrogen in blood, this occurs rapidly. The clearance curves, which can be obtained either from electrodes in venous blood or in tissue, are analysed in the same way as those obtained with the radioactive Xenon methods, see for example Aukland (1968). The main advantage of the method is that regional cerebral blood flow can be measured at a number of sites and measurements can be repeated frequently, although the comments made with regard to Xenon partial pressure gradients limiting the size of the region being resolved, also apply in the case of hydrogen. Technical difficulties can also be encountered due to damage of brain tissues surrounding implanted electrodes.

Heat Clearance Technique

With this method (see for example Betz (1968)), thermistors (small solid state devices whose electrical resistance changes with temperature) are placed on brain tissue. A bolus of hot or cold saline is given intra-arterially and the step function changes in temperature and subsequent clearance is monitored by the thermistors. Provided there is no change in body temperature during the study, the rate of clearance of heat from the area of brain under investigation will be proportional to regional cerebral blood flow. The main disadvantage of this method is that heat is not a physiologically inert tracer and that any changes in body temperature will affect the result.

The heat clearance method may also be used to measure blood velocity in vessels and a bolus injection of hot or cold saline is again used. One thermistor is intermittently heated (every five to fifteen seconds) and the second thermistor acts as a temperature sensor. The temperature of the second thermistor depends on the velocity of blood flowing past it. Changes in temperature of the blood do not affect the results in this case, but movement of the thermistors introduces artefacts and blood clot formation around the thermistor can distort the results.

Electrical Impedance Method

When a high frequency signal is passed through the body, it is modulated due to changes in impedance between the electrodes. One of the factors producing these changes is the pulsatile blood flow (Hadjiev, 1972). In this method an attempt is made to correlate measured impedance changes with cerebral blood flow. The curves are analysed measuring amplitude and rise and fall times. Unfortunately, analysis shows that a significant proportion of the wave form obtained results from extracranial blood flow and changes in cerebral spinal fluid.

Electro-Magnetic Flow Meter Measurements

The fundamental parameter measured by electromagnetic flow meters is velocity. Depending on the design of the flow probe, the velocity measurement can be related to flow. The probe is placed around the vessel under investigation (in cerebral blood flow work, this is normally the carotid artery). An electromagnet within the probe is excited by means of a square wave or a sinusoidal signal and, as a result, a magnetic field is set up at right angles to the direction of flow. When blood cuts the magnetic lines of force, an electric field is induced mutually perpendicular to the direction of blood flow and the magnetic field and this is detected by electrodes placed diametrically opposite on the vessel. The detected signal is then amplified and demodulated and displayed on a chart recorder. Calibration is carried out either before or after the investigation by passing a known amount of blood through the vessel. To permit good correlation between velocity and flow, the probe must produce a homogeneous magnetic field and for this reason the 'cuff' type is normally used.

The advantage of the method is that it will give continuous flow measurements in intact blood vessels, while the disadvantages are that the vessels have to be exposed and that only total blood flow in and out of the brain can be measured.

Ultrasonic Doppler Technique

When ultrasonic waves impinge on the blood stream, the frequency of the detected reflected waves from the moving blood particles is altered due to the Doppler effect, see for example Miyazaki (1972). The beat frequency (i.e. the difference in frequency between the transmitted and reflected sound waves) is proportional to the velocity of the moving particles. With this method, a probe which acts both as a transmitter and receiver is held against the neck at an acute angle to the direction of flow in the carotid artery and the Doppler beat frequency is detected. It is assumed that the diameter of the carotid artery does not change significantly and that blood velocity will vary in proportion to flow.

The advantages of the method are that it is completely atraumatic and dynamic changes in the carotid artery velocity patterns can be detected instantaneously. However, a great deal of controversy surrounds the design of probes necessary to give consistent results.

REFERENCES

Aukland, K. (1968). Measurement of local blood flow with hydrogen gas, in *Blood Flow through Organs and Tissues*, (eds. Bain and Harper), (Livingstone, Edinburgh).

Betz, E. (1968). Measurement of local blood flow by means of heat clearance, in *Blood Flow through Organs and Tissues*, (eds. Bain and Harper), (Livingstone, Edinburgh).

Gillespie, F.C. (1968). Some factors influencing the interpretation of regional cerebral blood flow measurements using inert gas clearance techniques, in *Blood Flow through Organs and Tissues*, (eds. Bain and Harper), (Livingstone, Edinburgh).

Hadjiev, D. (1972). Impedance methods for investigation of cerebral circulation, in *Progress in Brain Research, Vol. 35, Cerebral Blood Flow*, (eds. Meyer and Schadé), (Elsevier, Amsterdam).

Harper, A.M., Glass, H.I., Steven, J.L. and Granat, A.H. (1964). The measurement of local blood flow in the cerebral cortex from the clearance of Xenon 133, *J. Neurol. Neurosurg. Psychiat.*, **27**, 255.

Lassen, N.A. and Ingvar, D.H. (1961). The blood flow of the cerebral cortex determined by radioactive Krypton, *Experientia (Basel)*, **17**, 42-43.

Lassen, N.A. and Ingvar, D.H. (1972). Radioisotope assessment of regional cerebral blood flow, in *Progress in Nuclear Medecine, Vol. 1*, pp. 376-409.

Mallet, B.L. and Veall, M. (1963). Investigations of cerebral blood flow in hypertension using radioactive Xenon, inhalation and extracranial recording, *Lancet*, i, p. 1081.

Miyazaki, M. (1972). Studies on cerebral circulation by the ultrasonic doppler technique - with special reference to clinical application of the technique, in *Progress in Brain Research, Vol. 35, Cerebral Blood Flow*, (eds. Meyer and Schadé), (Elsevier, Amsterdam).

Oldendorf, W.H. (1962). Measurement of the mean transit time of cerebral circulation by external detection of an intravenously injected radioisotope, *J. Nucl. Med.*, **3**, 382-398.

Orr, J.S. and Gillespie, F.C. (1968). Occupancy principle for radioactive tracers in steady state biological systems, *Science*, **162**, 138-139.

Rowan, J.O. (1972). Radioisotopes in diagnosis, in *Scientific Foundations of Neurology*, (in press), pp. 316-327.

Rowan, J.O., Cross, J.N., Tedeschi, G.M. and Jennett, W.B. (1970). Limitations of circulation time in the diagnosis of intracranial disease, *J. Neurol. Neurosurg. Psychiat.*, **33**, 739.

Rowan, J.O., Harper, A.M., Miller, J.D., Tedeschi, G.M. and Jennett, W.B. (1970). Relationship between volume flow and velocity in the cerebral circulation, *J. Neurol. Neurosurg. Psychiat.*, **33**, 733.

Wolff, H.G. and Lennox, W.G. (1930). Cerebral circulation, effect on pial vessels of variations in oxygen and carbon dioxide content of blood, *Arch. Neurol. Psychiat.*, **23**, 1097-1120.

Zierler, K.L. (1965). Equations for measuring blood flow by external monitoring by radioisotopes, in *Circulation Research*, *Vol. 16*.

THE MEASUREMENT AND INTERPRETATION
OF CEREBRAL OXYGEN TENSION

I.A. SILVER

*Department of Pathology, University of Bristol,
Medical School, Bristol BS8 1TD, England*

INTRODUCTION

The oxygen environment of the central nervous system is both of fundamental interest and of practical clinical importance in that this is the most sensitive organ in the body to acute and chronic hypoxia and it has the least powers of recovery from damage of any tissue. It is also of interest that the CNS shows a differential regional sensitivity to hypoxia which appears to be related to the phylogenetic development of the different areas; the 'higher' and more recently developed centres being more sensitive to oxygen lack than the 'lower' centres. The reasons for this difference are not understood.

It is obvious that the normal oxygen tension in any organ will represent a balance between oxygen supply and local usage. The key to the supply is the vascular control mechanism and the key to the usage is the cellular metabolic activity. It cannot, however, be assumed that a measurement of the pooled cerebral venous PO_2 is a good reflection of the oxygen supply at the cellular level. The assumption that these two are easily equated might lead to considerable error in the assessment of patient status. The PO_2 of the brain as with other tissues is in a state of dynamic equilibrium and we do not yet know what are the physiological limits of this equilibrium, and neither do we know how far into the pathological range, PO_2 can stray in the short term and yet allow complete recovery. We do know something, on the other hand, about the long term results of hypoxia, but in the brain the 'long term' is measured in minutes.

There are four divergent approaches to the making of estimates of cerebral PO_2.

(1) Studies of gross blood flow and arterio-venous difference allow calculation of conditions within the brain and predictions as to the state at the cellular level; This method assumes a uniform intracerebral environment and an equal distribution of capillaries and flow which unfortunately does not exist.

(2) Another indirect method depends on 'instantaneous' measurement of capillary flow by means of radioactive markers and the subsequent calculation of the probable condition around the capillaries. This has the disadvantage that it gives no indication of the range of local variation and it is possible to do the necessary calculation satisfactorily since

the capillary architecture is asymmetrical and there is no agreed value for the O_2 diffusion coefficient in brain.

(3) Direct measurements more or less at the cellular level can be made with polarographic oxygen microelectrode systems and these can be modified to give either local or integrated information. The major disadvantage with this method is the uncertainty of what the electrodes are measuring and whether they themselves alter the cellular environment significantly. The method is most useful in combination with simultaneous recording of cellular activity by other means, e.g. electrical activity or intracellular redox states.

(4) The fourth general approach has been via computer simulation and model systems (see Reneau, Bruley and Knisely, 1967); Reneau, Bicher, Bruley and Knisely, 1970). The outcome of this approach depends on the accuracy of the input information and the complexity of the blood supply. While simulation is a useful exercise it is still in its infancy as regards predicting a cellular environment in the brain under varying circumstances. It is, however, an area of very rapid growth and as more information becomes available from electrode studies it should be possible to predict quite accurately areas of danger under different clinical conditions.

This paper will deal only with electrode studies since these present the only method at the moment for direct continuous readout of a dynamic situation, and it will try to show how these methods correlate with cellular activity and intracellular state.

METHODS

The original studies of Davies and Brink (1942) on the cat cortex with microrecessed electrodes showed the existence of very low PO_2 levels in the inter-capillary spaces on the surface of the brain, and they demonstrated steep inter-capillary oxygen gradients. They found that levels of as low as 2.0 mm Hg or less were frequently encountered. Davies and others working with larger electrodes in the brain showed responses to oxygen and nitrogen breathing and Davies and Rémond (1947) clearly demonstrated the dramatic falls in PO_2 that accompany massive synchronous discharge of large numbers of cells in Metrazole-induced convulsions, when sudden O_2 usage exceeds the ability of a local or general vascular regulatory mechanism to maintain a normal O_2 environment. The large electrodes used for these studies precluded the measurement of actual PO_2 in the brain since it is virtually impossible to calibrate large electrodes for use in tissues, owing to the many interfering factors which may affect the 'oxygen' current.

The development of a membrane covered electrode by Clark (1956) produced a tool that would measure absolute PO_2 continuously at surfaces of organs, including brain. At that time, and for some years afterwards, Clark-type electrodes had relatively large cathodes and could be used only for the measurement of general PO_2 over a relatively large area of tissue, which included several capillary beds, and therefore gave little information about local cellular environment. This method has been extended by the development of the multicathode probe of Lübbers (1969).

Cater and Silver (1961) introduced the microneedle oxygen electrode which they and many subsequent workers, notably Lübbers and his co-workers at the Max Plank Institute in Dortmund, have shown to give reasonably accurate information about the absolute PO_2 in very small volumes of fluid in tissues. Cross and Silver (1962) demonstrated steep PO_2 gradients within the brain as opposed to the gradients previously reported at the surface, and Chance, Schoener and Schindler (1964) showed that intracellular redox states as measured by the variation in ultraviolet fluorescence of pyridine nucleotides in the oxydised and reduced states could be correlated with cerebral arterial PO_2 monitored with a large Platinum electrode.

The essential characteristics of the Clark electrode and the needle electrode were combined by Silver (1965) who measured PO_2 gradients in brain and tried to correlate these with the structure of the capillary network, and he also showed that electrical activity of cells could be recorded simultaneously on the same electrode as PO_2. Similar dual recordings have been made in muscle by Kunze (1968) and the work on brain has been extended by Bicher and Knisely (1970) and Erdmann and Kunke (1972). The last authors have produced a multi-electrode which allows the recording of electrical activity from as many as 8 cells simultaneously while the PO_2 at the several monitoring sites is recorded concurrently.

The volume of fluid from which a 1μ microelectrode of the needle type draws its oxygen is a sphere of about 6μ diameter which is small in comparison with the size of most cells. It can easily be calculated that the O_2 consumption of the electrodes is also very small compared to that of an actively metabolising nerve cell. Thus it can be predicted that the presence of an electrode of this order of size is unlikely to upset the pericellular environment to any great extent. More positive proof of this can be obtained directly by advancing the electrode through the brain until the spontaneous action potentials of a single cell are detected (extra cellularly). The electrode is then slowly polarised and the output from it is divided into AC and DC components. It will be observed in almost all cases that the cell continues to fire at the same rate as it did before the polarising voltage was applied, thus showing that its signal generating and transmitting capacity has not been affected by the presence of the oxygen electrode. The exception to this is if the electrode has been inadvertently placed directly touching the cell membrane, in which case application of the DC voltage will affect the polarisation of the cell membrane and will consequently change its firing pattern. However, this is a direct electrical effect and not an effect of the oxygen diffusion zone generated by the electrode.

A method of demonstrating whether or not the presence of a microelectrode significantly affects the intracellular oxygen environment is to use a 10 micron ultraviolet spot to determine the redox state of a cell in terms of the pyridine nucleotide fluorescence. If the spot can be located over a cell body against which an electrode is placed, any drastic lowering of PO_2 when the electrode is polarised will be detected by an increase in the NAD fluorescence. However, it is the general experience that oxygen microelectrodes of tip sized less the 1.5µ behave in a reliable manner and do not unduly interfere with the conditions they are designed to measure.

Other microelectrodes may be used in combination with oxygen microelectrodes to increase the amount of information which is being obtained and to render the interpretation of that information more effective since it is obviously desirable to know the conditions in which oxygen is being used. It is now possible to make micro pH and micro PCO_2 electrodes with tip sizes of the order of 1 micron. Oxygen electrodes themselves may also be used for monitoring blood flow if they are covered with a layer of palladinum. They are used for measuring oxygen when polarised with a voltage of about -600 to 700 millivolts, and they are used as microhydrogen clearance electrodes when polarised at about 1.2 volts. The hydrogen clearance, following either injection of hydrogen-containing blood or a few breaths of hydrogen-containing air is an indication of blood flow rate in a small area of tissue. A multiple electrode system such as that described by Erdmann and Kunke (1972) may use alternate microelectrodes for hydrogen and oxygen measurement thereby giving continuous assessment of flow and oxygen tension within a very small region of tissues.

The question now arises as to what these electrodes are measuring and if it is of any significance either at the cellular, whole organ or clinical level.

THE MEANING OF CEREBRAL OXYGEN MEASUREMENTS

With regard to large electrodes, i.e. anything with a diameter of more than 5µ and more particularly those greater than 10µ, the diffusion zones around the electrode are larger than the intercapillary spaces and therefore while these electrodes will detect temporal changes in PO_2 they are unable to resolve spatial changes except of a relatively gross kind. They do not give information about the variations in cellular environment due to diffusion gradients but they will give information about generalised changes of oxygen availability in a region, which may arise as a result of changes in blood flow or changes in blood gas tension. They will also detect gross changes in PO_2 due to massive alterations in O_2 uptake in their vicinity, for instance as a result of poisoning or inhibition of activity on the one hand, or sudden increases of metabolic rate on the other, e.g. changes which occur during convulsions (Davies and Rémond, 1947).

As a very generalised and therefore easily contested statement, it may be said that the output from large PO_2 electrodes in brain varies mainly in response to major changes in regional blood flow or to changes in blood gas tensions. It may, however, give useful indications of general conditions. For instance, the current from a 'large' probe should be derived from an integrated PO_2 covering several capillary and cellular fields and should approximate to the statistical mean of multiple values obtained with microelectrodes. This has been shown to be the case in the kidney by Strauss (1972) and surface measurements of cerebral cortex with large or multiwire electrodes appear to give the same overall picture as microelectrode readings. Unfortunately we do not know the limits of normality but the statistical mean of cerebral cortical PO_2 in grey matter appears to be about 20-25 mm Hg with a range from almost 0 to about 95 mm Hg.

With regard to readings from microelectrodes, provided that the system is reasonably reliable, can be calibrated and does not interfere with normal function, the interpretation of the information obtained is easier, although its significance may well be open to question. The essentials of the data from microelectrodes are as follows:

(1) The electrode strictly measures its own micro-environment which is bound to be slightly different from that of the cell.

(2) The information is extremely localised and must therefore be treated in terms of microanatomical position.

(3) The readings vary with time both in regard to cellular activity and as regards blood flow dynamics.

(4) Measurements are being made at some point on a gradient and this gradient may change both in steepness and even in direction if new capillary patterns open and others close.

(5) Not all of the cell will be in the same O_2 environment as the part that is being measured by the electrode. This applies especially to nerve cells because of the ramification of their processes. We do not know if some parts of the cell are more sensitive to oxygen lack than others. We also do not know if extra-cellular debris, caused by penetration of the electrode, significantly alters the cell activity.

(6) Inflammatory changes in tissue start immediately a foreign body is inserted. This has two major phases, the vascular and the cellular. Luckily in the brain the inflammatory response is slow and somewhat reduced compared with that in other tissues. Nevertheless its presence must be taken into account.

(7) The electrode itself may alter the environment by its O_2 usage to such an extent that the local cellular activity is changed. This is very unlikely when small electrodes are being used. However, the shaft of the electrode may throw what is best described as an oxygen 'shadow' in the

region of its tip if the main source of oxygen diffusion was from the direction now occupied by the electrode shaft.

(8) The electrode may compress the normal capillary supply and give rise to an abnormal diffusion field.

(9) Irritation from the electrode may enhance or reduce the local vascular adjustments.

(10) The electrode itself may be unreliable due to breakdown in insulation at the tip owing to hydration of the insulator or to electrochemical poisoning or physical alteration of the diffusion field by deposition of protein on the sensitive surface.

These difficulties must always be considered but most of them are easily recognisable in practice from the type of response that is obtained from the electrode when changes in blood PO_2 are imposed.

Some relatively constant findings in brain PO_2, as measured by microelectrodes, are as follows:

(a) Vascular dynamic changes at the arteriolar and capillary level which are correlated with local contraction and expansion have a periodicity of about 1-3 minutes and can be observed as waves on the oxygen trace.

(b) Changes due to systemic blood pressure alteration are usually very noticeable in the central nervous system. Rises or falls in blood pressure are almost always reflected in increased or decreased cerebral PO_2 respectively.

(c) Changes due to increased or decreased blood PCO_2. Increased PCO_2 is always accompanied by increased cerebral blood flow unless vessels are maximally dilated already, whereas decreases in local PCO_2 tend to be accompanied by vasoconstrictions especially if high PO_2 is present. PCO_2 increases are much more effective in raising cerebral PO_2 than is the administration of pure oxygen to breathe. It is usually found that when an animal is given pure oxygen the oxygen tension in the brain rises rapidly for a short period until the new PO_2 level is about 25-60% above the original level when it settles down to a new plateau which it maintains until the ambient oxygen tension in the respired air is altered. If, however, additional CO_2 is given at the same time as the increased oxygen, then the oxygen tension will rise to maybe 2, 3 or even 4 times the original level. High CO_2 levels in inspired air will cause a rise in oxygen tension in the brain even if the oxygen tension of the inspired air remains constant. This is due to vasodilatation and increased blood flow. Conversely, increases in oxygen tension without increase in CO_2 or with decrease of CO_2 leads to cerebral vasoconstriction, reduction in blood flow and a limitation of increase of cerebral oxygenation. This appears to be a protective mechanism. It is of course merely a reflection of the general sensitivity of blood vessel smooth musculature to oxygen.

(d) Changes due to sudden fluctuations in metabolic activity can often be observed and more rarely one can see changes due to generalised metabolic activity. For instance, during falling blood sugar levels due to high insulin concentrations the PO_2 of the brain rises because of increased blood flow and reduced oxygen uptake.

(e) Changes due to variations in local activity. If one is recording the oxygen tension in the vicinity of a single cell and obtains a value of say 15 mm Hg and the cell is then stimulated to fire fast, the oxygen tension at the cell surface will drop after a lag of about 0.5-1 second and recovers to the original level in about 1.5 seconds, provided that the cell continues to fire at its new rate. When the cell stops firing or returns to its original resting firing rate the process is reversed so that about 0.5 to 1.0 second after cessation of firing there is an overshoot in the direction of increased PO_2 which lasts for about 1.5 seconds when the PO_2 returns again to the resting level. Thus it appears that there is a 'set point' of PO_2 to which the vasculature is adjusted and to which it makes every effort to return the PO_2 whatever the circumstances. We do not know what is the significance of the level of this 'set point' since it obviously varies from place to place in the brain. Furthermore it does not stay constant for hours on end even in one place, although it does stay constant in a short term. We do not know the limits between which the set point can fluctuate in normal circumstances and we do not know about its extreme limits in the short term which are compatible with survival of the cell. The control of the cellular environment clearly depends on the vascular reaction upstream from the cell and we have to postulate that some feedback mechanism which can go as it were against the bloodstream, and can do so quite rapidly, must exist. The most likely candidate at the moment is the diffusion of CO_2 from the area of activity back to the arteriolar ends of the capillary where the adjustments are made.

(f) Changes in hypoxia. These are very important clinically and we do not yet understand what is the precise difference between the cerebral cortex and the brain stem which makes the former so much more susceptible to hypoxia than the latter and what makes both of these structures so much more susceptible than most other organs in the body. Why is the cortex at risk? Are the levels of PO_2 here low or is the consumption excessively high and is the feedback mechanism from the vasculature inadequate to cope with the demands that may be thrust upon it in a stressful situation?

(1) Measurements suggest that the cerebral PO_2 does not fall more or faster than elsewhere in the brain during an hypoxic episode.

(2) Pyridine nucleotide measurements with ultraviolet fluorescence indicate that cortical cell bodies become reduced at the same time as cells in the brain stem.

(3) Electrical activity in brain stem is correlated with this pyridine nucleotide reduction, i.e. as the NAD and NADH change occurs, electrical activity in the respiratory centre fades, but in the cerebral cortex electrical activity ceases long before there is any reduction in NAD.

(4) Cortical cells lose the ability to transmit impulses before they lose polarisation of their cell membranes.

(5) Cortical cells lose polarisation when NAD is fully oxidised and they can even die while this state is maintained if they are kept in a low oxygen environment for 10-15 minutes which still just allows spontaneous respiration.

(6) Brain stem cells do not lose transmission ability or polarisation of cell membranes until the NAD is about 30% reduced and they do not die unless the NAD is kept reduced for many minutes. Spontaneous gasping respiration can occur for a relatively long period during a 20% reduction. This corresponds to external oxygen tension at the cell surface of about 1 mm Hg or less.

This raises the question as to what is the 'soft' structure in the cortex which is most easily damaged by hypoxia. The transmission failure and some other evidence (Grossman and Williams, 1971; Chalazonitis et al., 1966; Silver, 1972) suggests that the synapse is the point most at risk in cerebral cells during hypoxia. It is not at all clear why this should be. Are some synapses in a dangerous position anatomically from the point of view of availability of oxygen? Is the oxygen uptake at the synapse very high? We know that the production of synaptosomes is an oxygen utilising mechanism but why should cerebral cortical synapses be apparently so much more sensitive than those in the brain stem? Maybe it is merely a reflection of the vascular architecture and the size of the cells. It may also be due to much more imponderable factors which are somehow inherent in the specialised cells of the cortex as opposed to the more 'primitive type' of cells which are found in the brain stem.

What is the cellular mechanism that is critical in hypoxia? From most cells it is energy production and this carries on unimpaired down to levels of about 0.001 mm Hg at the intracellular level due to the activity of cytochrome A3. What determines the critical oxygen tension below which oxygen uptake falls off? This differs in different circumstances, for instance in Longmuir's brain slices (1972) there is a fall in O_2 uptake with oxygen pressure from several hundreds of millimetres of mercury, but in vascularised tissues the critical oxygen tension below which oxygen uptake begins to fall off is around 1 to 2 mm Hg, and this is the point at which NAD fluorescence changes in most cells. This suggests that there is an oxygen gradient of about 100-1 from the cell surface to the surface of the mitochondria.

CONCLUSION

We are still very much in the dark as to the meaning of oxygen tension measurements in brain. For instance how do diving mammals protect themselves from cerebral damage. We know that they change their cerebral vascular perfusion pattern during the dive, but however good their oxygen stores may be it is clear that an animal such as the Weddell seal which can swim for 5 miles under water, cannot but have an extremely low cerebral oxygen tension at the end of such a journey. We need to know what is the danger point at the cellular level and which particular organelle is most at risk in the cerebral cortex before we can make a rational attempt to apply oxygen measurements in the brain to the clinical situation and then be able to act on information obtained. We must have information about the reversible pathology of cerebral hypoxia and we must be able to recognise from electrode readings when irreversible changes start to occur. When we have this knowledge it may become possible to delay the onset of irreversible damage, or to arrest and reverse what at present is a progressive deterioration.

REFERENCES

Bicher, H.I. and Knisely, M.H. (1971). *J. Appl. Physiol.*, **28**, 387.
Cater, D.B. and Silver, I.A. (1961). In *Reference Electrodes*, (eds. Ives, D.J.G. and Janz, G.J.), (Academic Press, New York).
Chalazonitis, N., et al.. (1966). *C.R. Séanc. Soc. Biol.*, **160**, 1020.
Chance, B., Schoener, B. and Schindler, E. (1964). In *Oxygen in the Animal Organism*, (ed. Dickens, F.), (Pergamon, Oxford).
Clark, L.C. (1956). *Trans. Amer. Art. Int. Org.*, **2**, 44.
Cross, B.A. and Silver, I.A. (1962). *Proc. Roy. Soc. B*, **156**, 483.
Davies, P.W. and Brink, F. (1942). *Rev. Sci. Instrum.*, **13**, 524.
Davies, P.W. and Rémond, A. (1947). *Res. Publ. Ass. Nerv. Ment. Dis.*, **26**, 205.
Erdmann, H. and Kunke, K. (1972). In *Tissue Electrodes*, (eds. Kessler, M. et al.), (Urban and Schwartzenberg, Munich).
Grossman, R.G. and Williams, V.F. (1971). In *Brain Hypoxia*, (eds. Brierley, J.B. and Meldrum, B.S.), (Heinemann, London).
Kunze, K. (1968). In *Oxygen Transport in Blood and Tissue*, (eds. Lübbers, D.W. et al.), (Georg Thieme Verlag, Stuttgart).
Longmuir, I. (1972). In *Tissue Electrodes*, (eds. Kessler, M. et al.), (Urban and Schwartzenberg, Munich).
Lübbers, D.W. (1969). *Prog. Resp. Res.*, **3**, 112.

Reneau, D.R., Bicher, H.I., Bruley, D.F. and Knisely, M.H. (1970). In *Blood Oxygenation*, (Plenum Press, London and New York).

Reneau, D.R., Bruley, D.F. and Knisely, M.H. (1967). In *Chemical Engineering in Medecine and Biology*, (Plenum Press, London and New York), p. 135.

Silver, I.A. (1965). *Med. Electron. Biol. Engng.*, **3**, 377.

Silver, I.A. (1972). In *Tissue Electrodes*, (eds. Kessler, M. et al.), (Urban and Schwartzenberg, Munich).

Strauss, J. (1972). In *Tissue Electrodes*, (eds. Kessler, M. et al.), (Urban and Schwartzenberg, Munich).

INTRACRANIAL PRESSURE MEASUREMENTS - A REVIEW
OF AVAILABLE METHODS

I.D. EVERSDEN

Atkinson Morley's Hospital, London, SW 20

INTRODUCTION

The presence of raised intracranial pressure (ICP) can be recognised clinically by progressive headache associated with progressive mental change and the development and progression of localising neurological signs. However, these clinical signs can be unreliable and methods are required to detect increasing pressure and distortion of brain tissue preferably by techniques that permit continuous recordings.

The advent of low displacement electromanometers led not only to present day techniques for continuous monitoring but also to an awareness of low frequency pressure changes superimposed upon those of cardiac activity and respiration. From as early as 1930 attempts have been made to incorporate some kind of membrane or bellows which can be displaced by pressure and the displacement measured indirectly. Guillaume and Janny in 1951 devised a special membrane connected to an iron bar which moved in an electromagnet, while Gerlach in 1952 made use of devices similar to the carbon microphone. Gilland (1965) made a detailed study of several recording systems used for the measurement of pressure changes within the lumbar sac using an implanted catheter connected to both inductive and capacitive low displacement electromanometers. His conclusion was that adequate response up to 6 Hz was all that was required and measurements by various authors with the needle, catheter, transducer system indicate that the response is flat to only 5 Hz dropping to 50% at ∼14 Hz.

MEASUREMENT OF LUMBAR PRESSURE

A catheter is connected between a lumbar puncture needle and the dome of a pressure transducer. Typically a lumbar needle is 0.75 mm in diameter and about 10 cm long. The PVC or silicone rubber catheter is about 2 mm in diameter to provide the necessary flexibility between the freely supported needle in the patient's back and the rigidly held transducer. It should be noted that it is possible to increase the range of flat response to 20 or 30 Hz but if the recorded events do not demand this fidelity the system merely becomes more sensitive to air bubbles and to external vibrations.

The technique is not without its drawbacks. It is not reasonable to ask a patient to lie still for very long periods of time and the danger of the patient rolling onto the protruding needle is alarming. Even the slightest movement of the needle with respect to the transducer produces artefactual changes in pressure.

Care has to be taken to ensure that the transducer is at a known height with respect to the needle. Since there is virtually no flow in the catheter there is a tendency for blockage to occur, regular flushing of the system being the only solution. The needle tip is especially prone to blockage and its position is critical in the maintenance of reliable measurements.

Under conditions of high intracranial pressure there is a real danger of causing a rapid deterioration in a patient's condition, particularly if there is already distortion of the brain tissues. Since the condition of high ICP is not easy to assess clinically, lumbar puncture has to be avoided if there is even a suggestion of high pressure. The relief of pressure that occurs perhaps not immediately if only a small amount of fluid is withdrawn, but slowly due to seepage after the needle has been withdrawn, causes an already formed tentorial or cerebellar cone to precipitate with a resultant rapid deterioration in the patient's condition.

MEASUREMENT OF VENTRICULAR FLUID PRESSURE

These difficulties may be overcome by introducing a catheter into the ventricular system inside the cranial cavity. This technique is now well established not primarily for the measurement of pressure but for the control of pressure by draining fluid from the ventricular system, and for radiographic technique of ventriculography. A burr hole is made in the skull, usually in the posterior parietal region and a probe used to locate a ventricular cavity. The needle is then removed and replaced by a soft rubber catheter. Pressure may be recorded continuously by connecting this catheter to a suitable pressure transducer. Again because of the compliance of the catheter tubing the frequency response is flat to no greater than 10 Hz.

However, this method has proved invaluable in establishing many features of increasing ICP. In 1951 Guillaume and Janny described spontaneous fluctuation in cerebrospinal fluid (CSF) pressure in patients with intracranial pathology, but it was not until 1960 when Lundberg, in a monograph which is a milestone in the history of the study of raised ICP, that these fluctuations were accurately documented. Recordings were made of intraventricular pressure for periods of days to weeks in 48 patients with intracranial tumours before operation. He described three types of pressure wave, which he termed A, B and C, but adds that other terms such as plateau wave might be more suitable. These were defined as follows:

> A-waves (Plateau wave) Increase in pressure to a height of 50-100 mm Hg lasting 5-20 minutes and followed by a rapid fall to basal pressure or below;
>
> B-waves Rhythmic waves with an amplitude of up to 50 mm Hg and a frequency of about 1 per minute;
>
> C-waves Rhythmic waves with an amplitude ranging form discernibility to 20 mm Hg and a frequency of about 6 per minute.

Without going into detail about the causes of these various waves it is sufficient to say that plateau waves develop when intracranial compensation for raised pressure is beginning to fail and therefore have undoubted clinical significance. B-waves often precede the occurrence of plateau waves, and, like plateau waves are probably the result of compensating changes in blood volume. C-waves are thought to be related to rhythmic variations in systemic arterial pressure and seem to be of little clinical significance.

Monitoring using a ventricular catheter has most of the shortcomings of recording with a lumbar catheter. Artefacts due to patient movement, the position of the transducer with respect to some fixed level in the patient, the tendency for the catheter to block and as with a lumbar catheter a risk of infection requiring attentive nursing care. A notable effect of lasting high pressure in the presence of ventricular pathway blockage is a reduction in size of the ventricles. Under these conditions it is often difficult to locate the ventricular cavities and when in position, the patency of the catheter is difficult to maintain.

Despite this formidable list of snags much of the information concerning intracranial pressure variations has been obtained with these methods showing that persistence with a known technique causes the shortcomings to be overcome and many centres still use an intraventricular catheter to measure pressure. Smaller transducers are now available which can be strapped to the scalp so removing some of the artefacts due to movement.

There are advantages over the other methods which we will come to shortly. It is possible to remove fluid for analysis and if necessary to reduce the ICP by removing fluid.

The catheter may be removed from the patient without resorting to a further excursion to the operating theatre.

Having looked in detail at two valuable and reliable techniques of measurement, it would be useful to consider just briefly the characteristics which are required of a device used to measure ICP continuously.

DESIRABLE CHARACTERISTICS OF AN IMPLANTABLE PRESSURE TRANSDUCER

(1) Low risk of infection and as little discomfort to the patient as possible:

    (a) Extradural implantation;
    (b) Minimal operative discomfort - single operation if possible;
    (c) Small physical size and low mass;
    (d) Telemetric transmission.

(2) Reliable recordings of pressure:

    (a) Pressure range -10 to +300 mm Hg;
    (b) Sensitive to pressure changes of 1 mm Hg or less;
    (c) Stable;

(d) Insensitive to changes in atmospheric pressure and temperature;
(e) Impervious to environmental conditions within the head.
(3) Inexpensive.

IMPLANTED DEVICES

The shortcomings of catheter techniques led to investigations of other ways of measuring intracranial pressure. Brain tissue being almost entirely fluid it had been assumed that pressure in the ventricles and sub arachnoid space was identical to that elsewhere in the brain. The ventricles offer a convenient way of transmitting this pressure via catheter tubing to external equipment. An alternative method is to provide a small man-made ventricle in the form of a fluid filled latex balloon connected as before by a catheter to a low displacement pressure transducer, a technique reported by Rothballer in 1963 and Hoppenstein in 1965. An important departure from previous methods was the position of the balloon. It was placed just under the dura. Provided the system remains absolutely leak free, reliable continuous recordings can be achieved with this technique, but it is still prone to movement artefacts and hydrostatic error due to the position of the transducer.

In 1966 Numoto and his colleagues described a small intracranial device comprising a 9 mm diameter silastic envelope enclosing two gold electrodes as the poles of a simple switch the leads of which are brought out by wires in a PVC tube. Gradually increasing air pressure is applied to the envelope until the switch opens. The pressure applied is then equal to the ICP.

The device is certainly cheap and its simplicity is appealing but the recording is not continuous and the fidelity of the reading may be likened to that of the lumbar puncture.

In the same year Hulme and Cooper (1966) reported the use of a miniature pressure transducer only 3 mm in diameter held at the base of the burr hole in a stainless steel housing attached to the skull, the wires and reference tube emerging through the scalp.

This was the first of several efforts to use miniature pressure transducers implanted either subdurally or extradurally.

Table I gives details available from the literature on six pressure transducers used to monitor ICP continuously. It is noticeable that many blanks appear and this may be because these aspects of performance have been thought to make a negligible contribution to the transducer response or been left to the reader to interpret for him or herself.

Like most measuring devices, pressure transducers are not perfect. The relationship between applied pressure and output signal is *not* perfectly linear and the transducer is affected by factors other than pressure.

TABLE I

Author and date (Transducer type)	Pressure sensitivity (mV/mm Hg)†	Change of pressure sensitivity with temperature (%/C°)	Change in pressure reading with temperature (mm Hg/C°)	Non-linearity and hysteresis (%F.S.)	Drift in pressure reading
Hulme & Cooper 1966¶ (Schaevitz Bytrex HFD-2)	0.007§	—	—	—	—
Jacobson & Rothballer 1967¶ (Scientific Advances MM-3W)	0.005	—	2.0	—	—
Coe et al., 1967¶ (Scientific Advances MM-3W)	—	—	—	—	—
Nornes & Serck Hanssen 1970 (Akers AE 830)	0.1	0.2	0.03	1.0 (0→300 mm Hg)	Maximum: 3.3 mm Hg in 5 days Minimum: 0.0 mm Hg in 5 days
Eversden 1970 (Ferranti ZPT 25 GA)	0.1	—	−2.0 → +1.0	—	‡ Maximum: 10 mm Hg in 12 hours Thereafter less than 5 mm Hg/day
Dorsch et al, 1971	0.2	1.0	0.3	—	‡ 1 mm Hg after 12 hours

† Applied bridge voltage 3V. ¶ Non-vented transducers. § Applied voltage not given. ‡ In situ calibration available.

All the transducers contain diaphragms whose distortion or displacement is measured with resistive strain gauges. If the displacement of the diaphragm was linear with applied pressure then the strain gauge output would vary linearly with applied pressure. Unfortunately the relationship is not linear and the non-linearity gets worse as the ratio between displacement and diaphragm thickness increases. The smaller the pressure range to be measured, the thinner the diaphragm has to be to give a measureable amount of displacement. For this reason high sensitivity strain gauge elements are required to measure the smallest possible diaphragm displacement for a given diaphragm thickness.

Semiconductor strain gauge elements have high sensitivities and enable transducers to be made having 50 times the output of wire wound types. They are, however, more sensitive to changes in temperature and it is these changes which contribute to the figures given in columns 3 and 4 of Table I. The effects of temperature are lessened by connecting the resistive elements in a Wheatstone bridge circuit and providing the transducer is vented these changes in bridge balance and sensitivity are small. For those transducers having a silicon diaphragm mounted in a stainless steel or titanium body, compensation is made for the difference in coefficients of thermal expansion of the two materials.

Hysteresis is caused by friction and since in most cases there is very little movement between the component parts of the devices this effect is very small. Assuming a pressure sensitivity of 0.1 mV per mm Hg at an excitation voltage of 3V, an acceptable value for temperature coefficient would be 1% per C° which would cause a discrepancy of 1 mm Hg per C° for an applied pressure of 100 mm Hg. A value of 1 mm Hg per C° would be acceptable for change of pressure with temperature while non-linearity and hysteresis should be no greater than 0.3% of full scale over the range 0-300 mm Hg.

Finally we come to pressure reading drift which at present probably accounts for the majority of concern regarding miniature pressure transducers. A transducer may appear to be adequately stable when tested in air prior to implantation but when immersed in body fluid changes can occur in pressure reading that cannot be attributed to changes in ICP.

Figure 1 shows a recording of ICP in a patient with a large intracranial lesion. The pressure apparently rises from 44 mm Hg to 70 mm Hg over a period of nearly 2 hours. The transducer is then recalibrated and apparently the pressure continues to rise a further 22 mm Hg in the following 2½ hours. There is no change in the amplitude of pulsation during this period of time, which, together with details of the patient's clinical condition strongly suggests that there was no real change in ICP.

There is little published about the drift of implanted transducers but it appears that inadequate protection is provided against the intrusion of body fluid or moisture in the atmosphere. Silicon diaphragm transducers become more stable if the transducer is run in a warm dry atmosphere. Eventual failure invariably occurs at either end of a resistive element which allows the device to be used in a half bridge form if required.

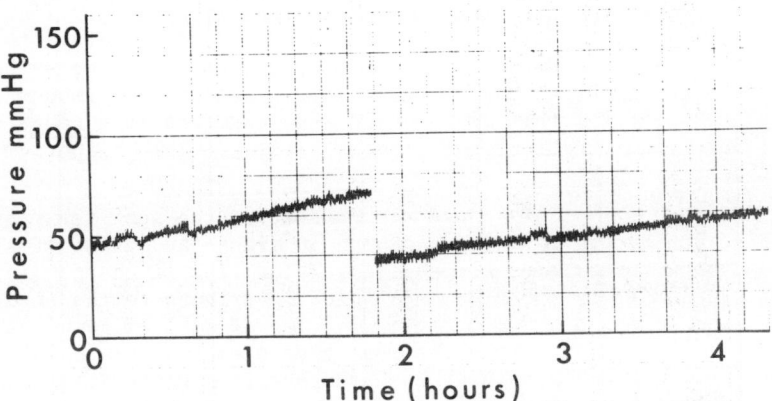

Figure 1 - Baseline drift of implanted pressure transducer.

Four transducers commercially available today are specified in Table II. The Kulite transducers consist of a monolithic integrated circuit Wheatstone bridge formed on a silicon diaphragm. They are only 3.2 mm in diameter and can be fitted neatly into the ends of standard sizes of catheter. The manufacturers claim that during the first 3-4 hours of implantation there may be a drift of 2-3 mm Hg but offer no details of drift during longer periods of implantation.

The Königsberg transducers consist of silicon strain gauges forming a Wheatstone bridge bonded to a titanium diaphragm. The diameter of the device recommended for ICP measurements is 7 mm in diameter and although guaranteed for 1 year against the intrusion of body fluid no details are given of pressure reading drift.

This Königsberg transducer is not vented to atmosphere. This is to prevent undue intrusion of water vapour to the transducer interior but makes the device susceptible to changes in atmospheric pressure. These changes can be as large as ±20 mm Hg but can with difficulty be compensated in the amplifying equipment.

The Sensatec transducer is similar in concept to the Königsberg, a Wheatstone bridge formation of silicon strain gauges being bonded to a stainless steel diaphragm. Again no details are available concerning drift and although there are no published details it is understood that after several hours of implantation the drift is appreciable.

Lastly the Norwegian produced Akers transducer consists of two planar resistors diffused on either side of a silicon beam forming a half bridge. The body of the device and hence the diaphragm can be made of silver plated brass or titanium. The device is rather large, 12 mm diameter but published reports of drift in two of

TABLE II

Transducer	Pressure sensitivity (mV/mm Hg)†	Change of pressure sensitivity with temperature (%/C°)	Change in pressure reading with temperature (mm Hg/C°)	Non-linearity and hysteresis (%F.S.)	Drift in pressure reading
Kulite (CQL 125 and CQL 080)	0.03	0.1	0.1	1.0 (0→300 mm Hg)	2→3 mm Hg during first 3→4 hours
Königsberg¶ (P.21)	0.01	0.2	0.1	0.5 (0→300 mm Hg)	—
Scientific Advances (Sensotec M-7BW)	0.05	—	0.2	0.5 (-100 → +300 mm Hg)	—
Akers (Guest International) (AE 830 A vented)	0.10	0.2	0.3	1.0 (0→300 mm Hg)	—

† Applied bridge voltage 3V.
¶ Non-vented transducers.

these devices after implantation for periods of up to 5 days, indicate drifts of no greater than 3.3 mm Hg over this period.

The cost of these devices in England is as follows:

           Kulite   £ 173
           Königsberg £ 256
           Sensatec   £ 188
           Akers   £ 49 or £ 75.

Figure 2 shows the relative size and shapes of the transducers available together with that of the Ferranti now no longer available.

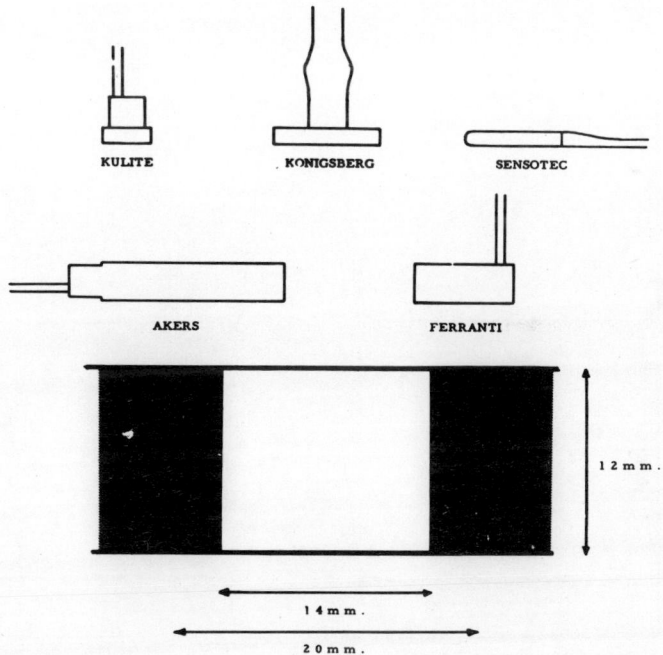

Figure 2 - Relative sizes of various transducers and burrhole.

A smaller version of the Akers transducers only 7 mm in diameter is now available, the cost of the titanium version being £ 195 but this may be reduced in the near future depending on demand.

In view of the continuing uncertainty of transducer stability it would seem sensible to add to the device an 'in situ' calibration chamber. This can be done by adding a thin flexible chamber to the face of the pressure sensitive diaphragm connected to atmosphere by fine tubing. The chamber is normally flattened against the transducer diaphragm and does not significantly affect the measurement of pressure. To check the calibration the fine tube is connected to an air filled syringe and sphygmomanometer. The air pressure is increased until it is sufficient to open the outer chamber. Readings on the sphygmomanometer should thereafter correspond to those indicated by the transducer if required; the zero pressure reading may be obtained by extrapolation or alternatively by applying equal pressure to both the outer chamber and the transducer venting tube.

Figure 3 shows the changes in pressure occurring during chamber inflation. The upper curve was obtained by replacing the sphygmomanometer with a calibrated pressure transducer and the lower curve that recorded by the implanted transducer.

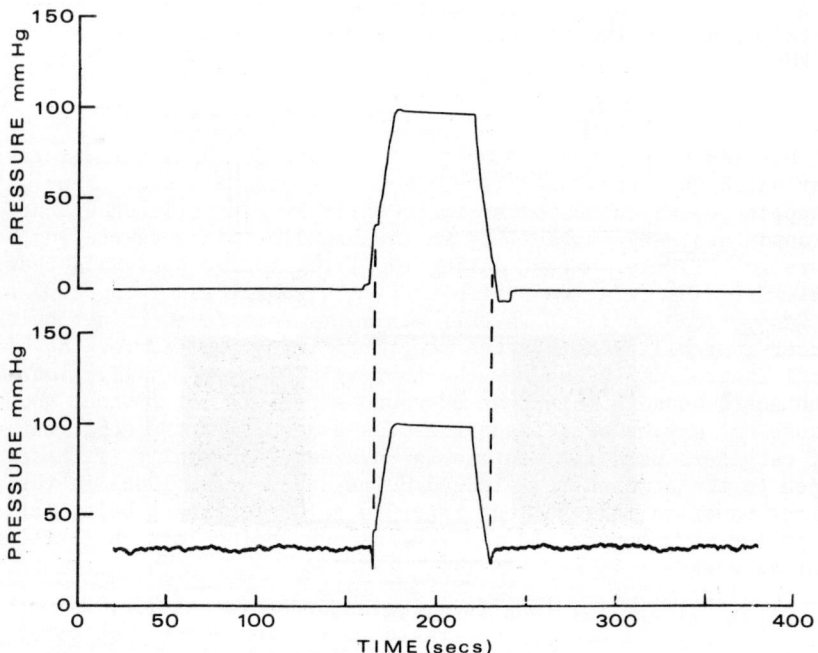

Figure 3 - Check of transducer zero by inflation of surrounding cuff.

In order to improve the durability of the modified device, the outer chamber now consists of a layer of 0.01 mm polythene film sandwiched between two layers of 0.03 mm silicone rubber film sealed to the transducer with silicone rubber adhesive. Fine silicone rubber tubing is used to connect both the outer chamber and the venting tube to a plug and the whole device covered with a thin layer of cold curing silastomer. The diameter of the modified transducer is 8-9 mm and the diameter of the lead 3 mm.

A similar facility is provided in a device reported by Dorsch and his colleagues (1971). Here a cylindrical block of epoxy resin fits snugly into a burr hole. It holds a berylium copper sensing arm to which are attached two p-type semiconductor strain gauges. The device is used extradurally, the sensing arm being separated from the dura by a 10 μ thick latex rubber membrane. By forcing air at a known pressure along the polythene venting tube the membrane is separated from the sensing arm to give the zero pressure reading. Ideally the tip of the sensing arm should be coplanar with the base of the transducer and this modification is, I understand, being incorporated at present.

The resonant frequency of this device appears to be below 1.5 Hz and cannot therefore be used for the analysis of the pressure waveform. This requires a device with a flat frequency response up to 20 Hz which is easily within the scope of the silicon and metal diaphragm transducers whose resonant frequency is well above 1 kHz.

DEVICES FOR LONG TERM IMPLANTATION

Until now the words 'long-term' concerning the length of time for which the transducer is planted have been avoided. From our experience, which has been almost entirely with silicon diaphragm transducers, any instability in the baseline pressure reading occurs to a limited extent during the first twelve hours and thereafter remains relatively stable for the remainder of the implantation period. A limit in this period is therefore set not by transducer instability but by the length of time required for the clinical control of ICP and by the increasing danger of infection at the scalp wound. This fear of wound sepsis is not without good cause but may be over exaggerated as a result of the negligent care of catheters used for ventricular drainage especially if these are open to the atmosphere. Indeed Hulme and Cooper (1966) in their first paper on this subject refer to gold electrodes being left in situ for many months and their transducer being left in position for 4½ weeks.

Nevertheless, for long term implantation for as long as perhaps as a year, it is clearly desirable to eliminate the problem of leads by telemetry from an implanted device through an intact scalp.

Such devices have been described by Watson et al. and Brock et al.. The latter consists of a capacitance pressure sensor, transmitter and battery all contained within a silastic coated container. What is described as an 'equaliser tube' maintains reference to ambient air but full details are not available and no extensive trials have been reported.

Batteries have a limited life and unless these are rechargeable and suitable circuitry included in the implanted package, the life of the pressure transmitter will depend upon the life of the battery.

The passive transensor is a delightful solution to this problem. Olsen (1967) has described the use of a 6 mm diameter 2 mm thick cylindrical capsule containing a pair of parallel coaxial Archimedian spiral coils. These form a resonant circuit whose frequency changes with coil separation, which in turn is affected by external pressure. The frequency of an external inductively coupled oscillation detector is repeatedly swept and the energy absorbed sensed through the intervening tissue. Although used successfully in animals there has been no report of routine clinical measurements with these devices. It is understood that the major problem is one of diaphragm creep, to the extent that glass has been tried as an alternative to the original mylar film.

This and other problems appear to have forestalled further attempts to create satisfactory transersors. Recently, however, Williams and his colleagues at the Royal Infirmary, Edinburgh, have designed a similar device which consists of a passive LC circuit in an implant which fits a 0.75" (19 mm) diameter burr hole. The inductance is varied by the pressure altering the air gap of a ferrite cone. The implanted tuned circuit forms the frequency controlling feedback path of an external oscillator. It is coupled to the oscillator circuit by two pairs of coils. The oscillator frequency has, by careful design, been made insensitive to exact positioning of the pick up coils over the implant.

Development problems have been the minimisation of the effect of inexact coil positioning, obtaining long term stability and selecting suitable materials for implantation. In passing it is pertinent to note that such a device, being isolated from atmosphere is susceptible to changes in atmospheric pressure and body temperature.

Before summarising I should like to comment briefly on the question of intra-dural versus extra-dural implantation. Dura is a tough layer of tissue which is firmly attached to the underside of the skull. Although described as elastic, or more correctly linearly viscoelastic, it does not readily stretch under stress. The degree to which this occurs can be observed when burr holes are made in a patient with high ICP - the dura bulges. Providing the dura is detached from the skull it will lie loosely over the surface of any small implanted device. It is doubtful if the dura follows the exact contour of the transducer which should therefore be as small and thin as possible. Being flexible the dura will lie in close contact with the transducer diaphragm provided there is positive pressure applied. Movement at the centre of the diaphragm is very small, usually less than 10^{-2} mm, and it is doubtful if the dura is in a stretched state or if it is held firmly enough at the edges to affect the diaphragm displacement. Clearly if placed at the base of a burr hole the entire surface of the transducer diaphragm must be in contact with the dura in order to comply with the conditions of transducer calibration.

Lastly, the incidence of infection in Lundberg's series of patients using intraventricular catheters was extremely low, 1-3%. With subdural or epidural transducers it should become almost negligible.

SUMMARY

It is reasonable to say that miniature pressure transducers are available whose size, shape and electrical characteristics are satisfactory for implantation. At Atkinson Morley's Hospital we prefer to add an outer chamber to all our transducers to enable us to check the calibration in situ, mainly perhaps to convince ourselves that the changes in pressure are bona fide and not a result of drift. It is also unnecessary to calibrate a transducer just prior to implantation which can be a serious drawback to routine clinical monitoring.

However, with the possibility of drift still existing a ventricular catheter connected to either standard or miniature externally mounted pressure transducers offers a reliable if somewhat troublesome alternative.

Certainly improvements are required in the stability of implanted devices and it is possible that the investigations involved in producing chronically implanted transensors may bring some advance in this respect. Meanwhile as much data as possible should be made available concerning the drift of transducers in use.

Hopefully there will be a move towards *smaller* devices which can be removed without a second operative procedure. The small diameter fibre optic probes being investigated for monitoring blood pressure could well have a rôle to play.

We still have much to learn of intracranial hypertension. The establishment of cheap, reliable, and simple to use pressure measuring techniques will undoubtedly hasten our advance in this field.

REFERENCES

Coe, J.E., Nelson, J.W., Rudenberg, F.H. and Garza, R. (1967). Technique for continuous intracranial pressure recording, *J. Neurosurg.*, **27**, 370-375.

Dorsch, N.W.C., Stephens, R.J. and Symon, L. (1971). An intracranial pressure transducer, *Bio-Med. Engng.*, **6**, 452-457.

Eversden, I.D. (1970). Modification to a miniature pressure transducer for the measurement of intracranial pressure, *Med. and Biol. Engng.*, **8**, 159-164.

Gerlach, J. (1952). Zerebraler Grenzdruck und Hirnpuls. Klinische Untersuchungen und Ergebnisse, *Acta Neurochir.*, **2**, 120-158.

Gilland, O. (1965). C.S.F. dynamic diagnosis of spinal block IV: Demands on electromanometric equipment, *Acta. Neurol. Scand., Suppl. 13*, **41**, 75-105.

Guillaume, J. and Janny, P. (1951). Manametric intracranience continue, *Rev. Neurol.*, **84**, 131-142.

Hoppenstein, R. (1965). A device for measuring intracranial pressure, *Lancet* i, 90.

Hulme, A. and Cooper, R. (1966). A technique for the investigation of intracranial pressure in man, *J. Neurol. Neurosurg. Psychiat.*, **29**, 154-156.

Lundberg, N. (1960). Continuous recording and control of ventricular fluid pressure in neurological practice, *Acta Psychiat. Neurol. Scand., Suppl. 36.*

Nornes, H. and Serck-Hanssen, F. (1970). Miniature transducer for intracranial pressure monitoring in man, *Acta Neurol. Scand.*, **46**, 203-214.

Numoto, M., Slater, J.P. and Donaghy, R.M.P. (1966). An implantable switch for monitoring intracranial pressure, *Lancet* i, 528.

Olsen, E.R., Collins, C.C., Loughborough, W.F., Richards, V., Adams, J.E. and Pinto, D.W. (1967). Intracranial pressure measurement with a miniature passive implanted pressure transensor, *Amer. J. Surg.*, **113**, No. 6, 727-729.

Rothballer, A.M. (1963). Continuous recording of intracranial pressure in man and animals, Presented at meeting of *Harvey Cushing Society*, Philadelphia, Penn., (April).

Watson, B.W., Riddle, H.C. and Currie, J.C.M. (1967). The measurement of intracranial pressure in man using radio telemetry, in *Proceedings of the 7th International Conference on Medical and Biological Engineering, (Stockholm)*, p. 91.

Williamson, D. (Private communication).

MICRO-ELECTRODE RECORDINGS IN THE HUMAN THALAMUS DURING STEREOTAXIC SURGERY

J. ANDREW

The Middlesex Hospital, Mortimer Street, London W1

N. DE M. RUDOLF

Charing Cross Hospital, Fulham Palace Road, London W6

Unit recordings during 77 stereotaxic thalamotomies were performed to determine the optimum site for the lesion. The procedure also provided the opportunity to correlate physiological localisation with the average position of nuclear boundaries and their variabilities.

There were 112 trajectories explored, using this technique, in 64 patients. 47 of these had Parkinson's disease, and the remaining suffered from other dyskinesias.

A multiperforated sphere designed by Watkins was fixed between plates near the coronal suture and approximately 4 cm from the midline using the Bennett-Rivers stereotaxic frame. The perforations in the sphere were 3 mm apart in the sagittal and coronal planes, allowing the exploration of an area 12×12 mm. Check X-rays were made. Subsequently, under local anaesthetic the electrode was passed through one or more of the perforations into the thalamus. The distance from the electrode tip to the vertical transverse plane through the posterior border of the Interventricular Foramen of Munro (IVF), the horizontal plane between the IVF and the Posterior Commissure (PC), and the mid-line could be calculated at any given point along its track.

A micrometer screw, fixed into the sphere, was used to propel the electrode. This was either one designed by Albé-Fessard, bipolar, with a tip of not more than 50 μ, or by Claude Bertrand which has a slightly smaller tip. Recording was usually commenced 20 mm proximal to the target point and continued down to 5 mm beyond. The insertion was halted at every millimeter from the target point and the activity observed and recorded and appropriate tests applied. If during the advance of the electrode any activity of interest was encountered additional halts were made. After amplification the signal was displayed on an oscilloscope at 20 μV/cm and on a second channel after an H.F. cut at 500 c/s or lower, in order to reveal rhythmic or semi-rhythmic components underlying the spike discharges. The signal was also played over an audio channel which gave a sensitive indication of the activity present and of any changes in it, either spontaneous or evoked by somatic stimulation.

Testing was carried out at most points at which the electrode was halted unless no unit activity was present. A record was kept of whether tests were applied, their nature and results. The face, upper limb and lower limb were usually examined for responses to skin stimulation, and joint and muscle stimulation. The face was always stimulated bilaterally; the leg on the side of the thalamus being investigated was sometimes examined (especially if a response was found in the contralateral leg), and the ipsilateral arm occasionally examined. In addition, tests of the thorax and abdomen, tongue, teeth-clenching, eye-opening and closing, eye movements and mental arithmetic were applied when appropriate. In a given thalamus recording may have been carried out along one, two or three trajectories.

When the total number of evoked responses from the head, arm and leg were plotted in 1 mm squares, and related to the coronal and midline planes only, it was clear that there was much overlapping of the somatotopic areas, which could be most satisfactorily explained by individual variability. However, there was a tendency for the leg to be most laterally disposed, the head medially, with the upper limb between them. (Figure 1).

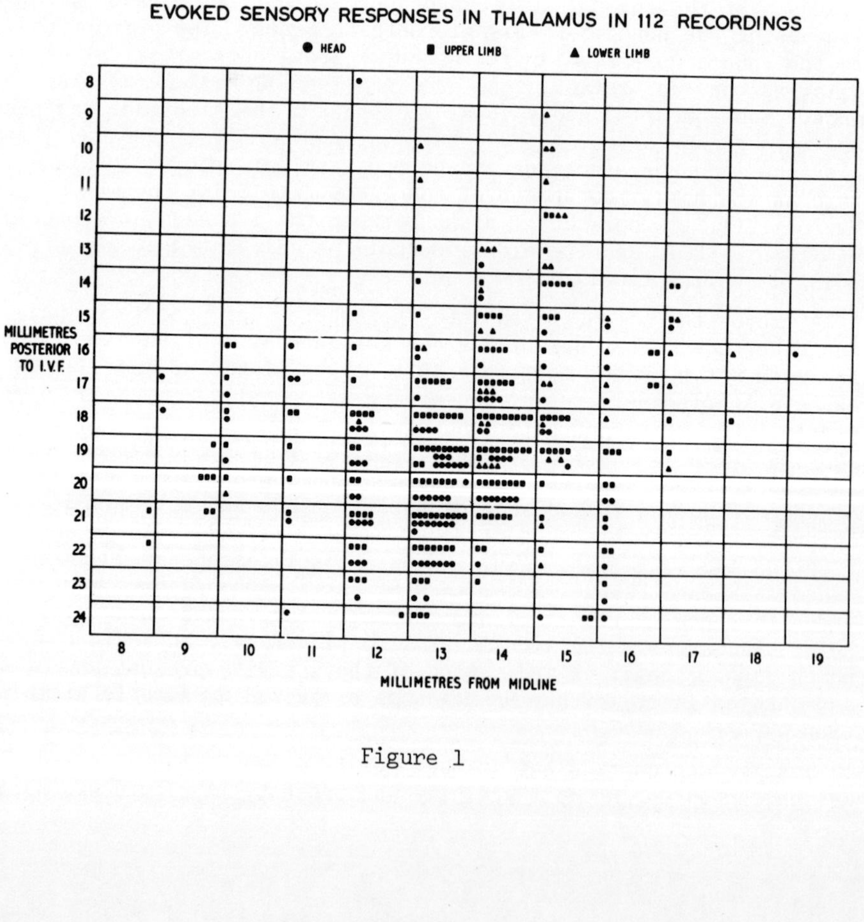

Figure 1

EVOKED RESPONSES FROM THE HEAD

It has been generally accepted that the ventralis caudalis internus nucleus (Vci) otherwise known as ventralis postero-medialis (Vpm) or the semilunar or arcuate nucleus, is the thalamic relay centre for the head. When the site of evoked responses from the head was related to the boundaries of this nucleus, a number was found to fall outside.

Although it has for long been known that there are variabilities in the position of the borders of the thalamic nuclei related to the reference points such as the commissures and the midline and the intercommissural plane, there was no detailed information as to these variabilities. Accordingly Andrew and Watkins (1969) prepared a variability atlas by measuring the boundaries of the thalamic nuclei and related structures to the Interventricular Foramen of Munro (IVF), which they believe to be the most reliable reference point, and to the plane joining this structure to the posterior commissure, and to the midline.

26 brains were cut in the coronal plane and 1 mm slices at right angles to the IVF-PC plane, and measurements made. A 'model' atlas was prepared for every 1 mm posterior to the IVF giving the average position of the nuclear boundaries and their distances from the reference planes. When the head responses were plotted on the appropriate charts at 1 mm intervals posterior to the IVF and in the coronal plane, it was found that 72% of them fell either within the Vci *or* the first standard deviation outside the mean position of its boundary. If all the head fibres relay in the Vci and the instrumentation and variability study were perfect, at least 83.5% of the responses should have fallen within this zone. (Figure 2).

Ipsilateral responses from the head were also obtained, and if there were no contralateral responses at the same point they were usually more laterally place in the thalamus; they were less often encountered more posteriorly. Responses from the tongue and lips tended to be more medial than those from the angle of the mouth and cheek. In a few of the anatomical specimens the anterior limit of Vci was found to extend forwards to 10 mm posterior to the IVF but of insufficient frequency for inclusion in the 'average thalamus'. At a given distance posterior to the IVF at least 40% of the specimens had to contain a structure before averages could be calculated. This would account for head responses occurring apparently in front of the anterior limit of Vci and also for some of the very posterior responses, of which a few could have been in the medial lemniscus. Figure 3 shows the antero-posterior disposition of the recordings and also the bias of the usual direction of the trajectories.

EVOKED RESPONSES FROM THE UPPER AND LOWER LIMBS

The responses recorded were to active or passive movements at individual joints or to deep pressure and light tactile stimulation of the skin. The responses were grouped into deep or superficial responses in the upper limb but deep responses only were obtained

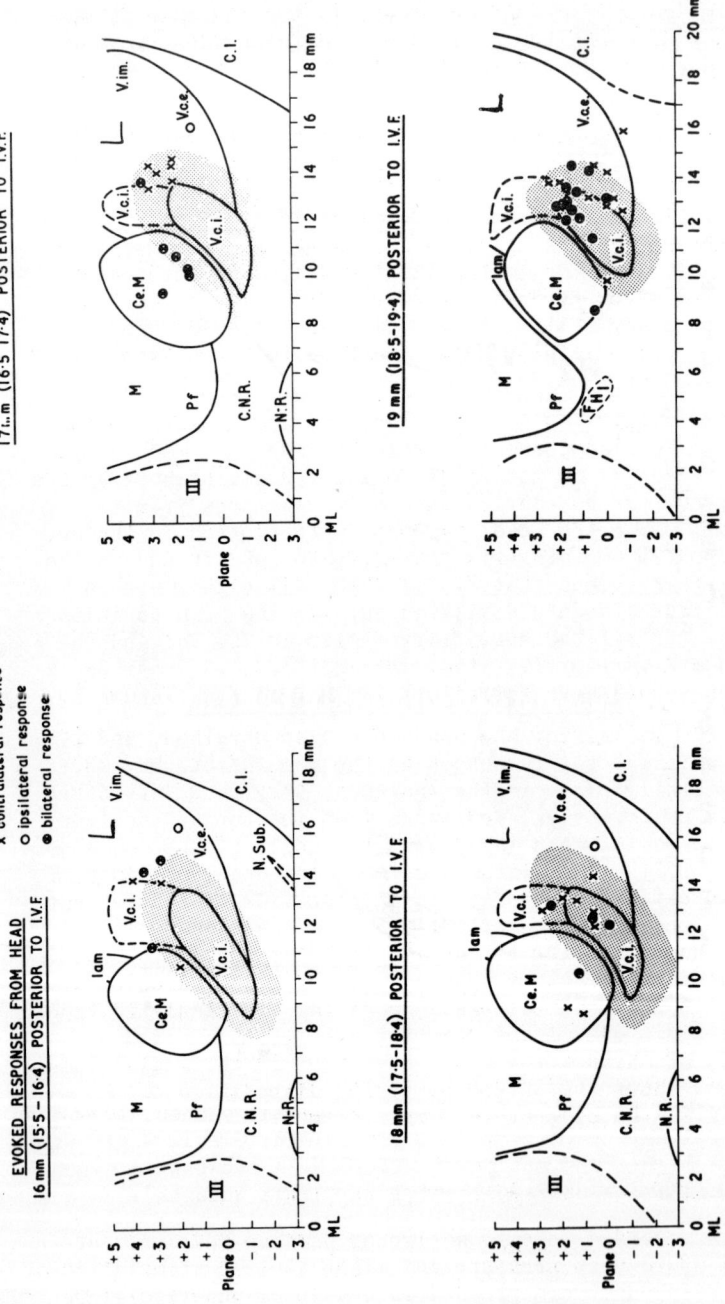

Figure 2 - Evoked responses from head. Coronal planes, 16 mm – 19 mm posterior to interventricular foramen. (Shaded zone denotes the Vci and the limit of its first standard deviation. III = third ventricle; C.I. = internal capsule; C.N.R. = capsule of red nucleus; Ce.M. = centro-medianum; F.H.I. = fasciculus habendulo-interpeduncularis; I.V.F. = interventricular foramen of Munro; L. = lateral thalamic mass; Lam. = internal medullary lamina; M. = medial thalamic mass; M.L. = midline; N.R. = nucleus ruber; N.sub. = subthalamic nucleus of Luys; Pf. = parafascicularis; V.c.e. = ventralis caudalis externus; V.c.i. = ventralis caudalis internus; V.i.m. = ventralis intermedius).

from the lower limb. The responses would be expected to occur in the ventralis caudalis externus (Vce). Precise localisation of this is only possible histologically. In the 1 mm slices the boundaries of this nucleus were inferred by the inner border of the internal capsule laterally, the lateral border of the ventralis caudalis internus and centro-medianum medially, and the lower margin of the thalamus below.

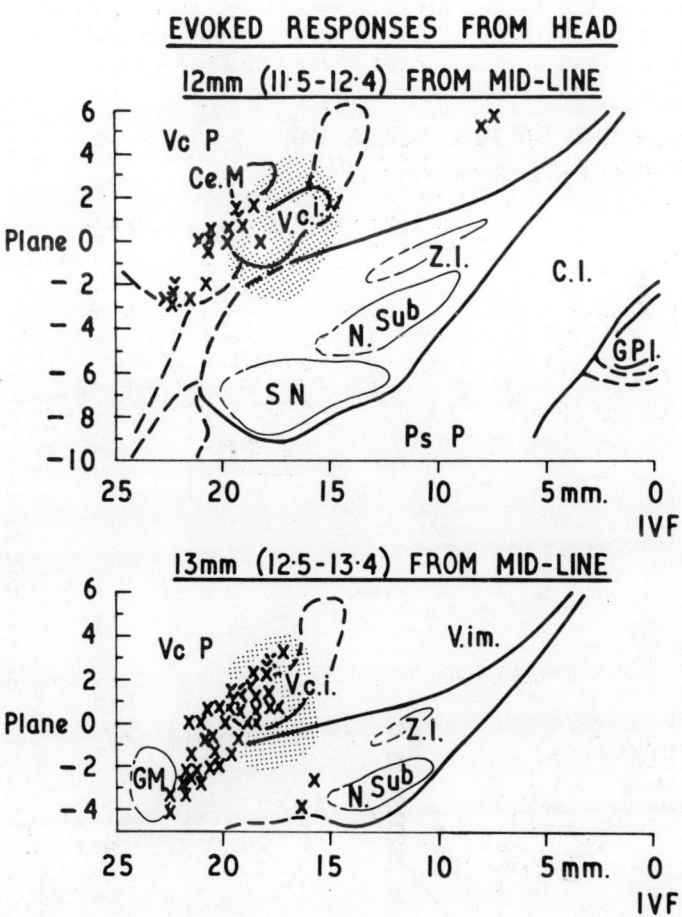

Figure 3 - Evoked responses from head. Sagittal planes, 12 mm - 13 mm from midline. (G.M. = medial geniculate; G.P.I. = globus pallidus crus 1; Ps.P. = pes pedunculi; S.N. = substantia nigra; V.c.P. = ventralis caudalis portae; Z.I. = zona incerta).

From histological studies, (Tomlinson, 1969) it is known that its anterior and posterior limits correspond to those of the Vci, which is visible to the naked eye. The small number of responses obtained more anteriorly to the position of the Vci as shown in the atlas is accounted for by the occasional more anterior limit of this nucleus.

The distribution of the majority of evoked limb responses in the coronal planes is shown in figure 4. 93% of the responses fell within the Vce and in the first standard deviation outside the mean position of its border. This compares favourably with the minimum number of responses expected there, which is 83.5%.

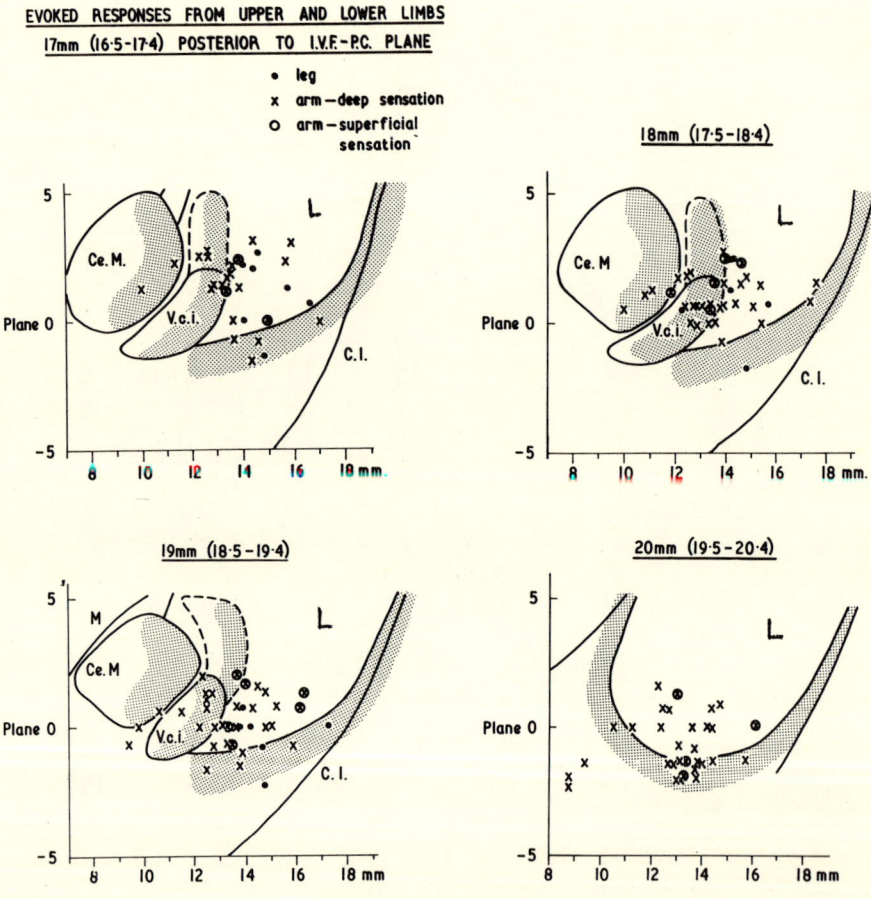

Figure 4 - Evoked responses from limbs. Coronal planes, 17 mm - 20 mm posterior to interventricular foramen. (The shaded zones indicate the medial limit of the first standard deviation for the lateral borders of CeM, Vci, the lateral limit of that for the lateral and inferior borders of L).

It will be seen that there is a tendency for the lower limb responses to be more anteriorly, superiorly and laterally placed than of those for the upper limb. Superficial responses appear to be evenly scattered in the limb responsive zones. The few ipsilateral lower limb responses have not been indicated, but they were found in the lateral part of the responsive area at an average distance of 15 mm from the midline.

In the sagittal profile (figure 5) there is again the suggestion that some responses may occur in the medial lemniscus; the directional lines of the trajectories are also seen.

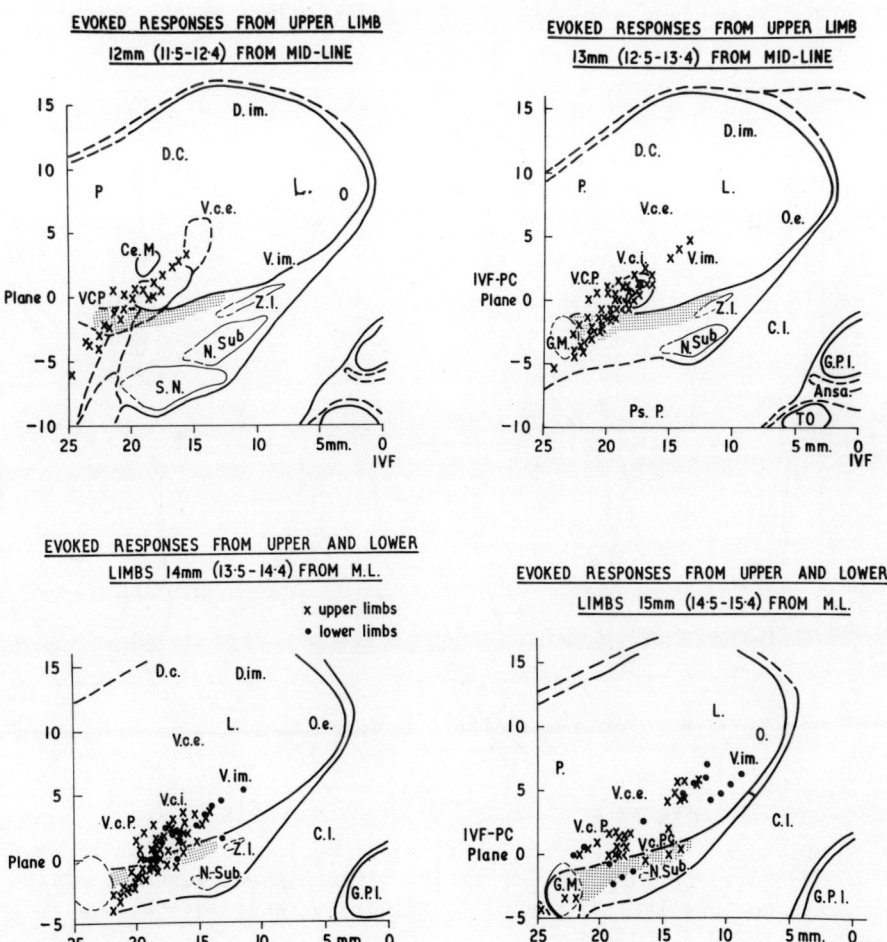

Figure 5 - Evoked responses from limbs. Sagittal planes 12 mm - 15 mm from midline. (D.c. = dorsalis caudalis; D.im. = dorsalis intermedius; L. = lateral thalamic mass; O. = oralis; O.e. = oralis externus; P. = pulvinar; T.O. = optic tract).

NORMALISATION OF RESPONSES

To eliminate such a bias due to some areas having been more frequently traversed than others, the antero-posteriorly disposed solid rectangular region containing all the tremor bursts and responses has been divided into 432 cubes with edges of 2 mm, so the results could be normalised. 162 of the 2 mm cubes have been stopped in, as well as others more proximally than the region of interest, that is, higher up the trajectories, and some more distally. The results from all patients are pooled and include both the right and left sides together. The responses are expressed as the percentage of positive results for the number of times stimulation has been applied while the electrode was stationary in a particular cube.

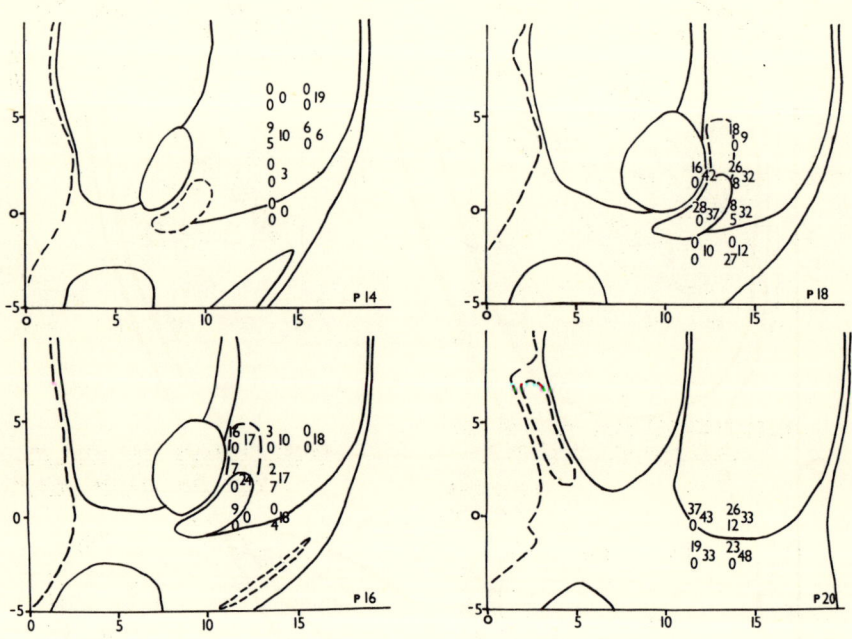

Figure 6   Figure 7

Figures 6,7,8 - Coronal sections at various distances in mm (denoted by P) posterior to IVF. (Abscissa = vertical scale in mm (0 = IVF - PC plane). Ordinate = medio-lateral scale in mm (0 = midline)).

In figures 6-8 only percentages based on 10 or more observations (that is, testings) have been entered. In each cube (group of 3 figures) the top left percentage is for the head, the centre right figure is for the upper limb and the lower left figure is for the lower limb. Each diagram applies to the layer of cubes centred on it.

The results are in general agreement with our conclusions from sites of responses shown above. At 20 and 18 mm posterior to the IVF the region near the lower limit of the *average* thalamus yields many responses, particularly in the ventralis caudalis parvo-cellularis and ventralis caudalis portae, although it is possible that some are outside the thalamus in afferent fibres terminating in those thalamic areas. Lower limb responses are situated laterally.

At 18 and 16 mm (figures 6,7) the encroachment of the upper limb area on the Vci is probably more apparent than real when one remembers the extent of the first standard deviation. Again the lower limb responses tend to be lateral while the head is more medial at 16 mm posterior. At 12 mm posterior to IVF (figure 8), where the Vci and Vce are not shown in the atlas, the variability data show that in nearly a quarter of the brains the Vci (and presumably the Vce) extends this far forward. This explains why there were some responses here.

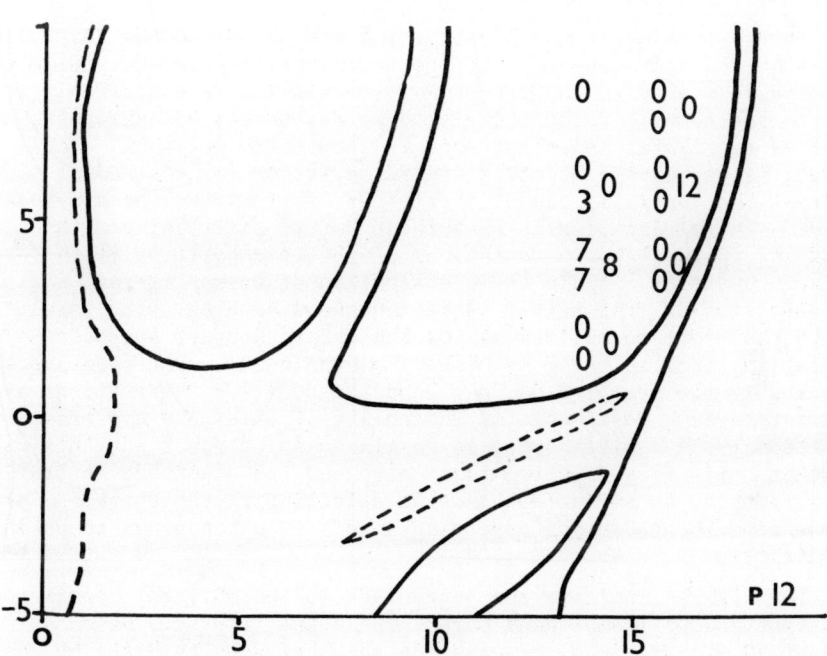

Figure 8 - See caption to figures 6,7 for caption and scaling.

TREMOR BURSTS

Tremor bursts were first described in the thalamus by Albé-Fessard, and Bates (1969) and others have confirmed these, and they also found them to be of two different types as in the present series. Firstly there are the spontaneous tremor bursts which are obtained anterior to the somatic relay zone. These are distinguished from tremor responsive bursts obtained in the somatic relay nuclei in the following manner. The spontaneous bursts cannot be modified by body stimulation. Also they may not be at the frequency of the observed tremor, or they may have a varying phase relationship with the tremor, although the bursts are usually in the tremor frequency range of 3-7 cycles per second; lastly the spontaneous bursts may persist after the tremor spontaneously disappears, or they may reappear before the tremor itself re-appears. Bursts of firing in the tremor frequency band were only found in patients with tremor, and occurred in 40% of the 55 cases.

Figure 9 shows the situation in the sagittal plane at different distances from the midline from which spontaneous tremor bursts have been obtained. The majority of these were between 13 and 15 mm from the midline and for the most part they were anterior to the sensory relay nuclei and well above the IVF-PC plane, and there were none below this plane. Some of the more medial bursts *appear* to be situated in the sensory relay nuclei. The directional lines of the trajectories again are seen.

The responsive tremor bursts which are influenced by body stimulation and are thought to be due to muscle stretch or tactile response secondary to the tremor were obtained more posteriorly mainly in the somatic relay nuclei. Some responses, however, were obtained fairly far medially, even in the centro-medianum. This would be beyond the second standard deviation for the medial border of the ventralis caudalis externus, that is for the arm relay area. One explanation is that these bursts occur between the second and third standard deviations of the mean position of the nuclear boundaries. Again the distribution of tremor firing, whether spontaneous or responsive, suggested sampling bias. The results were therefore normalised as for the evoked sensory responses by referring them to the 2 mm cubes (figures 10-12). For spontaneous bursts in the tremor frequency band the positive observations are expressed as a percentage of the number of times the electrode was stationary in a given cube, in Parkinsonism or other patients with tremor. (It is considered that only when the electrode is stationary is there an adequate chance of detecting rhythmic firing, since some time is needed for observing an effect which tends to be intermittent).

The figures indicate the percentage (or normalised) occurrence of spontaneous tremor band bursts where the result is based on at least 10 observations. It was thought that results based on less than 10 observations were liable to be quantitatively misleading. This distribution coincides quite well with the Vim but perhaps extends forwards into the oralis externus (figure 12).

There is a suggestion that unresponsive tremor rhythmic firing may also occur in the ventro-caudalis internus; however, examination of the succession of events along all trajectories in which tremor bursts occurred shows none occurring at a point at which responses could be elicited from the head, although they may be found as close as a millimetre to such a point. Therefore there is no *direct* evidence that the region with spontaneous rhythmic

RECORDINGS IN THE THALAMUS DURING STEREOTAXIC SURGERY 63

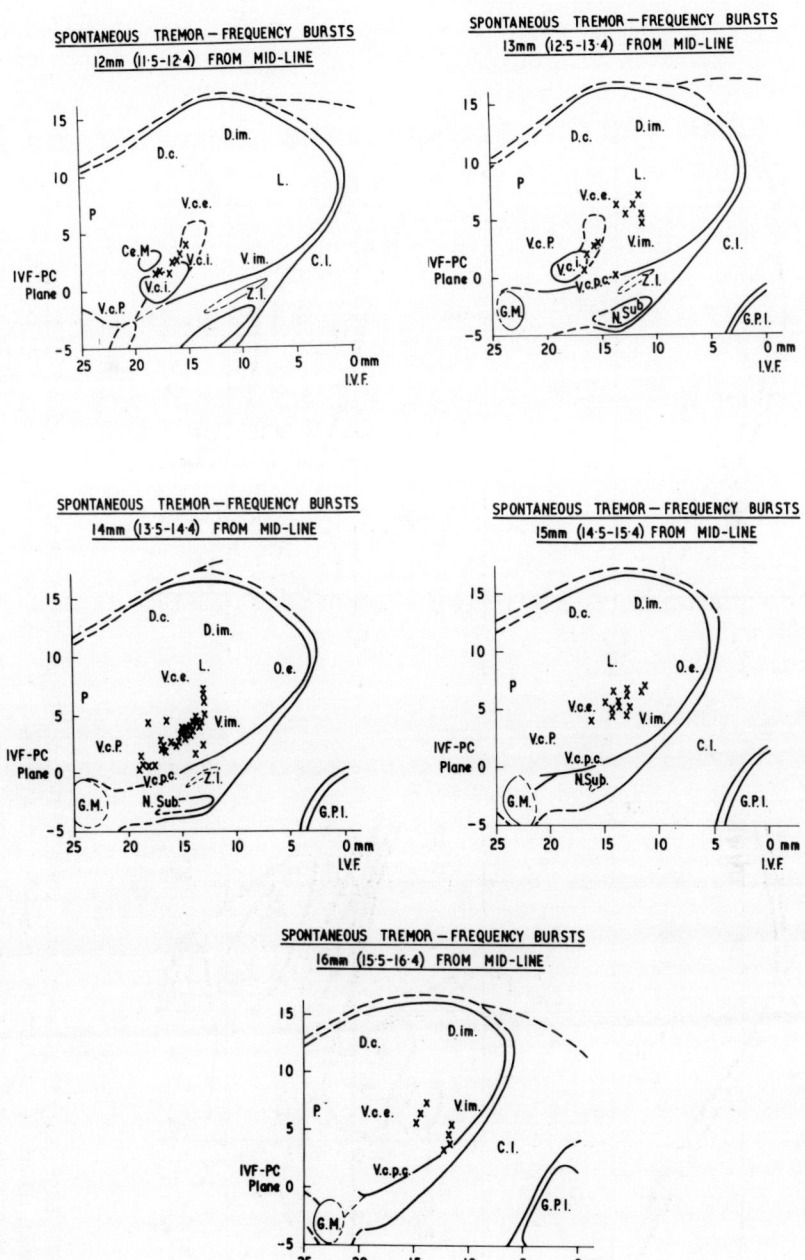

Figure 9 - Spontaneous tremor-frequency bursts. Sagittal planes, 12 mm - 16 mm from midline.

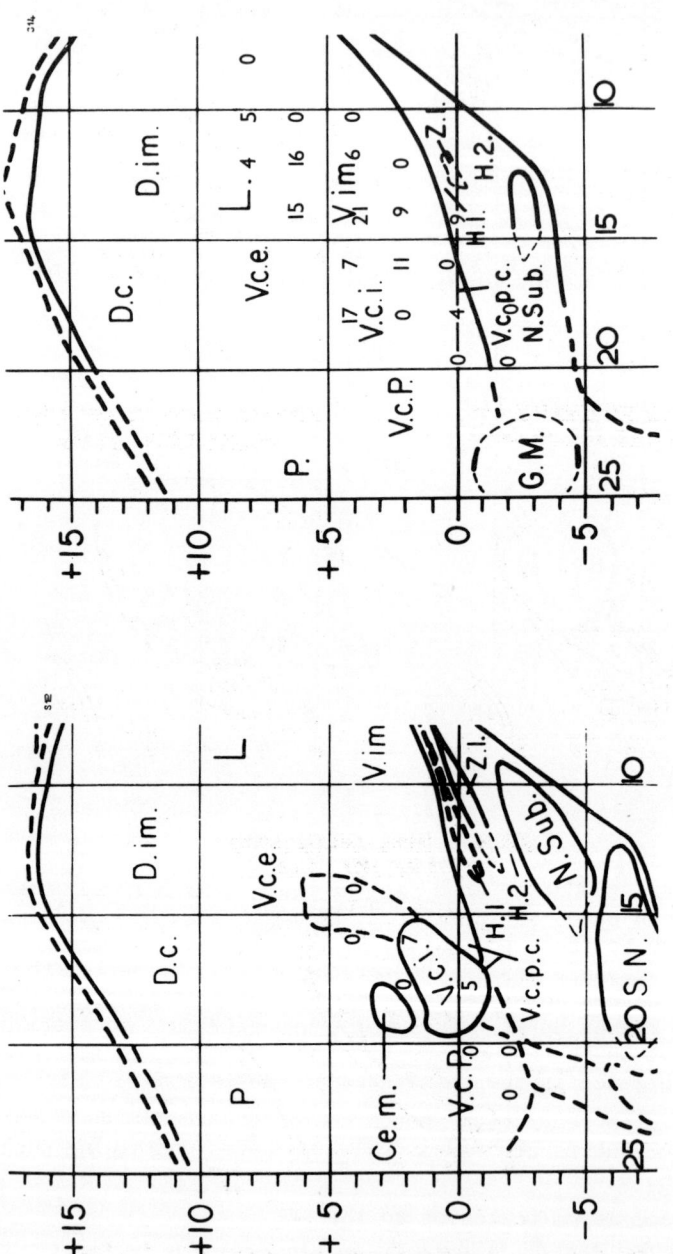

Figure 10

Figure 11

Figures 10, 11, 12 - Sagittal sections at 12, 14 and 16 mm (denoted by S) from midline. (Abscissa = vertical scale in mm (0 = IVF-PC plane). Ordinate = antero-posterior scale (distance in mm posterior to IVF). Anatomical abbreviations as before plus V.c.p.c. = ventralis caudalis parvo-cellularis. H.1, H.2 = fields of Forel).

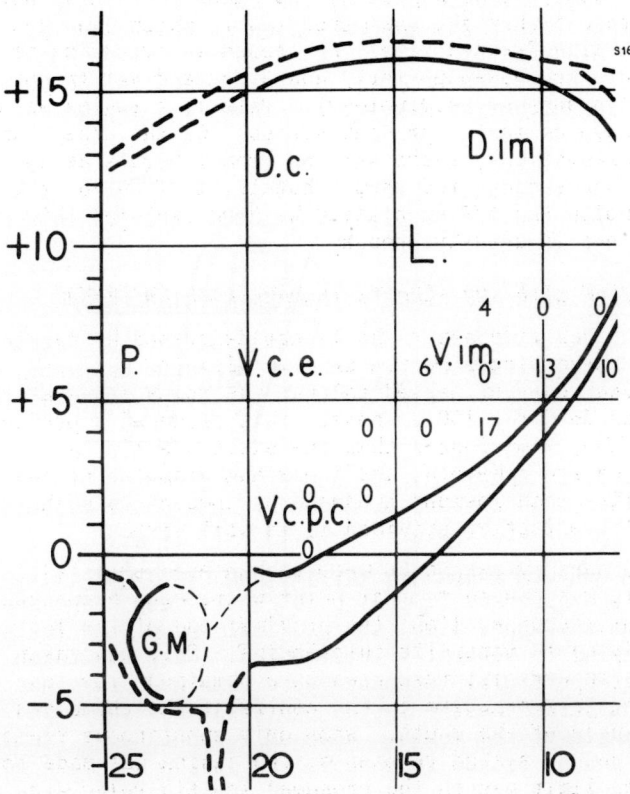

Figure 12 - See caption to figures 10,11 for caption and scaling.

firing overlaps the relay area for the head. Furthermore, tremor burst points in cubes at 12 mm from the midline might come from patients whose Vci does not extend as far laterally as the average; the mean and standard deviations for the lateral border of the Vci at these two places do allow this interpretation. However, there are just two tremor burst points which are difficult to attribute to Vim, except on the assumption of minor instrumental inaccuracy or their occurrence in the third standard deviation.

With regard to the region in the coordinate system where spontaneous tremor bursts are found, the 2 mm cubes containing such bursts are those whose centres are between:

 8 and 18 mm posterior to the FM;

 the FM-PC plane and 8 mm above it,

 and 12 and 16 mm from the midline.

Negative observations (many are not shown because they are less than 10 per cube) surround most of the cubes containing bursts, but it is of interest that the one direction in which they are few is one in which Albé-Fessard (1967) has found an extension of tremor bursts, namely postero-superiorly above Vce and Vci in dorso-caudalis (or LP in another terminology). This is a region which is inadequately covered in the present series. On the other hand, in but a few observations, there were no tremor bursts as low down as this author has encountered them, that is, in front of the relay nuclei but below the IVF-PC plane. We *have* explored this region, but perhaps not frequently enough.

LESION SITE AND RESULTS IN PARKINSONIAN TREMOR

The lesion was made after the manner described by Watkins (1955). A 5 or 6 mm bared electrode tip of 1 mm diameter was used, and a radio frequency current passed so that the temperature at the electrode tip was 66°C for 150 seconds. This produced a predictable discrete lesion, 1 mm longer than the electrode tip, and with the shape of an oblate spheroid, and a maximum diameter of 3-4 mm. This is smaller than lesions produced by some other authors, but can be equally effective provided it is well sited.

When only sensory responses were encountered this lesion-making electrode tip was passed to that point where deep responses were obtained from the upper limb; the proximal end of the lesion would usually be lying in ventralis intermedius. Care was taken to avoid a site where superficial responses were obtained, for fear of causing permanent paraesthesiae in the contralateral thumb and index finger and angle of the mouth. When only spontaneous tremor bursts were found, and no evoked responses, the lesion was made so that its posterior limit was in the presumed somatic relay area, but its anterior limit in the tremor band zone. When both spontaneous tremor bursts and evoked deep responses from the upper limb were found and were separated by less than 5 mm, a lesion was made to extend into both zones, making its length up to 7 mm long.

If there were neither spontaneous tremor bursts nor sensory responses, our target was sought by electrical stimulation, the site being that where paraesthesiae were produced in the upper limb but not in the face. A unipolar electrode with a tip 1 mm long and 1 mm in diameter was used with a 0.5 volt since wave at 50 c/s.

RESULTS

In general the early results were good but there were some relapses. However, if a lesion was made in the zone of spontaneous tremor firing the early result tended to be less good than if the lesion was known to include the responsive region, and a further lesion or even two lesions had to be made. In the 18 cases when the lesions had to be placed after electrical stimulation had located the upper limb relay zone, or even by relying on anatomical probability, the results were intermediate (Table I). The tentative conclusion is that lesions in the appropriate region for deep responses are effective in relieving Parkinsonian tremor while those in the spontaneous tremor firing zone may be less so, although there may possibly be an advantage in including this zone in the lesion.

TABLE I

Results in Cases of Parkinsonian Tremor from Lesions Made at Different Sites. 47 Patients.

Location of lesion	Number of cases	Result	
Lesion extending posteriorly into muscle stretch responsive area	16	Tremor abolished Tremor much reduced Late relapse	12 4 2
Lesion in spontaneous tremor firing zone	5	Tremor abolished Tremor reduced Late relapse	2 3 0
Lesion straddling responsive and tremor firing zones	8	Tremor abolished Late relapse	8 3
Lesion made in zones inactive on recording, and based on the result of electrical stimulation and anatomical probability	18	Tremor abolished Tremor reduced Late relapse	12 6 2

SOMATIC REPRESENTATION IN THE THALAMUS

Our findings are consistent with the concept of medio-laterally lying homunculus, with the head medially, which occupies the Vci and Vce and probably some regions such as the ventralis caudalis portae and ventralis caudalis parvo-cellularis below.

Another point our analysis brings out, from the generally higher percentages for upper limb responses than for head or lower limb, is that the upper limb is more richly represented in the thalamic relay zone.

It has been pointed out on a previous occasion (Rudolf, 1969) that many of our trajectories do not conform with this relatively simple pattern. It was also realised that the succession of events along trajectories gives precise information about the relations between different relay areas in a given thalamus. Further analysis has therefore been undertaken, starting with thalami in which multiple penetrations were made, since these would give a greater amount of somatotopic information. Scale diagrams were made of the events found along the individual trajectories of multiple-trajectory explorations of a given thalamus. One series was for trajectories lying in sloping transverse planes and the other for those lying in parasagittal planes, as exemplified in figure 13.

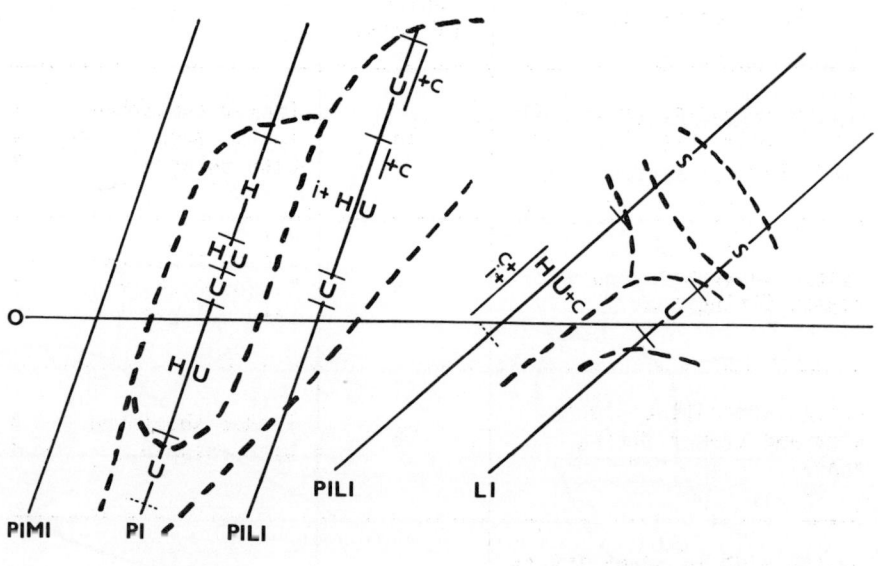

Figure 13 - Trajectories through perforations in the spherical electrode guide are designated as follows: P1M1 = 3 mm posterior and 3 mm medial to the central hole (CH); P1 = 3 mm posterior to CH; P1L1 = 3 mm posterior and 3 mm lateral to CH; L1 = 3 mm lateral to CH: O = IVF-PC plane; H = head; U = upper limb; S = spontaneous tremor bursts. If response ipsilateral as well as contralateral, i is added; if cutaneous as well as deep, c is added. Solid line crossing trajectory = known limit of responsive zone. Fine interrupted line crossing trajectory = distal point of electrode passage. Heavy interrupted lines = probably boundaries of head, upper limb and spontaneous tremor burst regions.

Putative mutually exclusive areas for the spontaneous tremor burst, upper limb and lower limb regions were then drawn on sheets of tracing paper placed over each multiple-trajectory diagram, in the way indicated.

Support for such division of areas, rather than for drawing areas of combined representation (e.g. head plus upper limb) is given by a count of points having single, double or triple responses, which showed that of the 304 responsive points, only 16% were multiple (nearly all double; only 1 was triple). This indicates that multiple representation occupies at the most only a small volume of the sensory relay region. The relatively few multiple points found may often result from the electrode entering presumably narrow junctional zones where activity from two regions (e.g., for head and upper limb) can be detected.

The IVF-PC plane was also drawn on the two series of tracing paper sheets, and each series was then separately superimposed and transilluminated, with respect paid more to aligning the spontaneous tremor burst or responsive areas than the IVF-PC plane. The two oblique-transverse and parasagittal superimposed series, showed good internal agreement, and one could therefore draw a common diagram of each series (figure 14).

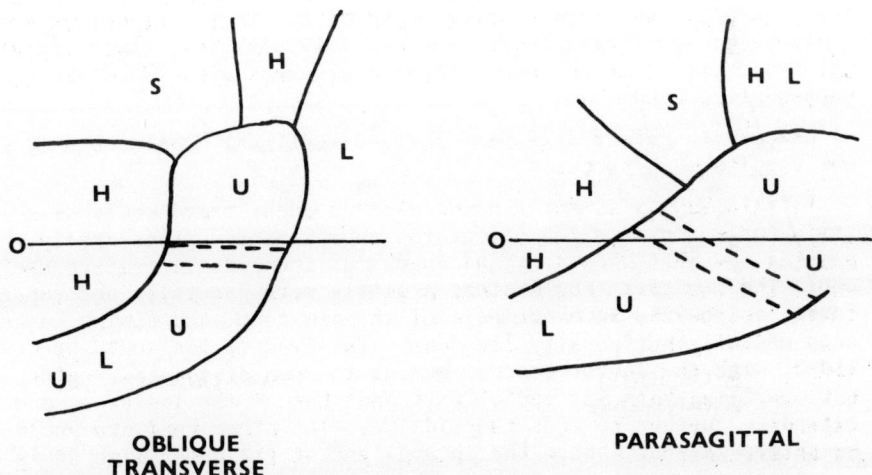

Figure 14 - O = IVF-PC plane; H = head; U = upper limb; L = lower limb; S = spontaneous tremor bursts. Interrupted lines enclose probable unresponsive band.

In the oblique transverse diagram, the right thalamus is viewed from behind, so the top is further away than the bottom, the average slope being 43° to the FM-PC plane. Tha parasagittal diagram, in which we are looking at the right thalamus from the right, slopes only slightly inwards from top to bottom, (the mean angle to the vertical being 10°) and from front to back.

It can be seen that the two diagrams agree fairly well, the oblique transverse one lying at right angles to the parasagittal one and roughly parallel to its long axis. The tremor burst region is no doubt more medial than posterior to the uppermost responsive region, for the electrode advance is slightly medial as well as downwards and backwards.

The next stage was to consider single trajectories (those which had been the sole trajectory in a given thalamus) and see if, as a test of the hypothesis, these were compatible with the same arrangement of regions. It transpired that out of 35 positive single tracks, only 4 did not readily fit; they all contained spontaneous tremor burst and lower limb entries, usually in that order going down the trajectory. This seems to indicate that the two lower limb regions may be linked by a similar region; perhaps, since it is fairly closely associated with the tremor burst region, lying just in front of the upper limb area.

Distorted but nevertheless continuous homunculi are found, e.g., in the cerebral cortex. It does not seem possible to subsume the present findings in one such homunculus, although they might be more consistent with two, one with its head medially, leg laterally and arm in an intermediate position, while the other sloped downwards and medially from its head to its legs. Both would be more anterior laterally, and more posterior medially. Their respective arms would be close to each other, but possibly separate, since individual trajectories often show a divided arm area with an intervening unresponsive band.

However, a rather different three-dimensional model seems to fit our results much better.

In this, which is not a homunculus as such, there would be a strip for the upper limb orientated approximately transversely, but sloping somewhat backwards and downwards from its lateral to medial end. The leg strip would start a little more laterally and superiorly, follow the anterior edge of the arm zone, and finish rather less medially but equally low down. The head region would be divided, with the larger section medial to much of the arm region, but overlying both its medial part and that of the leg area, and extending further towards the midline. The other head are would be antero-lateral, above the lateral end of the upper limb strip.

Spontaneous tremor band bursts, if present, seem to come from a zone superior and anterior to the arm and leg strips, partly between the two sections for the head. These latter are probably also separated by part of the arm representation. Mountcastle made a similar observation in the monkey.

Such a model does not contravene the notion of the Vci representing the head, and the Vce the limbs, since, as we have suggested, the V.c.portae and parvo-cellularis may take part in limb representation, and explain the presence of limb responses near the Vci.

Our findings may be compared with those of Mountcastle and Hennemann (1952) in the monkey, and of Gilles Bertrand, Jasper and Wong (1967), of Tasker and Emmers (1969) and of Mme. Albé-Fessard et al. (1967) in man. Tasker and Emmers use electrical stimulation, but the others derived their results from recordings similar to ours.

Most of these authors have found in man a discrete tactile area posteriorly in the Vci and Vce with the various deep modalities situated in front, and possibly encroaching on the Vim where the spontaneous tremor bursts are recorded. Our results reveal a *mixed* superficial and deep representation posteriorly, but do show only deep responses in the antero-superior part of the sensory relay zone. Single trajectories may encounter, going downwards and backwards, deep, superficial, deep plus superficial and then again deep responses, for example.

Many have considered that the arrangement in man corresponds to that in the monkey, that is, a single homunculus lying roughly medio-laterally. Only Tasker and Emmers, basing their conclusions on electrical stimulation, needed to propose two homunculi, such as those which could partially explain our results. Their vertical homunculus was, however, a bilateral representation of the body, and we do not have evidence of this.

ACKNOWLEDGMENTS

The authors wish to thank Dr. A.J. Hewer and the Department of Clinical Measurement at the Middlesex Hospital, as well as Miss K. Miller of the EEG Department, Oldchurch Hospital, for much assistance in carrying out the recordings. Mr. A.E. Booth, F.R.C.S., analysed the surgical results and these will be fully reported in a subsequent communication.

REFERENCES

Albé-Fessard, D., Arfel, G., Guiot, G., Derome, P. and Gilbaud, G. (1967). Thalamic unit activity in man, in *Recent Advances in Clinical Neurophysiology, (Supplement No. 25 to Electroenceph. Clin. Neurophysiol.)*, (Elsevier Publishing Co., London, Amsterdam and New York), pp. 132-142.

Andrew, J. and Watkins, E.S. (1969). *A Stereotaxic Atlas of the Human Thalamus and Adjacent Structures. A Variability Study*, (Williams and Wilkins Co., Baltimore).

Bates, J.A.V. (1969). The significance of tremor phasic units in the human thalamus, in *Third Symposium on Parkinson's Disease*, (E. & S. Livingstone Limited, Edinburgh and London), pp. 118-124.

Bertrand, G., Jasper, H. and Wong, A. (1967). Microelectrode study of the human thalamus: functional organisation in the ventrobasal complex, *Confin. Neurol.*, **29**, 81-86.

Mountcastle, V.B. and Hennemann, E. (1952). The representation of tactile sensibility in the thalamus of the monkey, *J. Comp. Neurol.*, **97**, 409-439.

Rudolf, N. de M. (1969). Somatic representation in the human thalamus, *Electroenceph. Clin. Neurophysiol.*, **27**, 709.

Tasker, R.R. and Emmers, R. (1969). A double somatotopic representation in the human thalamus. Its application in localisation during thalamotomy for Parkinson's disease, in *Third Symposium on Parkinson's Disease*, (E. & S. Livingstone Limited, Edinburgh and London), pp. 94-100.
Tomlinson, J.D.W. (1969). In Andrew and Watkins (1969), ibid..
Watkins, E.S. (1955). (Personal communication).

INTEGRATION TECHNIQUES FOR LOCALISATION DURING STEREOTAXIC EXPLORATION OF THE THALAMUS AND BASAL GANGLIA

M.A. ARMSTRONG-JAMES

Department of Physiology, The London Hospital Medical College, Turner Street, London, E1 2AD

INTRODUCTION

One considerable problem presenting itself to the neurosurgeon using stereotaxis is the problem of accuracy in placement of his lesion.

In the past, stereotaxis relied for accuracy upon the supposition that relative positions of cell masses are constant from brain to brain and that these cell masses are equivalent in size. Clearly, differences between brains occur, and such an occurrence may well lead to a 'hit or miss' situation in the placement of a lesion.

Andrew and Watkins significantly improved the accuracy of technique by estimating statistical probabilities of the electrode tip being within a particular nucleus or portion of a nucleus.

Until recently, however, physiological tracking methods applied to the human brain have been restricted to observations on the oscilloscope of amplified activity recorded from the electrode tip. Alternatively, the signals were played through an audio monitor and the surgeon, too, relied on his ability to distinguish the different 'sounds' that occur in passage of the electrode from grey to white matter.

The work that I shall present has sought to improve physiological tracking procedures in two ways:

(1) Evolution of a technique for quantitative evaluation of neuronal activity at all levels of an electrode trajectory.

(2) Determining whether firing patterns of individual neurones within different areas of thalamus and subthalamus differ from one another in a qualitative and quantitative fashion.

METHODS

Collection of Data

During the past two years at The London Hospital under the guidance of Professor Watkins, we have carried out stereotaxical investigations on the brains of some twenty patients during the course of operations for the release from conditions such as epilepsy, intractable pain and Parkinsonism. Using tungsten microelectrodes with 10-20 micron tips, we have been able to record from single cells within the thalamus, subthalamus and basal ganglia. The spontaneous activity of several hundred cells was recorded on magnetic tape and the data so collected was then treated for analysis by replaying through a Biomac computer. On line treatment of data was also carried out utilising a gated frequency meter device constructed in the laboratory. The output was recorded on paper using a pen recorder.

Digital events in the central nervous system may be analysed in a number of different ways. Broadly speaking, the data can be divided into signal and noise, the signal being near neuronal activity, and the noise being compounded of a number of components such as electrode noise, very distant neuronal activity and low amplitude synaptic events (waves). Our interest has centred around the analysis of neuronal activity within a 200 microns or so of the electrode tip, and the activity of single neurones.

All of our electrode penetrations were orientated in such a way as to pass through the thalamus initially; normally routes through the VIM were taken. Subsequently after passing through subthalamic white matter, the electrode often has the opportunity to pass into the Red nucleus or the Substantia Nigra. The opportunity therefore arose to compare the integrated and unitary activity of VIM with Substantia Nigra or Red nucleus. The following report will substantially be related to these sites.

Data Analysis

Figure 1 shows a block diagram of the set-up used for each investigation. Activity at the microelectrode tip was fed into a unit gain operational amplifier (ug) from whence it passed to a

DATA ACQUISITION

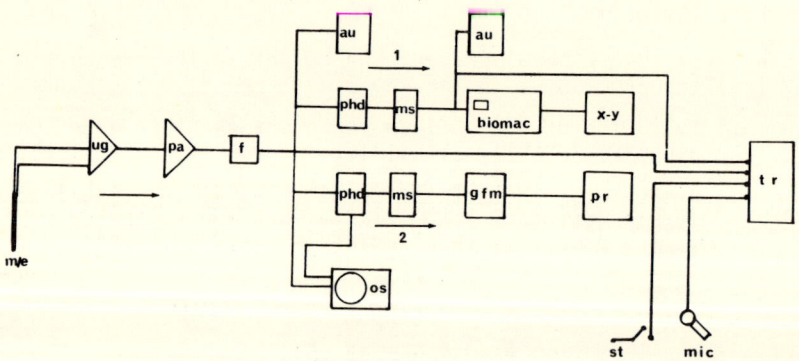

Figure 1 - Diagrammatic illustration of Data Acquisition. Signals from the microelectrode (m/e) are processed by the instrumentation outlined above. Further details are described in the text. ug: unity gain amplifier; pa: preamplifier; f: filter; au: audio unit; phd: pulse height discriminator; ms: monostable multivibrator; x-y: x-y recorder; gfm: gated frequency meter; pr: paper recorder; os: oscilloscope; tr: tape recorder; st: stimulus marker; mic: microphone.

Grass preamplifier (pa); set at a gain of about 20,000. The amplified signal was then filtered at f to pass a band width of 100 Hz to 5 kHz, thus eliminating slow brain potentials and 50 Hz pick up, as well as most of the electrode and amplifier noise. The activity was then divided into five routes. 1) Directly recorded on magnetic tape (tr). 2) Displayed on one beam of a Tektronix 502A oscilloscope (os). 3) Monitored on an audio unit (au). 4) Passed into a pulse height discriminator (phd 1). 5) Passed into another pulse height discriminator (phd 2). One channel of the tape recorder was used for recording speech (mic), a further channel was used for stimuli pulses (st). On the route 1 through phd 1, action potentials from a single unit triggered 5 volt 100 μsec pulses each time the cell fired (figure 2). The temporal sequence of these pulses therefore perfectly copied the temporal sequence of action potentials from a single cell.

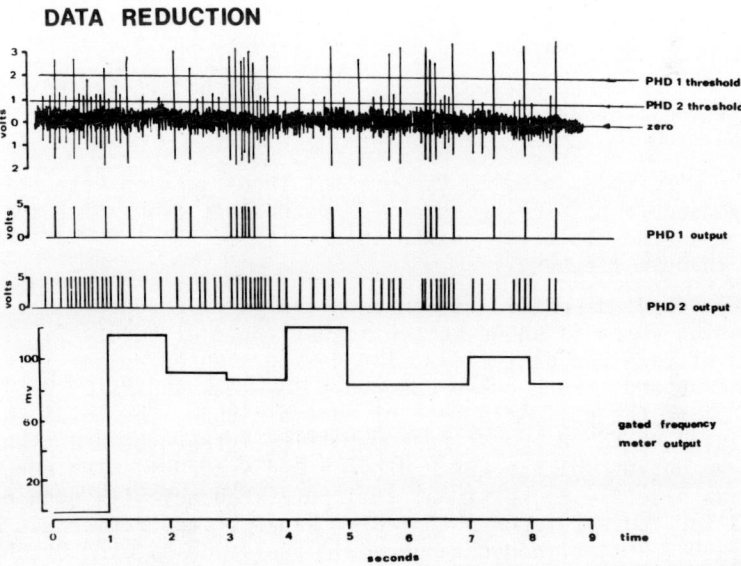

Figure 2 - Method for data reduction. Logic pulses from phd 1 and phd 2 are derived from the microelectrode recording (top trace). Threshold for phd 2 is set at 1 volt to measure mean recorded activity. phd 1 selects single cell activity. Lower trace shows mean neuronal activity derived from phd 2 pulses by the gated frequency meter. Further details in text.

This data was then analysed on the biomac computer in terms of distribution of intervals between sequential action potentials (interval histogram analysis). The results were plotted out on an x-y recorder. More commonly the output of phd 1 was recorded on magnetic tape and treated at a later date by the biomac.

Figure 2 shows how activity passing into phd 2 was discriminated in such a way that all neuronal activity exceeding 1 volt in amplitude produced logic pulses of 5 volts lasting 100 μsec. Hence the frequency of the output of phd 2 was determined by the frequency of action potentials exceeding an amplitude of 1 volt. It was possible for more than six cells to contribute towards the generation of logic pulses from phd 2. The frequency of the output of phd 2 was therefore determined by the following factors:

(1) The proximity of active units to the tip of the microelectrode;
(2) The size of the neurones which may influence the recordable amplitude of action potentials;
(3) The frequency of cell discharge.

Factor 1 is of particular interest since it is determined largely by the cellular packing density of the recorded zone. Since action potentials are electrotonically conducted in extracellular space to the recording microelectrode, then neuronal activity at a distance of some 200 microns or so from the electrode tip would not be expected to be recorded and discriminated by phd 2.

It follows that nuclear zones where cell bodies are most densely packed would produce the highest frequency of logic pulses from phd 2.

The electrodes used in the present investigation were not generally capable of picking up action potentials from white matter. Thus when the electrode passed into white matter the phd 1 output fell to zero frequency.

The output of phd 2 was fed into the gated frequency meter, the output of which is shown in the lowest trace of figure 2. The operation of this was as follows: The device counted pulses in a period of one second. Each pulse charged a low leak capacitor by a fixed quantum of charge. At a rate of once a second, the total charge was gated on to an operational amplifier integrator and transformed into an output voltage which drove a pen recorder. The output voltage was directly proportional to input frequency within an accuracy of 2% for the worst possible case. Range of the device was normally set at 0-3 kHz, although range could easily be altered by changing the duration of phd 2 logic pulses.

GENERAL OBSERVATIONS

1. *Thalamic Activity*

Individual action potentials from neurones close to the recording microelectrode were characterised by high amplitude spikes of long duration. Spikes generally lasted 2-4 msec and often had notches on the descending phase. A further common occurrence was the presence of moderately high amplitude wave activity which had to be filtered out for unitary analysis. Neurones had a strong tendency to fire in bursts of discharges lasting a few milliseconds at burst frequencies of 2-10 per second. Discrimination of single units was found to be relatively easy compared with other sites in the CNS since the cell most proximal to the recording electrode often gave considerably higher amplitude spikes than other cells. On this evidence it was considered that neuronal packing density in the thalamus is relatively low compared with other nuclei that we have encountered. On the other hand, injury potentials on advancement of the microelectrode through the thalamus were profound. Extracellular recordings from single cells were possible for periods exceeding five minutes.

The output of the frequency meter when the electrode was in the thalamus was therefore moderately high, and on electrode advancement often increased to saturation level during injury discharges.

2. *Red Nucleus Activity*

Action potentials from cells close to the electrode were of moderately high amplitude, the largest being about 1/2 to 2/3 of the amplitude of thalamic spikes. The form of the action potentials was quite different from those of the thalamus, being of very short duration (about 1 msec) with sharply defined peaks and no notches on the descending portion of the spike. Discrimination of single units was more difficult than in the thalamus since invariably the activity of several units was simultaneously recorded within a short distance of the recording microelectrode. These observations led us to believe that Red nucleus cells were smaller than thalamic cells, and that the packing density of neurones was considerably higher. Upon electrode advancement injury discharge was minimal and often not encountered. As a consequence of this type of activity, the frequency meter output voltage remained relatively steady at a very high level, at 20 to 100% greater levels than when the electrode was dwelling in the thalamus. Due to the lack of injury potentials on electrode movement, the output of the frequency meter showed little change.

3. *Subthalamic White Matter*

When the electrode was in the subthalamic white matter spike activity was minimal to zero. At white matter/nuclear boundaries stray cells were occasionally picked up, and these were characterised by a very high signal to noise ratio. White matter activity was therefore normally compounded of uniform white noise under the recording conditions, and the threshold level for both pulse height discriminators was not reached. Furthermore, on advancing the microelectrode no injury potentials were recorded. The output of the frequency meter was, of course, zero.

4. *Trajectories*

All trajectories of the microelectrode were calculated from the work of Watkins and Andrew, which was strictly based upon statistical anatomical data from a large number of sections from postmortem material. At any particular position of the microelectrode there was therefore a statistical probability of the tip being in a particular place. In the first instance, activity from the microelectrode indicates whether the tip is located within a cellular mass or within white matter. Hence boundaries between white matter and cell masses were normally clearly shown by the recordings and in particular, by the output level of the gated frequency meter. An example of a clearly defined trajectory is shown in figure 3. Correlation between the anatomical data of Watkins and Andrew was normally very good. On occasions, however, the thalamic borders

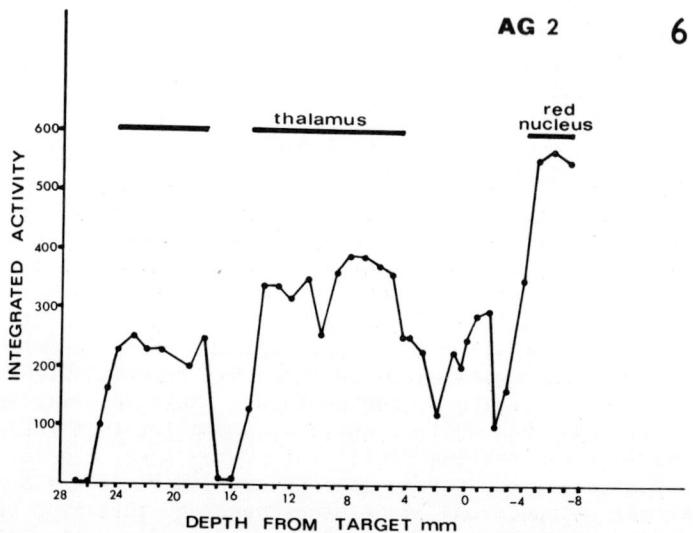

Figure 3 - Gated frequency meter output (integrated activity) at 38 points during passage of microelectrode through a trajectory within caudate nucleus, thalamus, red nucleus and intervening white matter boundaries.

in particular were found to be lower than expected from the statistical data of Watkins and Andrew. We considered this to be due to some regressive changes in the brain whereby the whole thalamus sank as a single structure. The physiological tracking procedure was therefore invaluable in such situations where this occurred.

5. *Interval Distribution Analysis*

On certain trajectories, the frequency meter output was difficult to interpret with regard to cell mass boundaries. An example is shown of a trajcetory taking us sequentially through VIM, zona incerta, and substantia nigra or red nucleus (figure 4). Clearly the changes in the level of the output of the gated frequency meter are not quite adequate for determination of the boundaries of these cell groups.

The need therefore arose for a more sophisticated method for determining the difference between the activities of neurones within each cellular mass. For this, the Biomac computer was used to analyse the interval distributions between action potentials recorded at different sites, from single units.

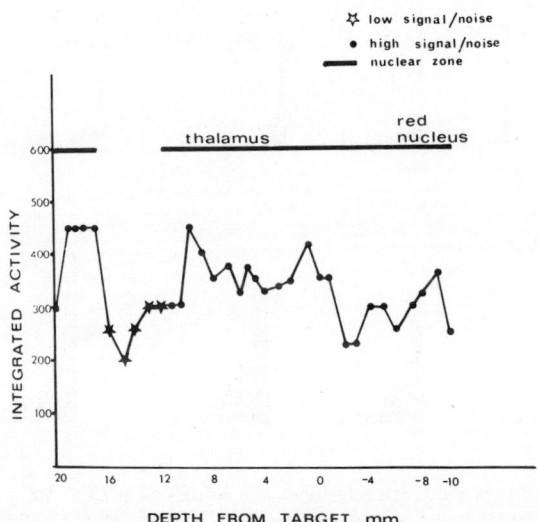

Figure 4 - A further example of gated frequency meter readings in a trajectory where cell boundaries are difficult to estimate by this method alone. For further details see text.

It was necessary to ascertain that the firing frequency of single cells was relatively constant for a minute or so whilst analysis of interval distributions was carried out. Interval analysis was carried out only in the absence of stimulation and during periods when the spontaneous firing frequency was relatively constant.

Figure 5 shows interval distribution analyses for single v.i.m. units and Red nucleus units respectively. The abscissa of each profile shows the group times of intervals in 1.28 msec bins, from 1.28 msec to approximately 100 msecs. The ordinate indicates the number of such intervals occurring within each time bin.

For most thalamic neurones, intervals are strongly grouped at the short end of the interval spectrum, at about 2 to 6 msec, often with an even dispersion of longer intervals. Alternatively, two clear peaks occur within the interval distribution curve, one at 2-6 msecs, the other at 20-40 msecs (figure 6). On the other hand, Red Nucleus cells show a different pattern of interval distributions. In common with thalamic cells there is a major peak for red nucleus cells at 2-6 msecs, but progressively decreasing numbers of intervals occur from 6 msecs onwards (figure 5). The peak at 20-40 msecs is absent or very poorly defined, as a notch on the falling phase of the interval histogram. Interval histogram distributions for thalamic neurones fall to one half of their maximum bin count at

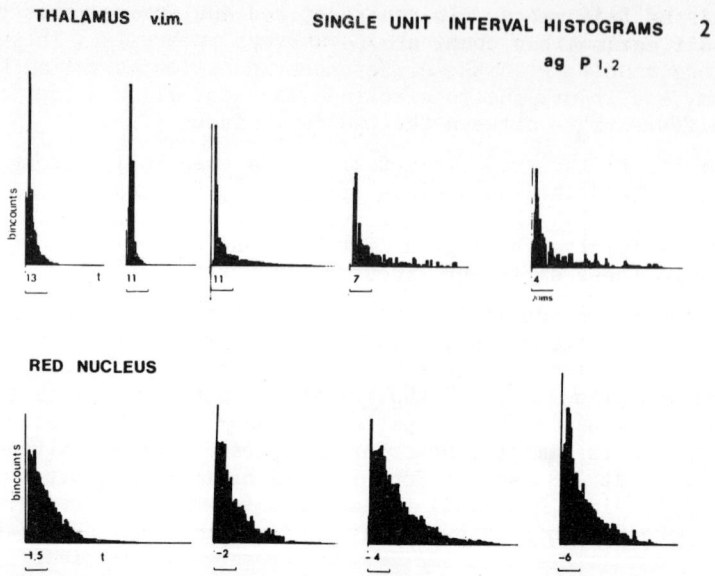

Figure 5 - Interval histograms of single units in a single subject to illustrate the different firing patterns of thalamic (vim) and red nucleus units.

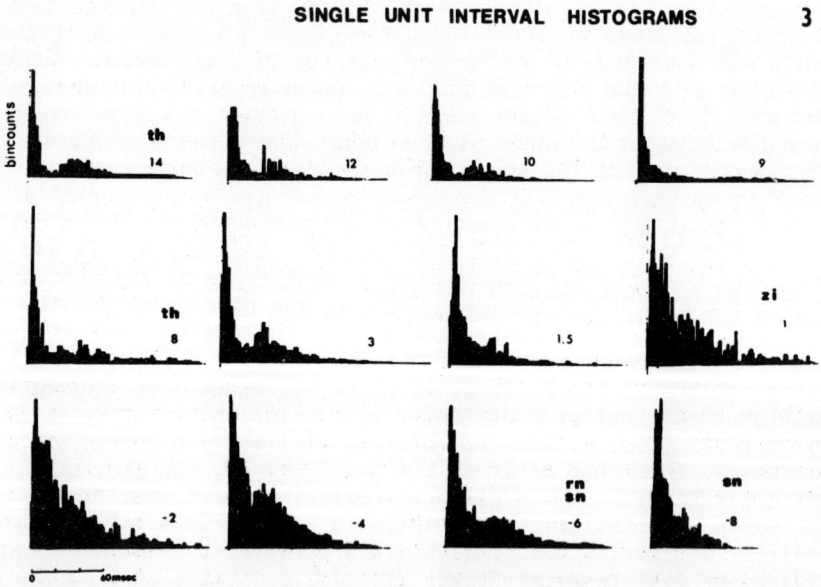

Figure 6 - Interval histograms from trajectory shown in figure 4. Further details are found in the text.

intervals of 3-10 msecs. In contrast, red nucleus neurones exhibit a one half maximum bin count at 20-40 msecs intervals. These observations coupled with the differences in action potential height and form, and injury due to electrode movement allow us quite clearly to differentiate between the two cell masses.

Returning to the trajectory taking us sequentially through v.i.m., zona incerta and the red nucleus (figure 4), the analysis of interval histograms shows how these zones can be distinguished. Figure 6 shows the interval histogram distributions of cells randomly chosen from these different sites, in such a trajectory.

Thalamic v.i.m. cells (th) show the expected distribution of intervals noted beforehand, with a single early peak followed by a later peak or not as the case may be. On passage of the electrode into the zona incerta (zi), the interval histogram distribution changes to quite a different pattern (lines 2-3). The decay of the histogram is almost linear for the first 20 msecs, although the peak remains at 2-8 msecs. Zone incerta histograms typically exhibit a long right hand tail of longer intervals compared with S.N. or R.N.. Coincidentally injury discharges grew less and action potential amplitudes were smaller and of shorter duration.

On passage of the electrode into the red nucleus substantia nigra boundary, the changes were more subtle. Action potentials were considerably shorter in duration and less injury discharges were apparent. The interval histogram distribution changed once again to give a sharper fall and a shorter tail reaching the substantia nigra at -8.

During our investigations upon the discharge intervals of thalamic cells from v.i.m., a further type of cell was found. About 5% of single cells we recorded from gave totally different interval histogram profiles. These cells were characterised by a low frequency discharge at a fairly steady rate. There was no tendency for these cells to fire in bursts of activity. The bottom row of figure 7 shows that interval histograms assumed a nearly normal distribtution as opposed to the skew distribution of all other cells. The peak of the interval histogram was at 20-30 msecs. It can be seen that the interval histogram for these types of cells occupies the same position for the later peak in the histograms for the commonest type of thalamic v.i.m. cell. The earlier peak at 2-6 msecs is totally absent. Thus the frequency of discharge of the commonest types of cell with two peaks in the interval histogram could be construed as being compounded of two frequencies; a fast and slow component. Such a situation has been previously noted in somatosensory cortex cells of the cat in the investigations of Smith and Smith (1965). The slower component was found by these workers to be most easily influenced by cell body depolarisation, leaving the fast component unaffected. The fast component is envisaged by Delisle Burns (1968) as being generated by E.P.S.P.'s on remote dendrites, and the slow by axosomatic synapses. Clearly, there is an opportunity for investigating the two processes in response to sensory stimulation, and it would be of interest to know which component is most easily influenced within the human thalamus. We are investigating this at the present time as part of our general project.

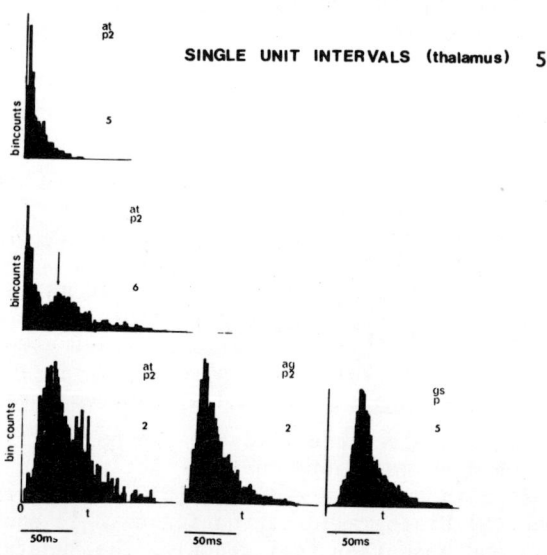

Figure 7 - Interval histograms of thalamic units showing a strong tendency for one of two modal interval values to predominate. For further details, see text.

In summary, it is felt that if profiles of interval histogram patterns and integrated activity patterns are stored and recognizable, then very fine delimitation of cell mass boundaries will be possible on-line. Such data could be of considerable value in the operating theatre when decisions for placement of electrolytic lesions are made.

REFERENCES

Andrew, J. and Watkins, E.S. (1969). *A Stereotaxic Atlas of the Human Thalamus and Adjacent Structures*, (William and Wilkins, Baltimore).

Burns, B. Delisle, (1968). *The Uncertain Nervous System*, (Edward Arnold (Publishers) Limited).

Smith, D.R. and Smith, G.K. (1965). A statistical analysis of the continual activity of single cortical neurones in the cat unanaesthetized inlated forebrain, *Biophys. J.*, **5**, 47-74.

~~UPON THE POSSIBLE~~ ROLE AND ORIGIN OF RHYTHMIC ACTIVITIES ~~OBSERVED IN~~ PARKINSONIAN PATIENTS' THALAMUS

D. ALBE-FESSARD

Laboratoire de Physiologie des Centres Nerveux,
4 avenue Gordon-Bennett, 75016 Paris, France

In patients suffering from Parkinson's disease rhythmic activities at the frequency of the tremor can be recorded in a thalamic region which surrounds superiorly and anteriorly the specific somatic relay (figure 1). This thalamic area, was first recognized for its posterior zone (LP in figure 1) in 1963 (Albe-Fessard et al., 1963). The anterior position was studied later (Albe-Fessard et al., 1966; Jasper et al., 1964, 1966).

The results presented here are deduced from the examination of recordings and stimulations performed in more than 240 Parkinsonian patients. Two hundred and twenty of them were recorded with the group of Dr. Guiot, the others with Drs. Le Beau and Dondey. Experiments performed on cats, monkeys and chimpanzees, and having as an aim the understanding of Parkinson's disease will also be discussed.

§(1): RHYTHMIC THALAMIC ACTIVITIES ARE NOT ONLY EVOKED BY THE RHYTHMIC PERIPHERAL MOVEMENTS

That the rhythmic activities seen in the thalamic region just described do not all originate from primary cells driven by the peripheral movements seems to be now a fact generally accepted (see references in Choh-Lu-Li and van Buren, 1972; Raeva, 1972; Ohye and Narabayashi, 1972; Lucking et al., 1972).

However, one has to think that, in its anterior part, cells from the somatic relay nucleus devoted to the representation of movement are intermingled with these rhythmic cells. The independence of some of the rhythms from evoked potentials was suggested on the basis of several different sorts of studies.

(a) For neurosurgical groups which have, like ourselves, recorded rhythms only from human brains, the evidence was based on the comparison of these rhythmic activities with the electromyograms from the peripheral limbs presenting tremor.

In all Parkinsonians, the central burst frequency was almost invariably highly correlated with the tremor frequency. However, in most of the rhythmic thalamic area, the central burst frequency is slightly slower than the peripheral frequency. It is only at the inferior limit of the area (VL-Zi) that the inverse is true (see figure 2).

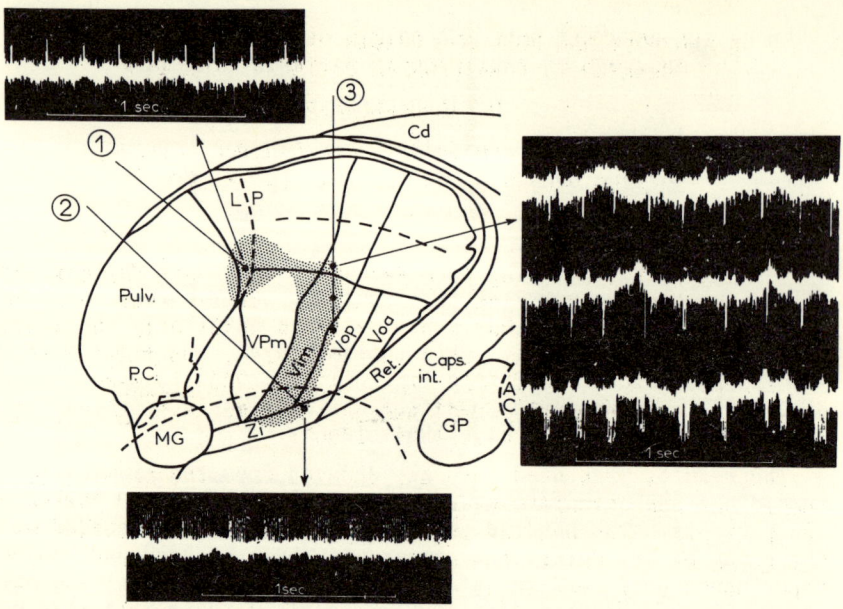

Figure 1 - On a schematic sagittal (lat. 15) section of a human brain (slightly modified form Schaltenbrandt and Bailey, 1959), the limits of the medial portion of nucleus ventralis posterior (VPm) are represented. Medial Geniculate (MG), Zona Incerta (Zi), n. Reticularis Thalami (Ret), Internal Capsula (caps. int.), Globus Pallidus (GP), n. Caudatus (Cd), Pulvinar (Pul.), n. Lateralis Posterior (LP). The three different regions which, taken together, constitute in Man the approximate homologue of n. Ventralis Lateralis (VL) in Monkeys are designated: Ventralis intermedius (Vim), Ventralis oralis posterior (Vop), Ventralis oralis anterior (Voa). The projections on this plane of the position of the posterior commissure (PC) and the anterior commissure (AC) are shown.

Recordings of rhythmic units were made during the process of the progression of the recording electrodes. For trajectories 1 and 2, a posterior approach was used (top and bottom of the picture). Units recorded during a vertical exploration (trajectory 3) are shown at right. The three cells presented for trajectory 3 were encountered in a man at three different levels of the same track. In grey is designated the position of the region where the same type of rhythmic cells can be encountered.

Note that duration of burst in zona incerta is longer than the one of cells placed more superiorly.

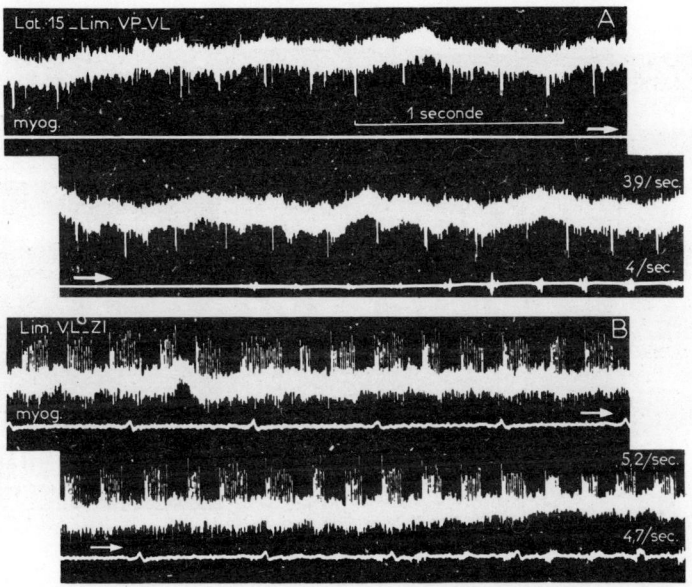

Figure 2 - Two examples are given of simultaneous recordings of central rhythmic units (superior lines) and electromyogram (myogr., inferior lines). These records were taken from two different patients (neuroleptanalgesia) during a period when the state of the patient is changing from drowsiness towards alertness.

An example is taken at the limit between VP and VL, another at the limit between inferior Vim and zona incerta.

The mean frequencies of the central burst (superior numbers) and of the electromyogram (inferior numbers) were calculated on longer time records. Note that, in both cases, the rhythmic activity of the central unit appears before the rhythmicity in electromyogram can be detected. On the inferior electromyogram, the slow rhythmic wave is an artefact due to a cardiac derivation.

These rhythmic central units showed regular rhythmic activities only during alertness, thus appearing under the same conditions as Parkinsonian tremor. Other rhythmic activities encountered in the thalamus undergo opposite variations (figure 3).

Following the release of the tremor due to voluntary movement, or to drowsiness of the patient, the rhythmic activity reappeared at the level of the central unit before the muscular burst reappeared in the electromyogram.

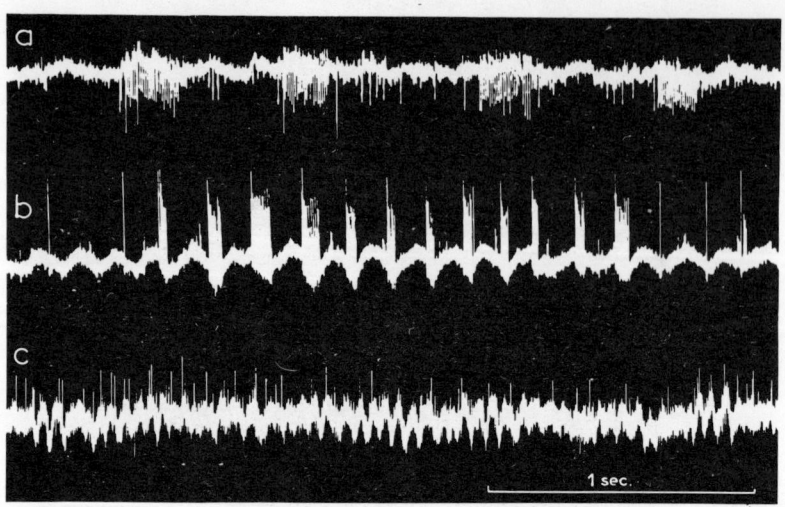

Figure 3 - Rhythmic activities encountered in three different structures in brains of patient during phases of drowsiness: (a) posterior pulvinar; (b) pulvinar near Lateralis posterior; (c) Vim. These types of rhythmic activities disappear during alertness while, on the contrary, the rhythmic bursts of units presented in figures 1 and 2 disappear during drowsiness and reappear during wakefulness.

When a voluntary movement is performed, as a general rule the central unit is inhibited as is the tremor. The inhibition of both phenomena occurs during the phase of preparation for movement and during the movement itself. This fact, demonstrated in figure 4, was published elsewhere (Albe-Fessard et al., 1966). Raeva (1972) in a careful study of this phenomenon, has shown that 90 per 100 of the rhythmic cells that she has encountered in VL are thus inhibited.

When the inhibition occurring during the preparation for a voluntary movement started, the last central burst occurred just before the last peripheral electromyographic burst (see figure 4).

(b) The indisputable proof that the central unit is at the origin of the tremor and is not produced by it, was, however, established in the monkey by Lamarre and Cordeau (1964, 1967). These authors have utilised monkeys having experimental tremor produced by lesions in or around the substantia nigra (Cordeau et al., 1960) and which are quite

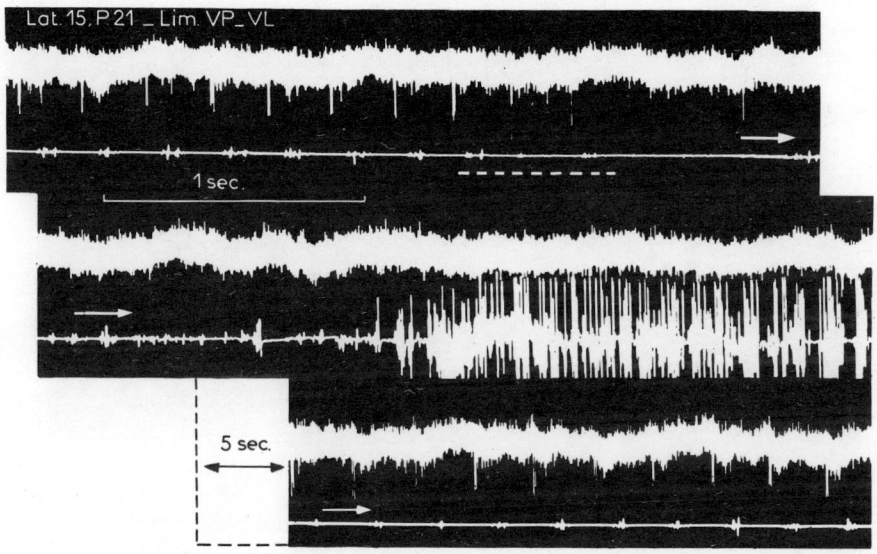

Figure 4 - Simultaneous recordings of central unit activity (upper traces) in a Parkinsonian patient. Rhythmic bursts can be seen initially in the two traces (top left). Rhythmic central activity and tremor cease when the patient is preparing to initiate a voluntary movement (top right). During the whole movement, the bursts of central units are suppressed, they both reappeared after 5 seconds.

perfectly identical to Parkinsonian tremor (in particular frequency of 5±1 c/sec). They have shown in these animals that the rhythmic activity of thalamic neurons can be recorded under curare.

§(2): A FEEDBACK LOOP SYNCHRNOIZES THE PULSATING CELLS

Rhythmic burst at 5/sec ±1 can appear in thalamus of patients having no tremor or in thalamus or motor cortex of chimpanzees having small doses of tranquilizer or of anaesthetics (Albe-Fessard, 1971). However, these bursts do not appear as regularly as the ones encountered in trembling Parkinsonian patients. When passive or active movements of the limbs are produced, a train of these bursts can appear (Albe-Fessard et al., 1966).

In Parkinsonian patients, during the time of non-tremor, in the so-called tremorogenic thalamic regions, different cells can be recorded at the same time. They beat at about 5 per sec but are not in phase. On the contrary, during tremor, the different central units become in phase.

These observations reveal that some pathway coming from the periphery arrives at the tremorogenic zone. This pathway is not able alone to evoke regular 5 per sec activities, but its action can synchronize the different pulsating units.

§(3): *ROLE PLAYED BY THE THALAMIC TREMOROGENIC REGION*

The tremorogenic impulses seem to be transmitted to the pyramidal tract via the motor cortex. The thalamic region where rhythmic cells appear is connected in monkeys with motor cortex (see references in Albe-Fessard et al., 1966).

> Lesions of motor cortex or of pyramidal tract are known to suppress tremor in Parkinsonians.

> By cooling the motor cortex of monkeys having experimental tremor and where rhythmic units can be recorded (Cordeau et al., 1960), Jasper et al. (1972) were able to suppress the rhythmic tremor.

> It was shown in addition that the stimulation of this thalamic area at a relatively high frequency inhibits the peripheral tremor (Alberts et al., 1966; Albe-Fessard et al., 1970).

These findings will be detailed here. They were an unexpected result of a series of experiments performed in order to recognize if different rôles can be played in sensation by different zones of the primary somatic relay.

Different regions can be recognized in the VP nucleus on the basis of the type of receptors that evoked cell activities at this level, in monkeys as well as in Man (Poggio and Mountcastle, 1963; Albe-Fessard et al., 1966). Schematically, if as in figure 1 a sagittal section through the thalamus is considered, the inferior part of VP receives tactile afferents only, while superior and anterior parts receive messages provoked by movements (figure 5). On the basis of the type of stimulus able to drive the cells, the position in nucleus VP of the recording electrode can thus be recognized.

We have profited from this observation to stimulate different zones of characterized cells to observe what sort of sensation can be evoked (see also Libet et al., 1972). To this end, we have determined in advance the optimal stimulating conditions and recognized that trains of shocks (0.5 to 1 msec), at frequency of 200 per sec and during more than 0.1 sec, give threshold responses for minimal current intensity. We have thus searched for the threshold of effect produced by such trains delivered through the same bipolar electrodes as the one through which activity was recorded. Systematic explorations were performed, in which recording periods were intermingled with stimulating periods (figure 6).

In the region where cells are driven by tactile stimuli, stimulation near threshold gave rise to a tactile sensation in the exact peripheral zone from where the cells were driven and, to give rise to a movement, the stimulus had to be greatly increased. On the

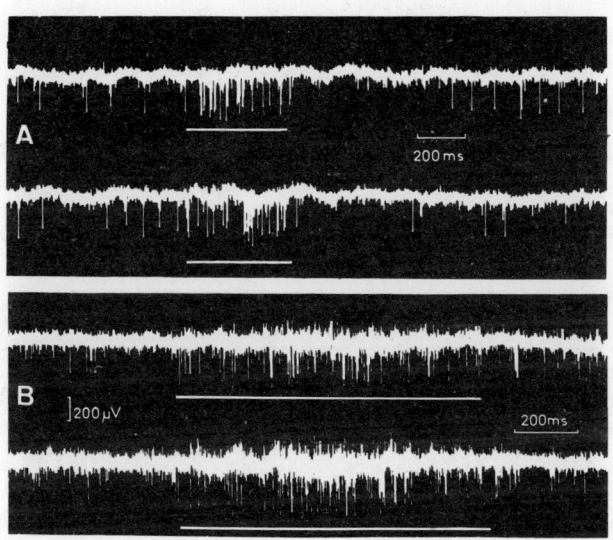

Figure 5 - (A) Activities of units driven by a tactile stimulus (light pressure of upper contralateral lip) (solid line); (B) Activity evoked by an active flexion of the contralateral index finger (solid line). Each response is presented twice to show its reproducibility.

contrary, in the regions where cells were driven by passive or active movement, threshold stimulations provoked in certain patients a sensation of movement, but a slight increase of the stimulus always gave rise to the movement itself. Thus these experiments showed that the supero-anterior part of VP is not only probably involved in movement sensation but can also drive movements and must correspond to the motor thalamic region previously described by Hassler (1959).

When a slight change of position of the recording electrode makes it leave the region of evoked activity and attain the tremorogenic zone, another effect of stimulation is obtained. Threshold stimulation provokes an arrest of the tremor which does not appear either posteriorly in the VP itself, or anteriorly in the anterior regions of VL (figure 6). To explain these findings we have proposed that a stimulation at 200/sec desynchronized the activities of the tremorogenic cells. However, another explanation of these findings can also be advanced: our stimulation is putting in action the same inhibitory pathways which are activated during the voluntary movements.

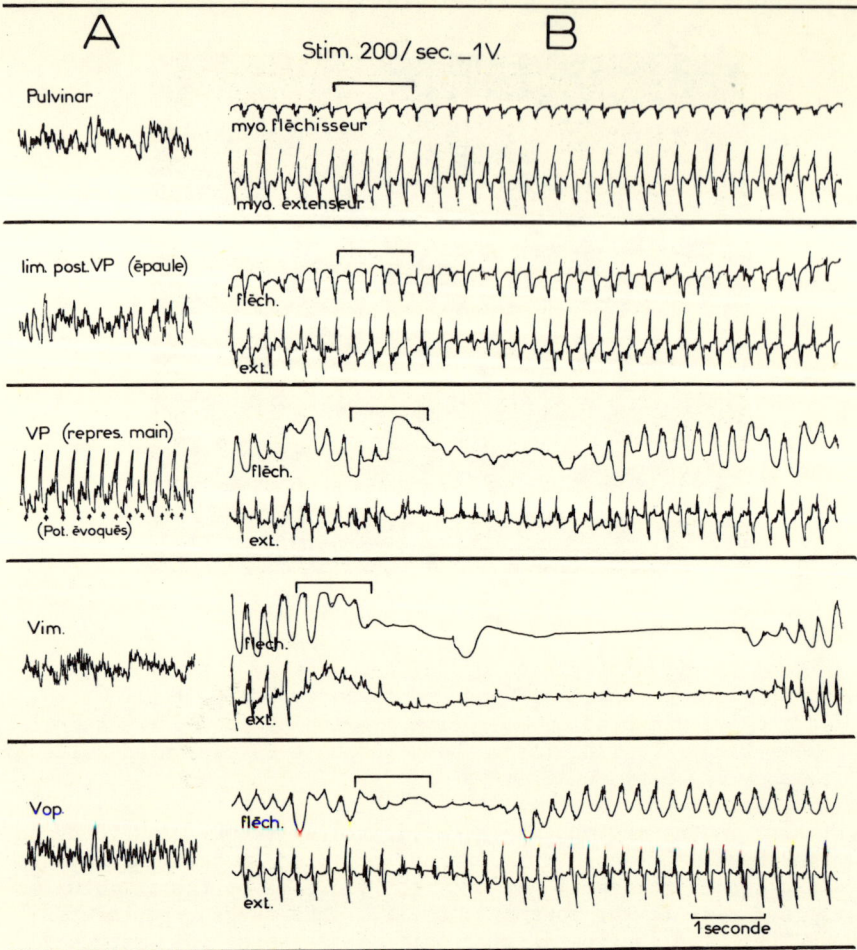

Figure 6 - In a patient recordings and stimulation were performed alternatively during the progression of the electrode (top to bottom). (A) The thalamic activities recorded on an ink-writer are presented with the position of the recording electrode deduced from the types of spontaneous activity and response to natural stimulation obtained at this level.
(B) Records of the electromyogram of the flexor and extensor muscles of a trembling arm during stimulation of the region of which the recording is presented in A in the corresponding row. Note that stimulation by trains of shocks (0.5 msec; 200 per sec: 1 volt; 1 second duration) has different effects when applied at different levels. Maximal inhibition is obtained when the region at the limit between VP and posterior VL (Vim) is stimulated.

§(7): RELATIONS BETWEEN THE APPEARANCE OF TREMOROGENIC ACTIVITIES AND THE PARKINSONIAN BRAIN DISTURBANCES

The fact that the majority of clear rhythmic cells are found in the thalamus (see Raeva, 1972) has to be reconciled with the fact that the Parkinsonian disease seems to be accompanied by a cellular destruction in Substantia Nigra and a depletion in dopamine content of the Substantia Nigra and striate centres. These findings, that seem to be very far one from the other, have given rise to an important group of studies.

That a dopaminergic connection exists between SN and striatum was demonstrated on the basis of fluorescence technique by Anden et al. (1966). The anatomical demonstration of the existence of SN-Caudate connection (Mettler, 1970); Moore et al., 1971) was parallelled by its electrophysiological one (Frigyesi and Purpura, 1966, 1967; Albe-Fessard et al., 1967; Albe-Fessard, 1971). Two types of caudate units can be affected by SN stimulation. Units of the first type are activated, the others are inhibited. The units that are inhibited by SN stimulation are the same as the ones inhibited by dopamine iontophoresis (MacLennan and York, 1967; Connor, 1968, 1970; Herz and Zieglgänsberger, 1968), (see figure 7).

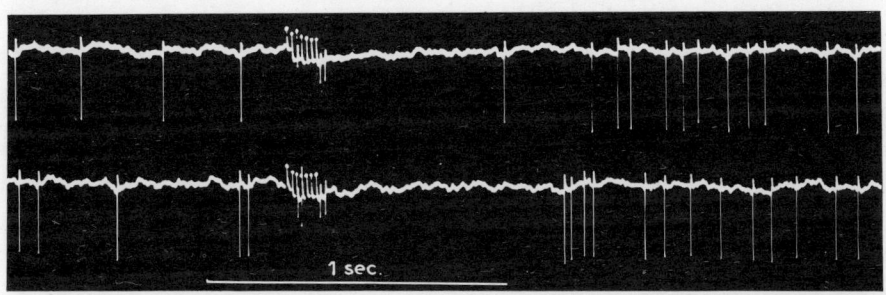

Figure 7 - In a cat under local anaesthesia, two units are simultaneously recorded in the head of n. Caudatus. Trains of stimuli are applied to the substantia nigra, the artefacts of stimulation are each designated by a white dot. Note that one unit (large amplitude) is inhibited and the other (small amplitude) is excitated. Two examples are given.

On the contrary, the units which are activated are not sensitive to dopamine and even are still driven after a large depletion of the dopamine content produced by intraventricular injections of 6-hydroxydopamine (Feltz and De Champlain, 1972). Thus two pathways exist between SN and Caudate which use different mediators, the dopaminergic pathway being essentially an inhibitory one. This permits one to suppose that, in a normal man, the cells in n. Caudatus are generally inhibited by afferents coming from Substantia Nigra; this inhibition is certainly lacking in Parkinsonian patients and this lack must be, at least in part, responsible for the syndromes recognized in these patients.

In this case, it must be that normally a facilitatory influence is coming from caudate that permits the rhythmic activities of tremorogenic cells to be present. This influence is suppressed by an inhibition originating in Substantia Nigra.

However, the connection of Substantia Nigra with n. Caudatus is not the only one that may be suppressed by nigral lesions. In fact, connections of SN were also described with Putamen, Pallidum and Ventralis Lateralis (Cole et al., 1964; Mehler, 1969; Kemp, 1970; York, 1970) and descending influences were observed on SN cells from cortex (Rinvik, 1966), n. Caudatus, Putamen and Pallidum (Voneida, 1960; Szabo, 1962; Kemp, 1970; Niimi et al., 1970; Goswell and Sedgwick, 1971). An inflow to VL from cerebellum is also well known. We have tried to summarize all these connections in figure 8.

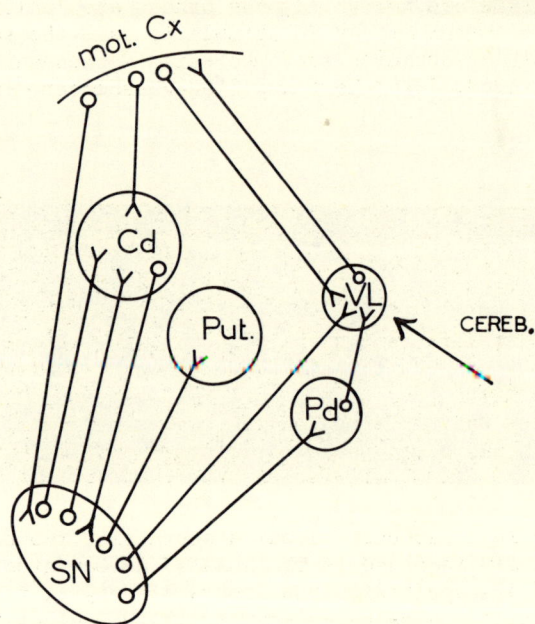

Figure 8 - Schematic drawing showing part of the connections which were demonstrated by various anatomical or electrophysiological techniques between different regions of the brain that may be involved in Parkinson's disease: Substantia Nigra (SN), n. Caudatus (Cd), Putamen (Put), Ventralis Lateralis (VL), Globus Pallidus (Pd), motor and somatomotor cortex, Cerebellum (Cereb.).

A clear understanding of the rôle of these different loops has not yet been attained. Certain observations by other authors and ourselves are, however, to be mentioned.

The connections between SN and VL, described by anatomists, can be demonstrated by electrophysiology (Frigyesi and Machek, 1971). These connections are complex and, in VL, three types of cells can be recognized by using the effect of SN stimulation. Certain cells are driven at short latencies, others are inhibited, others present a succession of excitation, inhibition, excitation, the rhythm in this case being not very different from 5 c/sec, (Deniau and Lackner, unpublished).

When, in cats, the somato-motor cortex is ablated on one side, all the cells which respond to SN are rhythmically activated (figure 9). The number of rhythmic cells is far smaller on the side which has still its cortico-somato-motor regions intact. The same observation was made by Jasper et al. (1972) in the monkey.

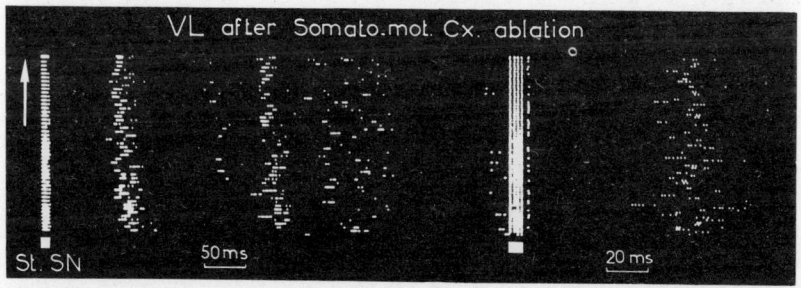

Figure 9 - At left, dot display showing the rhythmic organization of unit responses provoked at VL level by stimulation of Substantia Nigra (SN) when a cortical ablation of the somamotor cortex was performed on the same side. At right, the response is shown at a more rapid speed to permit observation of the short latency excitatory response (from Lackner and Deniau, unpublished data).

Thus, the somato-cortex seems to exert in a normal animal a damping effect on the rhythmic VL units. This damping effect passes possibly through the cortic-caudate pathway which is known to exist (Albe-Fessard et al., 1960; Kemp and Powell, 1970). The lack of this damping effect in Parkinsonian patients, due to the change of responsiveness of caudate neurons after dopamine depletion could be at the origin of the appearance in VL of the abnormal rhythmic units.

The control exerted through cerebellum is also of interest. From recent results published by Lamarre (1972), it seems that this control is normally inhibitory. In monkeys where 5/sec rhythmic units are developed after destruction of Substantia Nigra, the rhythmicity increases in the thalamus after cerebellar lesions. These experiments thus show that cerebellum has, like motor cortex, a damping effect on the tremorogenic zone. These results could possibly explain why, in monkeys having a tremor at rest following cerebellar lesions, L-Dopa administration suppresses the tremor (Goldberger and Growden, 1971). The lack of cerebellar control is in this case possibly replaced by an increase of the cortico-caudate control.

In conclusion, we wish to underline that the complexity of the control loops which have been described until now may explain why tremor can react very differently from one patient to another to L-Dopa administration.

REFERENCES

Albe-Fessard, D. (1971). Tentative d'explication neurophysiologique de la pathologie du Parkinson, in *Monoamines, Noyaux gris centraux et Syndrome de Parkinson*, (ed. Ajuriaguerra, de, J.), (Georg et Cie, Geneva), pp. 243-262.

Albe-Fessard, D., Arfel, G., Derome, P. and Dondey, M. (1970). Electrophysiology of the human thalamus with special reference to trigeminal pain, in *Trigeminal Neuralgia*, (eds. Hassler, R. and Walker, A.E.), (Georg Thieme Verlag, Stuttgart), pp. 139-148.

Albe-Fessard, D., Arfel, G. and Guiot, G., (1963). Activités électriques caractéristiques de quelques structures cérébrales chez l'homme, *Ann. Chir.*, **17**, 1185-1214.

Albe-Fessard, D., Guiot, G., Lamarre, Y. and Arfel, G. (1966). Activation of thalamo-cortical projections related to tremorogenic processes, in *The Thalamus*, (eds. Purpura, D.P. and Yahr, M.D.), (Columbia University Press, New York and London), pp. 237-253.

Albe-Fessard, D., Oswaldo-Cruz, E. and Rocha-Miranda, C., (1960). Activités évoquées dans le noyau caudé du chat en réponse à des types divers d'afférences. I. Etude macrophysiologique, *Electroenceph. clin. Neurophysiol.*, **12**, 405-420.

Alberts, W.W., Feinstein, B., Levin, G. and Wright, E.W. Jr., (1966). Electrical stimulation of therapeutics targets in waking dyskinetic patients, *Electroenceph. clin. Neurophysiol.*, **20**, 559-566.

Anden, N.E., Dahlstrom, A., Fuxe, K. and Larsson, K. (1966). Functional rôle of the nigro-neostriatal dopamine neurons, *Acta Pharmacol.*, *(Kbh)*, **24**, 263-274.

Cole, M., Nauta, W.J.H. and Mehler, W.R. (1964). The ascending afferent projections of the Substantia Nigra. *Trans. Amer. Neurol. Assoc.*, 74-78.

Connor, J.D. (1968). Caudate unit responses to nigral stimuli, evidence for a possible nigro-neostriatal pathway, *Science*, **160**, 899-900.

Connor, J.D. (1970). Caudate nucleus neurones: correlation of the effects of Substantia Nigra stimulation with Iontophoretic Dopamine, *J. Physiol.*, **208**, 691-703.

Cordeau, J.P., Gybels, J., Jasper, H. and Poirier, L.J. (1960). Microelectrode studies of unit discharges in the sensorimotor cortex. Investigations in monkeys with experimental tremor, *Neurology, (Minneap.)*, **10**, 591-600.

Feltz, P. and Champlain, de, J. (1972). Persistence of caudate unitary responses to nigral stimulation after destruction and functional impairment of the striatal dopaminergic terminals, *Brain Research*, (in press).

Frigyesi, T.L. and Machek, J., (1971). Basal Ganglia-Diencephalon synaptic relations in the cat. II. Intracellular recordings from dorsal thalamic neurons during low frequency stimulation of the caudatothalamic-projection systems and the nigrothalamic pathway, *Brain Research*, **27**, 59-78.

Frigyesi, T.L. and Purpura, D.P. (1966). Electrophysiological analysis of nigro-caudate evoked activities, *Trans. Amer. Neurol. Assoc.*, **91**, 236-238.

Frigyesi, T.L. and Purpura, D.P. (1967). Electrophysiological analysis of reciprocal caudato-nigral relations, *Brain Research*, **6**, 440-456.

Goldberger, M.E. and Growden, J.H. (1971). Tremor at rest following cerebellar lesions in monkeys: effect of L-Dopa administration, *Brain Research*, **27**, 183-187.

Goswell, M.J. and Sedgwick, E.M. (1971). Inhibition in the substantia nigra following stimulation of the caudate nucleus, *J. Physiol.*, **218**, 84.

Hassler, R. (1959). Anatomy of the thalamus, in *Introduction to Stereotaxis with an Atlas of the Human Brain, Vol. 1*, (eds. Schaltenbrandt, G. and Bailey, P.), (Thieme Verlag, Stuttgart), pp. 230-290.

Herz, A. and Zieglgänsberger, W., (1968). The influence of micromimetics and procaine on synaptic excitation in the corpus striatum, *Int. J. Neuropharmacol.*, **7**, 221-230.

Jasper, H. and Bertrand, G. (1964). Exploration of the human thalamus with micro-electrodes, *Physiologists*, **7**, 167.

Jasper, H.H. and Bertrand, G. (1966). Thalamic units involved in somatic sensation and voluntary movements in Man, in *The Thalamus*, (eds. Purpura, D.P. and Yarh, M.D.), (Columbia University Press, New York and London), pp. 365-390.

Jasper, H.H., Lamarre, Y. and Joffroy, A. (1972). Physiological studies of the effect of local cooling of motor cortex upon tremor, voluntary movement and thalamic unit activity in the monkey, in *Corticothalamic Projections and Sensorimotor Activities*, (ed. Frigyesi, T.L.), (Columbia University Press, New York and London), (in press).

Kemp, J.M. (1970). The termination of strio-pallidal and strionigral fibres, *Brain Research*, **17**, 125-128.

Kemp, J.M. and Powell, I.P.S. (1970). The cortico-striate projection in the monkey, *Brain*, **93**, 525-546.

Lamarre, Y. (1972). Lower brain stem mechanisms of Parkinson-like tremor in monkey, in *Third Conference on Experimental Medecine and Surgery in Primates (Lyon, France)*, (in press).

Lamarre, Y. and Cordeau, J.P. (19). Activités des neurones centraux chez le singe porteur d'un tremblement postural expérimental, *J. Physiol. (Paris)*, **56**, 589-590.

Lamarre, Y. and Cordeau, J.P. (1967). Etude du mécanisme physiopathologique responsable, chez le singe, d'un tremblement expérimental de type parkinsonien, *Actualités Neurophysiologiques, 7ème Série*, (Masson et Cie, Paris).

Li, C.L. and Buren, van, J.M. (1971). Micro-electrode recordings in the brain of man with particular reference to epilepsy and dyskinesia, in *Proceedings of the International Symposium on Neurophysiology in Man*, (ed. Somjen, G.), (Excerpta Medica, Amsterdam), pp. 49-63.

Libet, B., Alberts, W.W., Wright, E.W. Jr. and Fernstein, B. (1971). Cortical and thalamic activation in conscious sensory experience, in *Proceedings of the International Symposium on Neurophysiology in Man*, (ed. Somjen, G.), (Excerpta Medica, Amsterdam), pp. 157-168.

Lucking, C.H., Struppler, A., Erbel, F. and Reiss, W. (1971). Stereotactic recording from human subthalamic structures, in *Proceedings of the International Symposium on Neurophysiology in Man*, (ed. Somjen, G.), (Excerpta Medica, Amsterdam), pp. 95-99.

MacLennan, H. and York, D.H. (1967). The action of dopamine on neurones of the caudate nucleus, *J. Physiol.*, **189**, 393-402.

Mehler, W.R. (1969). Connections of the extrapyramidal motor system, in *Bing's Local Diagnosis in Neurological Diseases*, (ed. Haymaker, W.), (C.V. Mosby and Company, Saint-Louis), pp. 405-409.

Mettler, F.A. (1970). Nigrofugal connections in the primate brain, *J. Comp. Neurol.*, **138**, 291-320.

Moore, R.Y., Bhatnagar, R.C. and Heller, A. (1971). Anatomical and chemical studies of a nigro neostriatal projection in the cat, *Brain Research*, **30**, 119-135.

Niimi, K., Ikeda, T., Kawamura, S. and Inoshita, H. (1970). Efferent projections of the head of the caudate nucleus in the cat, *Brain Research*, **21**, 327-343.

Ohye, C. and Narabayashi, H. (1971). Activity of thalamic neurons and their receptive fields in different functional states in Man, in *Proceedings of the International Symposium on Neurophysiology in Man*, (ed. Somjen, G.), (Excerpta Medica, Amsterdam), pp. 79-84.

Poggio, G.F. and Mountcastle, V.B. (1963). The functional properties of ventro-basal thalamic neurons studied in unanaesthetized monkeys, *J. Neurophysiol.*, **26**, 775-806.

Raeva, S.N. (1971). Unit activity in some deep nuclear structures of the human brain during voluntary movements, in *Proceedings of the International Symposium on Neurophysiology in Man*, (ed. Somjen, G.), (Excerpta Medica, Amsterdam), pp. 64-78.

Rinvik, E. (1966). The cortico-nigral projection in the cat - an experimental study with silver impregnation methods, *J. Comp. Neurol.*, **126**, 241-254.

Schaltenbrandt, G. and Bailey, P. (1959). *Introduction to Stereotaxis with an Atlas of the Human Brain, Vol. 2*, (Georg Thieme Verlag, Stuttgart).

Szabo, J. (1962). Topical distribution of the striatal efferent in the monkey, *Exptl. Neurol.*, **5**, 21-36.

Voneida, T.S. (1960). An experimental study of the course and destination of fibres arising in the head of the caudate nucleus in the cat and monkey, *J. Comp. Neurol.*, **115**, 75-87.

EEG ASSESSMENT IN CLINICAL MEDICINE

M.V. DRIVER

*Department of Clinical Neurophysiology,
The Bethlem Royal and Maudsley Hospitals,
London, SE5*

The use of the electroencephalogram (EEG) in medical practice has a history extending over 40 years, during the first quarter of which most of the observations of current clinical diagnostic value were made and the methods to be used in EEG assessment established. The account published by Davis in 1941 on technique and evaluation of the EEG might well pass with little comment in a modern introductory text. The appearance of such a paper in a journal of neurophysiology makes it clear that electroencephalography was then regarded as having scientific value; in its subsequent history, however, dominated as it was by endeavours heavily orientated to clinical and particularly psychiatric correlates, neurophysiologists played but a small part and little progress was made towards an understanding of the basic phenomena of the EEG. However, the past ten years have seen a resurgence of interest, not only involving neurophysiologists but also mathematicians, physicists and computer technologists. It is largely with the work of these that this session of the Congress is concerned.

My task is to introduce clinical electroencephalography as a preliminary to the work to be presented by later speakers. I shall also give some account of methods of processing EEG data developed in the past as a pointer to what the clinician hopes to achieve in the future.

Voltage-time curves can be obtained from different areas of the scalp and these in some way reflect processes occurring within the substance of the brain. Recordings obtained from healthy alert adult subjects are broadly similar to each other, and certainly much more so than they are to recordings from sleeping adults or infants, whether awake or asleep (figure 1). We can single out phenomena of different ages and states of alertness and define them in a rather elementary fashion. For example, the most obvious phenomenon of the relatively alert adult's EEG, the alpha rhythm, has been defined (Storm van Leeuwen et al., 1966) as a "rhythm, usually with frequency of 8-13 c/sec in adults, most prominent in the posterior areas, present most markedly when the eyes are closed, and attenuated during attention, especially visual". Similarly, sigma rhythm is defined as an "episodic rhythm at about 14 c/sec, usually diffuse, with a maximum near the vertex, usually occurring during certain stages of sleep". These definitions, bringing in as they do frequency, topography and the conditions under which the rhythms appear, are reasonably comprehensive, but theta rhythm, a common phenomenon in normal children, is defined merely as a rhythm with a "frequency of 4 c/sec to less than 8 c/sec". A potential source of difficulty becomes apparent when one notes that alpha rhythm in children and in drowsy adults may have a frequency of less than 8 c/sec. It would appear foolish to assert that under these conditions it should be called theta rhythm, and the point becomes important if one is interested in the possibility that the ratio of theta to alpha activity is a meaningful parameter in the study of EEG.

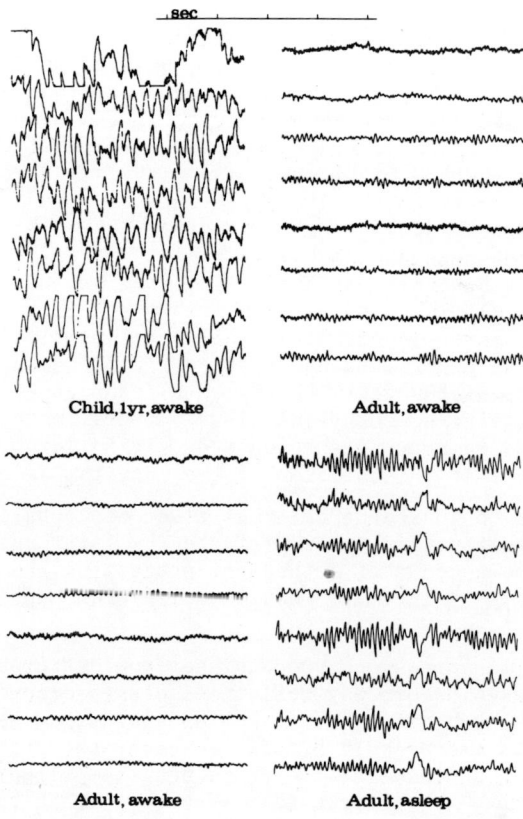

Figure 1 - Characteristic EEG's of a one-year-old normal child and two normal adults, all awake, and one sleeping normal adult, recorded at the same sensitivity and paper speed. In the child's record the channels are arranged from frontal to occipital, alternately right and left; in the remaining three records the first four channels are frontal to occipital from the right side and the second four similarly from the left. The child's record shows diffusely distributed waves mainly at at 4 to 6 c/sec; the awake adult's EEG's show little except for posteriorly distributed alpha rhythm at about 10 to 12 c/sec whereas the sleeping adult's record contains several activities of differing frequency, persistence and distribution.

A dozen or so recognizably different phenomena of the normal EEG can be so defined (figure 2). Many, if not all, of these may also be seen in the EEG of a patient with a cerebral disorder, for example a tumour, but it is not uncommon to see other phenomena, such

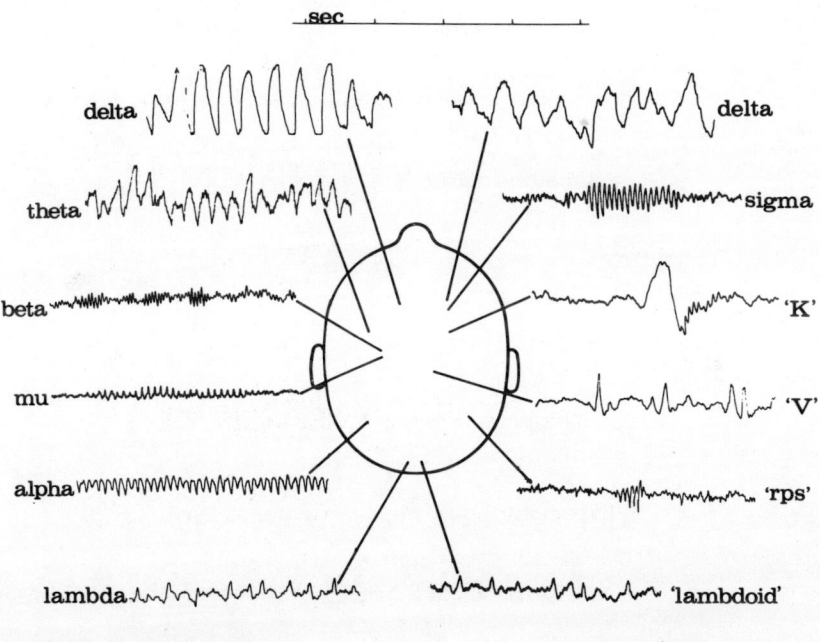

AWAKE   ASLEEP

Figure 2 - Samples of EEG activity recorded at the same sensitivity from healthy subjects, the lines pointing to the areas of the scalp where the individual phenomena are commonly most prominent. The delta activity on the awake side is from a hyperventilating adult, the theta from a 10-year-old child, the next three activities from adults lying at rest and the last, lambda, from an adult examining a pattern. All phenomena on the right were recorded from adults, the delta in very deep sleep, the remainder in lighter stages. The sigma activity, the K complex waveform and the V (vertex) waves may occur spontaneously or in response to a somatosensory stimulus. The abbreviation 'rps' signifies the 14 and 6 per second rhythmic positive spike phenomenon of light sleep.

as are never or but rarely seen in subjects without evidence of cerebral disease. These too can be defined in simple ways, for example a spike is a "wave distinguished from background activity and having a duration of 1/12 sec or less" and a spike and wave complex consists of "two waves, one with a duration of 1/12 sec or less (spike) and the other with a duration of 1/5-1/2 sec (wave)". Again about a dozen such phenomena can be recognized as sufficiently unusual in the healthy to make their appearance in an EEG acceptable evidence of cerebral disease (figure 3). The presence of one or

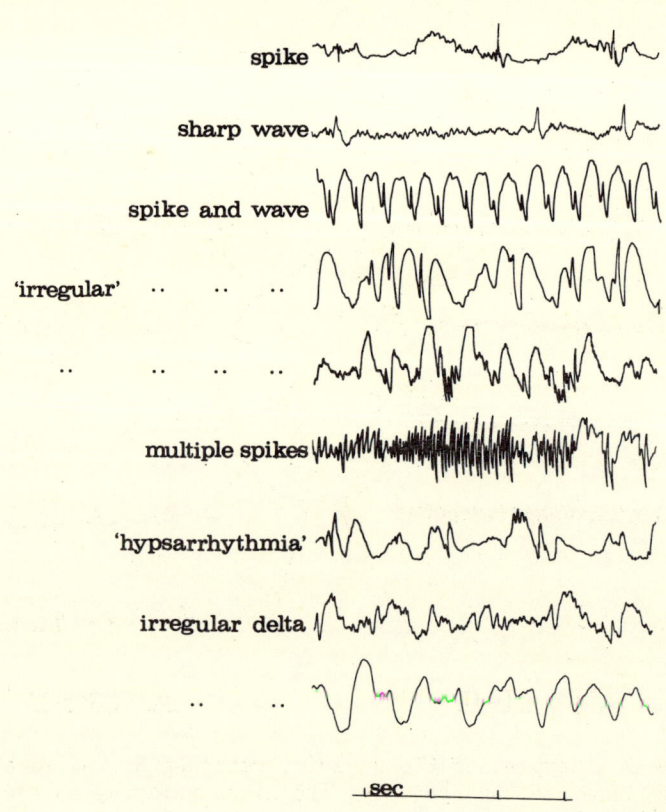

Figure 3 - Samples of EEG activity recorded at the same sensitivity from subjects with various cerebral disorders. The abnormal sharp waves are commonly distinguished from normal vertex waves (see figure 2) by reason of location, asymmetry, occurring during the waking state and so on, but distinction is occasionally very difficult. Irregular delta activity can usually be distinguished from the delta activities illustrated in figure 2 not only by its greater irregularity but by the inclusion within it of much slower wave forms than are seen in health. The other activities are readily identified as abnormal.

more of these features leads to the most definite diagnostic aid that can be obtained from the EEG. For example, localized irregular activity at about 1-3 c/sec implies definite cortical dysfunction in that area and, in the absence of a recent epileptic seizure or perhaps a recent blow on the head, indicates gross cortical damage as might be found with a tumour or acute abscess of the temporal lobe. In such cases the EEG can be very effective in lateralizing a lesion affecting one or other cerebral hemisphere and may also be sufficiently precise in localization within a hemisphere (figure 4). It is, however, of much less definite value in

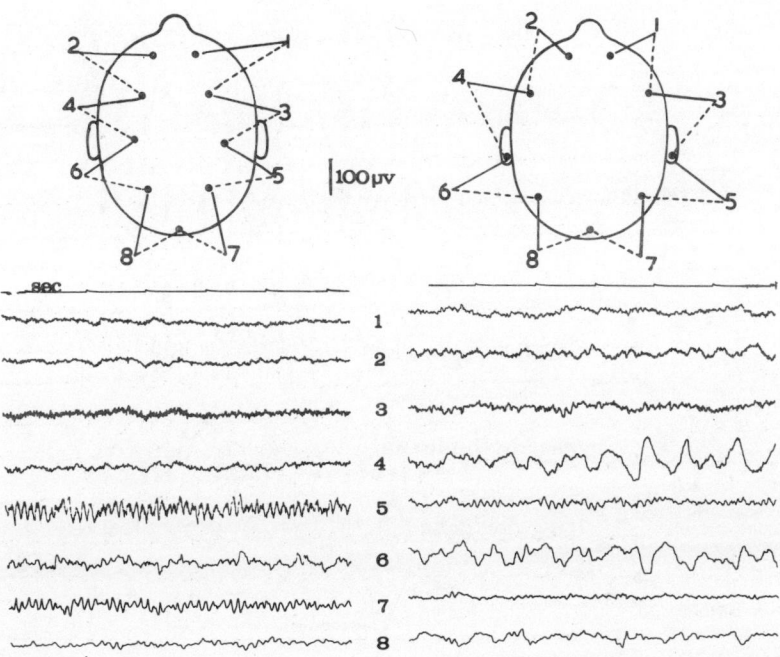

Figure 4 - Bipolar EEG recorded from parasagittal (left) and temporal (right) lines of scalp electrodes in a patient with an abscess of the left temporal lobe. It illustrates the two major signs of localized disease of the cerebral cortex: asymmetry of a phenomenon which is symmetrical in health (here the alpha rhythm: compare channels 5 and 6 in the left illustration), and the presence locally of a phenomenon not found in health (here the irregular delta activity of channels 4 and 6 in the right illustration).

relation to the pathological basis of the dysfunction. Recurrent bursts of rhythmic regularly formed waves at about 2-4 c/sec in one of the frontal regions may result not from a local area of cortical damage but indirectly from the disturbed function of a distant region providing afferents to that area, for example a deeply placed tumour near the midline. Wave forms containing spikes are commonly seen in epilepsy, being bilateral and synchronous in·

generalized seizures and localized in focal seizure varieties (figures 5,6).

Unfortunately, not all cerebral disturbances lead to such obviously unusual EEG phenomena. Patients with chronic and severely disabling diseases such as Parkinsonism and multiple sclerosis not uncommonly have what appear to be normal records. This is also

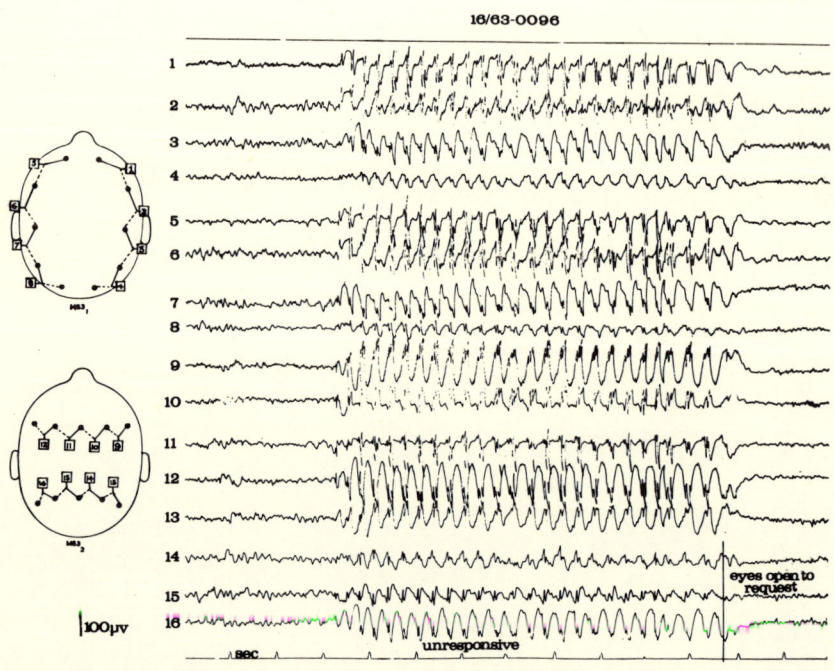

Figure 5 - Bipolar EEG recorded from a child with generalized epilepsy of 'absence' or 'petit mal' form, one brief attack occurring in this section. Note the apparent synchrony of onset and cessation of the spike and wave complexes on the two sides (channels 1 to 4 right, 5 to 8 left) and the similarity of wave form in homologous areas (e.g. channels 3 and 7, 9 and 12).

true of some of the major problems of psychiatry and in particular of chronic schizophrenia and the affective disorders. There exists a very large literature related to EEG findings in such patients, but little advance of fundamental diagnostic or prognostic usefulness has come out of it.

However, a number of observations have been made, for example that some psychotic patients show spiky wave forms and that others have generally low voltage records, and these tempt the psychiatrist to continue in his search for EEG significance. Is it possible, he asks, that the EEG of a psychotic patient, though not showing the obvious abnormalities of an epileptic, can yet yield

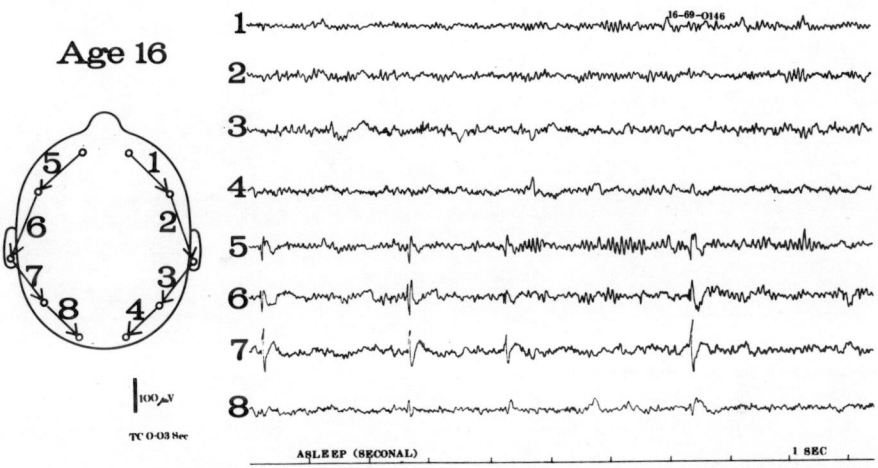

Figure 6 - Bipolar EEG recorded from a youth with a variety of focal epilepsy caused by disease of the left temporal lobe. The spikes appear at irregular intervals on the left and relate mainly to the two electrodes included in channel 6.

valuable information if it is assessed in the right way? Can there be, for example, an unusual variability or lack of variability in the EEG of a psychotic patient? (Figure 7).

Until the study of all night sleep became popular a few years ago the alpha rhythm was the only sustained normal EEG phenomenon readily assessable by simple methods and many attempts were made to differentiate psychotic and, in particular, shizophrenic patients from the normal on the basis of the amount of such activity.

In order to establish what was normal Davis and Davis in 1936 devised the *alpha index*, which was a measure of the percentage of time that a recognisable alpha rhythm appeared during a long sample of EEG recording. Using the levels of 25, 50 and 75% they divided their subjects, all normal adults aged 18 to 64, into 4 alpha categories: rare, mixed, subdominant and dominant. There appeared to be no significant difference in the numbers placed in each group, nor were any very convincing differences demonstrated in psychotic patients.

The use of methods of assessment involving concepts like the alpha index led to difficulties in practice, partly because of the subjective element and partly because of the failure of the alpha rhythm in many normal as well as abnormal subjects to show the necessary qualities of continuity and purity of wave form. What appeared to be necessary if progress was to be made was a form of assessment leading to the acquisition of both qualitative and quantitative data. As the EEG appeared largely to be composed of sine waves various attempts were made to resolve it into its components

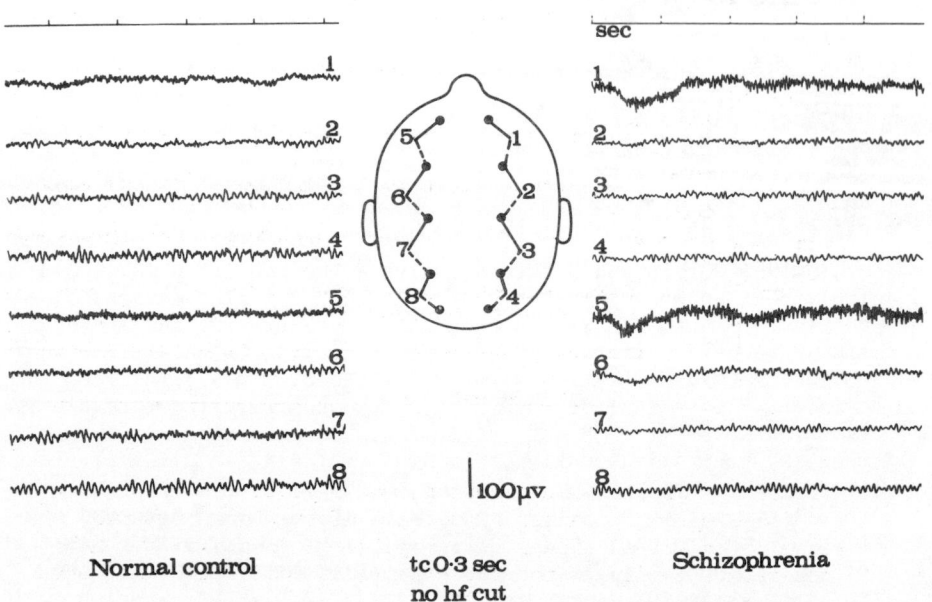

Figure 7 - Bipolar EEG's selected at random from a group of normal subjects (left) and a group of chronic schizophrenic patients (right). The records differ in alpha amplitude, frequency and distribution and possibly in other parameters capable of assessment by a computer. Do these differences represent true differences between the samples or are the records no more different than two selected from one group or the other, or from a mixed group?

by mathematical analysis. The experience of Russian and French investigators in the late 1930's that a few centimetres of EEG might take about a week to transform into sine waves of appropriate amplitude, frequency and phase may not have provided the original stimulus to automatic analysis but it probably hastened its development.

An early and quite successful method was reported by Grass and Gibbs in 1938. They recorded 30 seconds' worth of EEG on photographic paper via a mirror galvanometer, made it into a loop and passed it at 100 times the recording speed between a light source and a photocell. The resulting current fluctuations were analysed by a commercial sound wave analyser. The drawbacks of this type of analysis are obvious, major ones being the long time interval between recording and final presentation of the data and the fact that only a very limited portion of an EEG could be analysed economically. However, Gibbs analysed a large number of EEG's in this way and published studies not only related to diagnostic problems (Gibbs, 1939) but also to effects of changes in blood chemistry on EEG activity (Gibbs et al., 1940).

The tuned circuit analyser that followed, the best known of which was later produced in commercial form and commonly known as the Walter analyser, overcame many of the difficulties encountered by Gibbs and its use led to a number of interesting and useful observations during the next 20 or so years. These were to a great extent concerned with epilepsy, and in particular with petit mal and photically induced seizures, but studies on drug effects, endocrine disorders and many other subjects also appeared.

In 1955 Corbin and Bickford analysed the EEG of normal children. Their most interesting statement related not to the data obtained but to the fact that with 8 channels of EEG tracing and another of simultaneous Fourier analysis to contend with the observer's threshold of data assimilation might be exceeded. This reinforced the opinion of many analyser users, some of whom reverted to exclusive visual assessment of 8 and later 12, 16 or more channels, which remains, generally speaking, the state met with in clinical electroencephalography today. However, a few took up Corbin and Bickford's suggestion of simplification of the analysed data and continued with its use. One of the best known modifications was that of Lettich and Margerison (1961) who joined the summits of the analyser write out to produce relatively simple curves which could be compared between different subjects and also between different states in a patient with fluctuating symptomatology or under drug or other treatment.

Others, for example Shaw (1961), replaced the analyser pen by a digital display. This did not suffer from the non-linearity of the pen write out, nor was the sensitivity dependent on pen pressure. Above all, it did away with the time consuming measurement of the lengths of 20 to 40 pen deflexions repeating every 10 seconds for perhaps an hour or more. The device had become what could be regarded as a very specialized computer and with it the history of EEG reaches the present. We now have the use of many types of computer and numerous methods of analysis, data transformation, statistical processing and so on are available.

Broadly, the clinical electroencephalographer looks to computers to help him in two ways: firstly, to extend the accuracy and usefulness of his present methods of EEG assessment and, secondly, to provide him with information concerning certain neurological, psychiatric and other diseases in which traditional methods of EEG assessment have been on the whole fruitless. Ability to recognise differences in frequency, voltage, distribution and so on between the EEG phenomena of one side of the head and those of the other can be extended by computer analysis, provided the limits of differences existing in the normal can be ascertained; the recognition of abnormal wave forms may be refined if their characteristics can be adequately detailed and differentiated from those of normal wave forms. However, when we come to the application of data processing techniques to diseases in which the EEG has so far had very little success we are as though returning to the days of the Davises, Kennards and so on: we seize the available technologies and try them without necessarily having a very good reason.

We assume, from studies using microelectrodes within and in the immediate vicinity of neurones, that the voltage changes of the EEG represent summed depolarizing and hyperpolarizing postsynaptic potentials within the cerebral cortex and that they relate mainly to radially orientated neuronal structures. The EEG therefore probably receives a contribution from only a fraction of cells within the cortex. In addition, it may be that not all radially oriented neurones in the population under the electrode are behaving in a synchronized fashion, i.e. we are quite possibly recording averaged potential changes of cells engaged in different functions at any one time. We believe, following the work deriving from Eccles (e.g. Andersen and Sears, (1964); Andersen et al., (1967)) and others that the rhythmicity of electrocortical activity is largely an outcome of rhythmic changes arising in the thalamus. That is, the electrocortical rhythms are more dependent on what is happening in the thalamus than on what is primarily cortical. The cerebral cortex can be regarded merely as a projection area for the thalamus but it would not have developed as it has done in man without acquiring a much more important rôle, particularly in those aspects of cerebral function to disturbance of which the symptomatology of the psychotic patient may relate. The question to be asked, then, is does electrocortical activity as we record it in the EEG reflect in any significant way the complexities of cerebral cortical function or does it represent nothing more than a reflection of a primitive level of thalamocortical integration, such as may be found in lower animals. In the latter case it may well have some physiological, biochemical and pharmacological significance, though it would seem unlikely to bear directly on the major problems of psychiatry.

At present we cannot decide between these possibilities on the basis of our neurophysiological knowledge and it is difficult to see as yet how and to what extent computer studies of the scalp EEG can be of assistance.

The title of this Congress implies that the brain is to be the object of discussion, but it has been demonstrated in many recent publications that it is possible to discuss the EEG without thinking a great deal about the brain at all. Many concerned with the clinical use of EEG understand recent introductions in wave analysis and data processing only at a most elementary level and may feel that the outcome relates to questions not yet formulated or to unreal and perhaps unimportant problems. All would agree, however, that there are numerous possible computer applications of direct and immediate relevance to clinical medicine. The future development of electroencephalography will depend on the cooperative effort of physicians, scientists and technologists directed to an understanding of the workings of the brain in health and to an unequivocal appreciation of its disturbed function in disease.

REFERENCES

Andersen, P. and Sears, T.A. (1964). The rôle of inhibition in the phasing of spontaneous thalamo-cortical discharge, *J. Physiol.*, **173**, 459-480.

Andersen, P., Andersson, S.A. and Lomo, T. (1967). Nature of thalamolcortical relations during spontaneous barbiturate spindle activity, *J. Physiol.*, **192**, 283-307.

Corbin, H.P.F. and Bickford, R.G. (1955). Studies of the electroencephalogram of normal children: comparison of visual and automatic frequency analysis, *Electroenceph. clin. Neurophysiol.*, **7**, 15-28.

Davis, H. and Davis, P.A. (1936). Action potentials of the brain, *Arch. Neurol. Psychiat. (Chic.)*, **36**, 1214-1224.

Davis, P.A. (1941). Technique and evaluation of the electroencephalogram, *J. Neurophysiol.*, **4**, 92-114.

Gibbs, F.A. (1939). Cortical frequency spectra of schizophrenic, epileptic and normal individuals, *Trans. Amer. Neurol. Ass.*, 141-144.

Gibbs, F.A., Williams, D. and Gibbs, E.L. (1940). Modification of the cortical frequency spectrum by changes in CO_2, blood sugar and O_2, *J. Neurophysiol.*, **3**, 49-58.

Grass, A.M. and Gibbs, F.A. (1938). A Fourier transform of the electroencephalogram, *J. Neurophysiol.*, **1**, 521-526.

Lettich, E. and Margerison, J.H. (1961). Presentation of data from low frequency analysis to illustrate serial changes in the electroencephalogram, *Electroenceph. clin. Neurophysiol.*, **13**, 606-611.

Shaw, J.C. (1961). Further developments of a digital write out for the wave analyser, *Electroenceph. clin. Neurophysiol.*, **13**, 941-945.

van Leeuwen, W. Storm et al. (1966). Proposal for an EEG terminology, *Electroenceph. clin. Neurophysiol.*, **20**, 606-611.

CLINICAL ELECTROENCEPHALOGRAPHY AND COMPUTING

B.B. MacGILLIVRAY

*Royal Free Hospital
and The National Hospital for Nervous Diseases,
London.*

It is now twenty years or so since computers were first used in EEG analysis (Brazier and Casby, 1951) although they have only been more generally available in the last decade in the U.S.A. and for a rather shorter period in the U.K. and elsewhere. During this time the computer itself has changed from a roomful of valves to a relatively small box of considerably more power: five years is a long time in computer technology. Yet it is fair to say that the impact of this powerful technology on Clinical Electroencephalography has been, and is still, negligible. Why is this so? The clinical EEG, with its multiplicity of channels and wave patterns, is surely a computer man's paradise. Why aren't we all busy 'number crunching' and pattern recognizing?

Some of the answers to these questions relating to technology and costs are fairly obvious, but others, relating to what might be termed the philosophy of computing, the attitudes of the clinicians involved, the status of the EEG in the diagnostic hierarchy and the demand, are rather more elusive. The fact is that, whilst there is a considerable body of elegant and sophisticated work on the normal and some aspects of the abnormal EEG (see recent review in Schadé and Smith (1970), no one has implemented a practical scheme to deal with the everyday problems of the EEG clinic. We are still at the stage of dealing with limited and selected problems and most often in a laboratory atmosphere. Certainly there is no question of routine about any of these procedures.

From a technical point of view, despite an almost exponential fall in computing costs per bit, the clinical EEG still represents a fairly formidable challenge. The usual 10 minute, 16 channel clinical EEG trace is about 20 yards long and when digitized at a conservative 100 samples/sec yields some 10^6 10-bit numbers. Commonly used techniques for wave form analysis, such as spectral density (Walter, 1963) and pattern recognition based on these functions, and discriminant analysis techniques (Walter et al., 1967) are extremely expensive in computer time even on large machines. In a cost conscious world, only space biology or the demands of war can support such exercises. They have not been applied in any significant clinical sense and at present they are simply not cost effective, but they have shown the power of the machine to detect events in this complex situation beyond the range of unaided man.

The 'cost-effective' barrier, important though it is, is purely technological and likely to reduce in the fairly near future. Already the Fast Fourier Transform has dramatically altered computing times. 'Firm wired' (i.e. very fast permanently programmed, read-only, memory subsystems) hardware, capable of an incredible 5 million operations/sec, is already on the market and promises to revolutionize the speed at which such procedures as the Fourier transform are carried out, to the extent that they will become practicable on-line multi-channel operations. Whilst almost any procedure you can think of may well be carried out optimally by a little 'black box' in the future, this is not quite the same as 'think of any procedure' and carry it out - a malady not peculiar to computer technologists! It is this problem, 'I just thought of something else....' that keeps the cost barrier in being: no sooner has technology solved one problem than two more appear. Actually, such is the pace of technological advance that there is an inverse malady: 'I have a new technique, let's try it out', which is even more expensive, but lucrative for the manufacturer at least.

From the more philosophical point of view, in considering the problem of computing in the clinical enviroment, it is perhaps worth while returning to first principles: after all, we have not made that much progress so far. We may take it as self-evident (cautiously perhaps) that the clinical EEG, whatever one may think about brain waves in other contexts, is worth doing (*vide* the previous speaker) and that current practice can be considerably improved, simply by reducing observer error if nothing else, but hopefully with rather more substantial benefits. Every practising electroencephalographer is only too aware of the shortcomings of his art, and it can hardly be called a science.

What does the clinician demand of the EEG? The answer, finally and simply, is a 'diagnosis'; the terms is a relative one of course and must be defined in the context of its use. For my purposes, and having due regard for what I believe to be the potential of computing within the context of present technology and our current concepts of the brain and the electroencephalogram, I will define the diagnostic demand in general terms as *a statement of the presence (or non-presence) of a topographic or system dysfunction in the brain*. We cannot escape a definition of 'normal', i.e. the absence of dysfunction. This is a recurrent problem in medicine and we will adopt the usual operational device of listing the statistical distribution of the relevant properties of an arbitrarily defined group of the population, excluding subjects suspected, or known, to have any number of conditions which by consensus are classed as diseased states. The 'normal' or 'not abnormal' is thus a variable and generally diminishing set as knowledge progresses. The term 'system' is used to imply groups of neurones and their interconnections, postulated or known to behave in some related way, the effects of which can be observed in defined circumstances. For example, the 'blocking' of alpha activity reflects activity in the 'ascending reticular activating system'.

This is the ideal: we would like our patient to be put at one end of the machine, the diagnosis to come out of the other (leaving the patient relatively unruffled of course). Since the human operator is a relatively cheap, though slightly erratic, heuristically orientated, self-educating, self-reproducing and ambulatory device, he may be difficult to replace completely. We may have to settle for 'computer assisted' diagnosis. Is it worth doing? The answer is 'No', *unless* we can show substantial improvements on our present performance (which shouldn't be too difficult) and at reasonable costs (i.e. the sort of money one can squeeze out of grant-giving bodies - say £25-30,000, or less than $100,000 U.S.A.). Can it be done, now? I think the answer is again 'Yes', not today perhaps, but in a few years or so.

The use of 'diagnosis' as given above falls short of the usage usual in medicine in that it excludes 'causes' such as tumour, abscess, blood clot, etc.. This is because all our experience suggests that the abnormal EEG is generally non-specific and the aetiology cannot be deduced from EEG data alone. Given a modicum of additional data however, such as age, signs and symptoms and duration of illness, the position becomes quite otherwise and it is often possible to state that such and such a condition is more (or less) likely than some other possible condition, even to the extent sometimes of near certainty. There are in principle no reasons why such data should not be included in the computing process to expand the diagnostic statement defined above in a way which more nearly approaches clinical usage. However, to do so presumes that we can confidently make the limited primary statement about the EEG which is of more immediate concern. In practice, the clinician is very sensitive to the clinical data which come on the request form to carry out an EEG examination, and this should be taken into account should we want to mimic his behaviour in the computing process.

As is evident from the literature (see Brazier (1965), Stacy and Waxman (1965), Schadé and Smith (1970) for recent reviews) and from this conference, there are many ways of viewing the behaviour of the brain. All of them involve implicitly, if not explicitly, some sort of conceptual model. Of course we may choose to ignore any implied model and treat such observations as we make in a purely empirical way, and indeed this is common (and some would say the only) practice in clinical electroencephalography. We observe certain EEG patterns which correlate with particular clinical situations and we infer the latter from the former. On reflection, we all nonetheless have a model of some sort, even for the simplest abstractions.

Our conceptual model of the brain and the way in which the EEG is generated underlied the sort of questions asked of the data collected in an EEG record. The model I wish to use is quite conventionally based on current anatomical and neurophysiological concepts and may be briefly summarized as follows: the active elements are neurones which conduct information by means of brief spike trains along their axons to synaptic junctions on the cell bodies and dendrites of other neurones; the synaptic junctions conduct only in one direction and the effect of impluses at the synapses is to produce graded slow potentials (up to some hundred milliseconds or longer: post-synaptic potentials (PSP's)) in the recipient cell and its dendrites; these potentials are either depolarizing (exciting) or hyperpolarizing (inhibiting) and respectively increase or decrease the probability of the recipient cell discharging a spike along its axon to the next cell. In engineering terms, the synapse acts as a digital to analogue converter, information is processed in analogue terms and the output from the neurone is digital, in the form of a spike generated by the analogue to digital function of the cell body. These slow post-synaptic potentials in cortical neurones have been shown to correlate extremely well with the electrocortigram recorded from the surface (see reviews by Morrell (1967), Creutzfeld (1969)). The scalp EEG is thus conceived as reflecting the statistical behaviour of some hundreds of thousands of cortical neurones. The slow potentials reflect the information transactions occurring at the cellular level: when there is a high information input, in the alert state for example, the group behaviour becomes more random and the EEG tends to zero. On the other hand, in the resting state (and in the case of synchronous inputs such as occur when eliciting evoked potentials) greater synchronization occurs and slow and high voltage EEG waves are recorded. Alterations of the input to the cortex, as by lesions or changes in synaptic activity by drug or metabolic effects, will effect changes in the pattern of post-synaptic activity, thus altering the shape and amplitude of EEG waves. It is on this basis that EEG interpretations are made.

It is a remarkable observation that, despite all the possible variables when an EEG is recorded, including such factors as the precise location of a scalp electrode to the underlying cortex, the brain waves in the resting adult (though different in each individual) appear to be invariant from day to day, and year to year, under similar conditions. Furthermore, the EEG's in monozygotic twin pairs are virtually identical (Dumermuth, 1968). That is, the resting EEG pattern is apparently genetically determined and does not reflect learning or acquired experience. The EEG nonetheless reflects very well, in non-specific ways, the degree of difficulty of performing a task, performance before and after learning in a stimulus-response situation (Adey, 1970) and such phenomena as anticipation (CNV, see Cohen (1969)), and of course sleep states.

We may say therefore that, provided the circumstances in which the EEG is recorded are known, changes in the patterns must reflect changes in functional connections, ultimately of cortical neurones, i.e. in so far as they are affected by sub-cortical afferents. If biochemical effects are excluded (they generally produce symmetrical changes) then we should be able to specify, given an adequate knowledge, the particular cortical afferent connections involved in producing these effects. The interpretation is strictly analogous to the neurologist's use of clinical signs. When several connections, or systems, are involved in the lesion, the results are complex of course, but it is in just this sort of situation that the power of the computer is likely to be most evident. Whilst some progress has been made in this direction (Brazier (1968) located changes in the EEG of parts of the temporal lobe cortex associated with epileptic discharges in particular areas of the hippocampus in man) human pathology tends often to be too coarse and it will be necessary to resort to animal studies to elucidate the effects of more discrete lesions.

Whilst such speculations may be interesting in suggesting a heuristic use for computation, particularly when combined with evoked potential studies to yield locations of 'wiring diagram' faults, they must remain a long term view. There is insufficient basic information at present about cerebral interconnections to support other than rather simple models. Nonetheless I believe this to be a valid long term objective and one that cannot be achieved without computer assistance. If, in the interim, we use a more empirical approach, then we should bear in mind the longer view and record and process the data in such a way that they will serve both these ends.

The long term view is all very well and we can keep it in mind, but the clinician (and his patient) want results now. How should we proceed?

The human brain is particularly good at detecting patterns, one letter from another, a particular wave amongst many, and we have in recent years become obsessed with pattern recognition which in a general way is what we want from our computer. The term is so broadly used as to be almost debased currency: as Ashby (1966) has remarked, "Any machine that loses information is a pattern recognizer". A computer can be programmed to 'pattern recognize' by various techniques such as matched filters and multiple correlation (Weinberg and Cooper (1972), see also Lloyd et al., this conference) and this has been done for the characteristic spike and wave complex of petit mal epilepsy (Bickford, 1959; Stark, 1961). These are considerable achievements of course and have obvious applications in particular circumstances. But are they of use in the everyday clinical situation? Further thought suggests that they are not, at least in this simplified form: they are fairly time consuming, and there are very many possible wave forms that we would like to recognize (or exclude), and this through all 10^6 numbers of our clinical record - a monumental task even for our super-fast systems. And of course that is not the end of it, for there are other things we would like to know as well.

There are ways out of this dilemma. In the particular case of the classical spike and wave, for example, and taking all EEG channels together (i.e. spatial distribution†), the occurrence of a symmetrical step change in amplitude is almost unique to this condition. It helps to know that there is an approximately 3 c/sec dominant frequency, together with some fast frequency components. These parameters can be defined by a number of simple procedures and even broad

† This is contextual information: the context in which an event occurs is extremely powerful in information terms, as here, and is commonly neglected in schemes for computer diagnosis.

band analogue filters perform quite well. Having found an area of interest, in this case by the large symmetrical and synchronous step amplitude change, we can then 'pattern recognize' by whatever means we choose to differentiate between the usually very limited possibilities (here, slow waves without spikes, with one spike and with more than one spike). By this simple approach we have not only reduced the relevant portions of the record by some orders of magnitude, but reduced also the likelihood of particular wave forms in the area of interest to relatively few possibilities. In this way we deploy valuable central processor time to maximal advantage and the initial problem then is to determine the simplest computing procedure which will yield a separation of records in the most effective way.

It is fairly obvious that with the massive data inputs represented by the clinical EEG record, central processing time (and therefore cost) is at a premium. Although the fast Fourier transform is now very fast, it is still a massive item for 16 simultaneous channels (and we want all 16 at least) and is best avoided if possible - we do need to do other computations as well. (The matter might be very different with a hard or firm wired preprocessor). Fortunately the clinical EEG is not infinitely variable - it has a limited band width and it varies in a reasonably limited number of ways. We do not therefore need an infinite computing capacity.

Generalizing some of the points already made, and bearing in mind that decisions between equally probable alternatives are maximally informative, we may conceive of a diagnostic procedure along the lines of figure 1.

The scheme is oversimplified as, clearly, the details become rather involved in practice. The general principle is to start computation with a simple parameter, e.g. amplitude, proceeding to greater detail with each node reached in the branching process. In this way computing time is minimized for each record. The 'not abnormal' record will probably take the longest time, as it requires an *exclusive* statement. Note that a simple statement that an EEG record is definitely abnormal, without any specification, is very powerful in the clinical context and this statement may be made at the first node.

The process is the reverse of logical induction: here we proceed from the most general to the specific. (It is rather doubtful that the human brain ever uses induction in the formal sense; we generalize instantly, even from a single exposure, probably by a process of association, and we have great difficulty in particularizing. To this extent the process mimics the human observer - which may be advantageous for developments, but is not an intended or necessary condition). The branching or sequential diagnostic process has some other benefits. We shall, from an early stage, obtain useful computing results on a proportion of records at least. The diagnostic process is evolutionary and always responsive to clinical demand: higher order nodes will be created wherever clinical information suggests it would be advantageous to establish sub-categories from the grouping reached at the last node. In this way, computing problems are thrown up by the diagnostic process itself rather than on the basis of *a priori* speculations as to what they ought to be. The success of a node is measured by appeal to the clinical conditions and the particular attributes used in differentiating categories at a node are in a strict sense irrelevant (although in practice of very great interest so far as they reveal properties of the EEG generators).

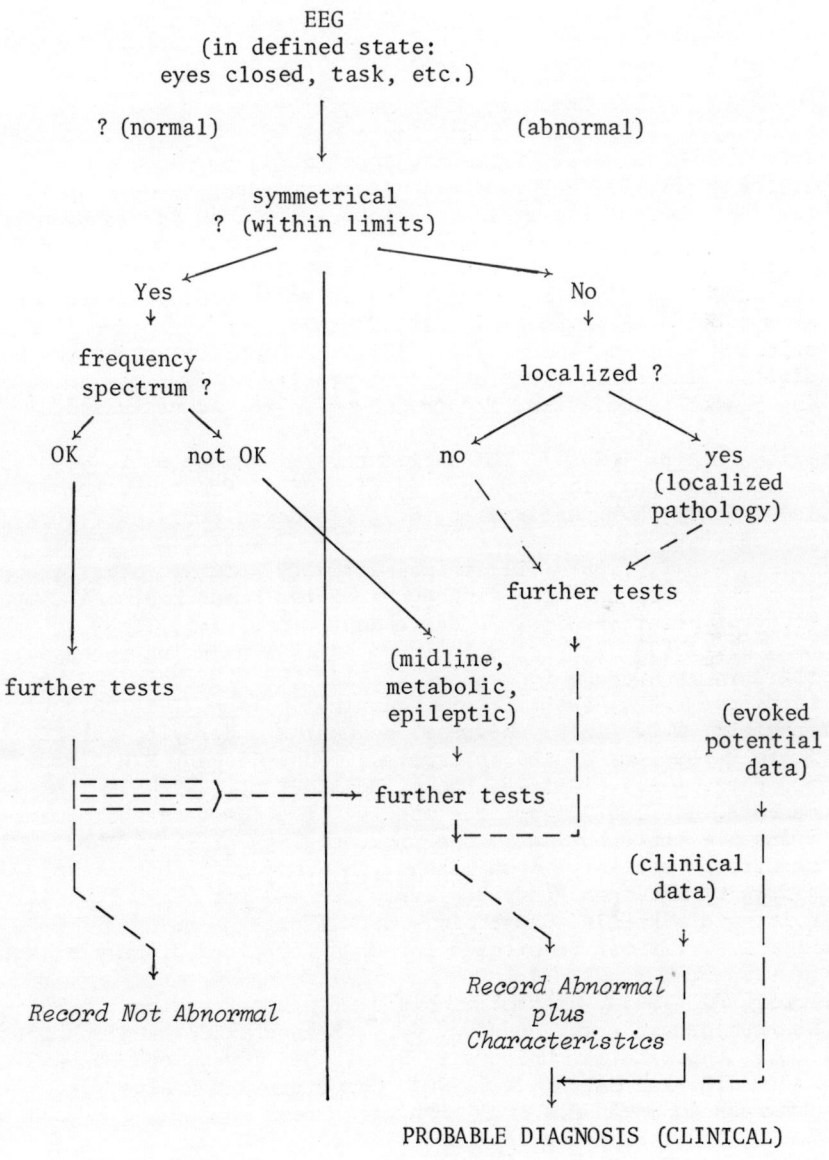

Figure 1 - Schematic diagnostic process.

It is likely that there are several possible implementations and there will be no unique decision tree, only more or less efficient ones. The sequential diagnostic process is well suited to the computer and economical (see Gorry (1968) for discussion). We are currently implementing a process along the lines discussed, with the hopeful intention of approximating the 'ideal' already mentioned. Whatever the outcome, we can be reasonably certain at least that our thinking about the EEG will be very different at the end of it.

REFERENCES

Adey, W.R. (1970). Computing devices of the second and third generations, in *Progress in Brain Research, Vol. 33*, (eds. Schadé, J.P. and Smith, J.), (Elsevier, Amsterdam), pp. 45-62.

Ashby, W.R. (1966). Mathematical models and computer analysis of the functions of the central nervous system, in *Annual Review of Physiology, Vol. 28*, 89-106.

Bickford, R.G. (1959). An automatic recognition system for spike-and-wave with simultaneous testing of motor response, *Electroenceph. clin. Neurophysiol.*, **11**, 397-398.

Brazier, M.A.B. and Casby, J.U. (1951). An application of the MIT digital electronic correlator to a problem in EEG: the EEG during mental calculation, *Electroenceph. clin. Neurophysiol.*, **3**, 375.

Brazier, M.A.B. (1965). The application of computers to electroencephalography, in *Computers in Biomedical Research, Vol. 1*, (eds. Stacy, R.W. and Waxman, B.), (Academic Press, New York), pp. 295-318.

Brazier, M.A.B. (1968). Electrical activity recorded simultaneously from the scalp and deep structures of the human brain. A computer study of relationships, *J. Nerv. Ment. Dis.*, **147**, 31-39.

Cohen, J. (1969). Very slow brain potentials relating to expectancy: the CNV, in *Average Evoked Potentials*, (eds. Donchin, E. and Lindsley, D.B.), (NASA SP-191, Washington), pp. 143-163.

Creutzfeld, O.D. (1969). Neuronal mechanics underlying the EEG, in *Basic Mechanisms of the Epilepsies*, (eds. Jasper, H.H., Pope, A. and Ward, A.A.), (Little, Brown, Boston), pp. 397-410.

Dumermuth, G. (1968). Variance spectra of electroencephalograms in Twins - a contribution to the problem of quantification of EEG background activity in childhood, in *Clinical Electroencephalography of Children*, (eds. Kellaway, P. and Petersen, I.), (Almqvist and Wiksells, Stockholm), pp. 119-154.

Gorry, G.A. (1968). Strategies for computer aided diagnosis, *Math. Biosciences*, **2**, 293-318.

Morrell, F. (1967). Electrical signs of sensory coding, in *The Neurosciences*, (eds. Quarton, G.C., Melnechuk, T. and Schmidt, F.O.), (Rockefeller University Press, New York), pp. 452-469.

Schadé, J.P. and Smith, J. (1970). Computers and brains, in *Progress in Brain Research, Vol. 33*, (eds. Schadé, J.P. and Smith, J.), (Elsevier, Amsterdam).

Stacy, R.W. and Waxman, B.D. (1965). *Computers in Biomedical Research*, *Vol. 1*, (Academic Press, New York), p. 562.

Stark, L. (1961). Pattern recognition for EEG diagnosis, *MIT Res. Lab. Electron. Quart. Prog. Rept.*, **61**, 215-219.

Walter, D.O. (1963). Spectral analysis for electroencephalograms: mathematical determination of neurophysiological relationships from records of limited duration, *Exp. Neurol.*, **8**, 155-181.

Walter, D.O., Kado, R.T., Rhodes, J.M. and Adey, W.R. (1967). Electroencephalographic machines in astronaut candidates estimated by computation and patter recognition techniques, *Aerospace Med.*, **38**, 371-379.

Weinberg, H. and Cooper, R. (1972). The recognition index: a pattern recognition technique for noisy signals, *Electroenceph. clin. Neurophysiol.*, **33**, (in press).

SIGNAL ANALYSIS

P. FENWICK

Institute of Psychiatry, De Crespigny Park, London SE 5

Meaningful analysis of the EEG depends on the assumption that the EEG signals contain information about the functioning of the brain. Both Dr. Driver, in the clinical field, and Dr. MacGillivray, from the theoretical standpoint of computer analysis, have indicated their belief and have demonstrated that information about brain function is contained within the EEG and that it is meaningful to attempt to recover this. Two main avenues of EEG analysis exist. Those which depend on a sophisticated statistical model of what the generation processes involved in the EEG are likely to be, and these methods allow precise statistical description of the EEG signals. Alternatively, no a priori assumptions about the EEG signal and its methods of generation need be assumed, and only an arbitrary set of parameters concerning the EEG signal are measured. These empirical methods suffer from the restriction that the information obtained from the EEG can only with difficulty be related to a theoretical statistical model, and thus their interpretation is difficult.

Which methods of analysis are used will depend entirely on the question to be answered, as all methods of EEG analysis, if they are to be successful, must be directed towards answering specific questions concerning the EEG signal.

Figure 1 shows a chart of the decision-making process, and attention should be drawn to the first branch of the tree, which ends in 'No'. This has been included because frequently the EEG is used in an attempt to answer questions which are much more suitably answered by other methods. However, should the EEG prove the system of choice, then various decisions as illustrated by the table have to be taken as to which aspects are required to answer the specific problem being considered.

Several of the following speakers will deal with the analysis of stimulus locked transient events in the EEG, such as the average evoked response and also transient spontaneous episodic phenomena, for example the high voltage spikes of epilepsy. The remainder of this talk will be devoted to a description of some methods of background EEG analysis, together with a discussion of the problems involved.

Figure 2 shows a table of the more usual methods of EEG analysis, which have been shown under three headings. Firstly, those methods which deal primarily with frequency and periodicity in the record (Blackman and Tukey, 1958; Brazier, 1961; Byford, 1965; Boldyrera, 1968; Elazar and Adey, 1967; Hannan, 1960; Liskie et al., 1967; Walter, 1966). Secondly, those which deal with the amplitude

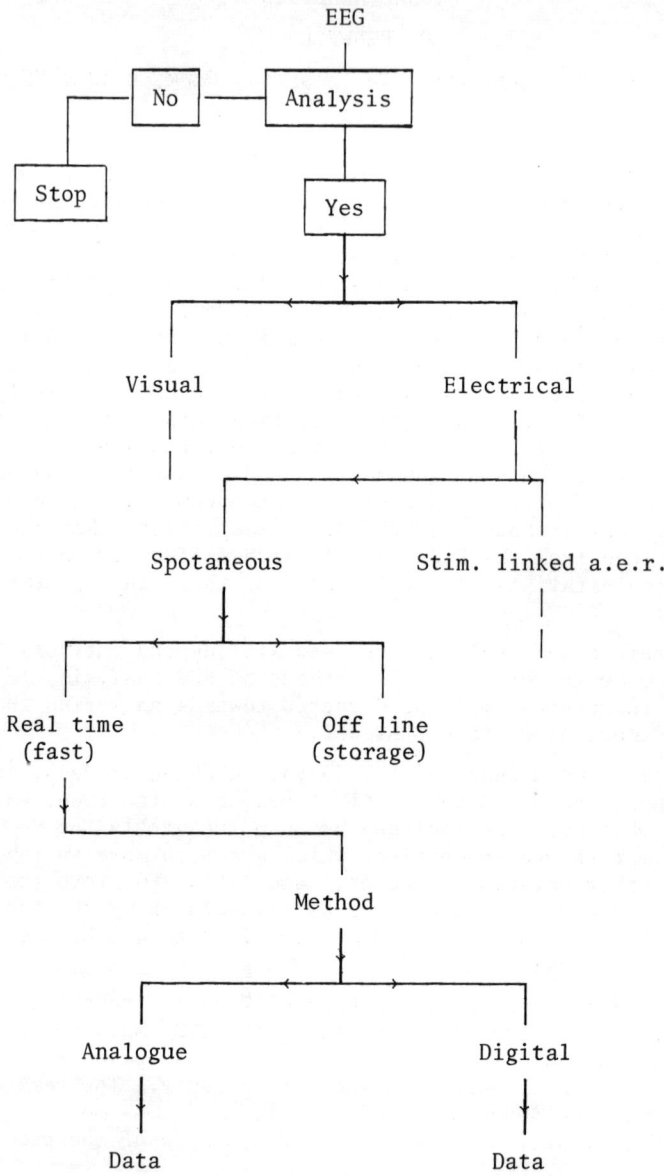

Figure 1 - Problem requires solution.

Figure 1 - Decision chart illustrating the pathway to be used when considering the use of EEG to solve a physiological problem.

SIGNAL ANALYSIS

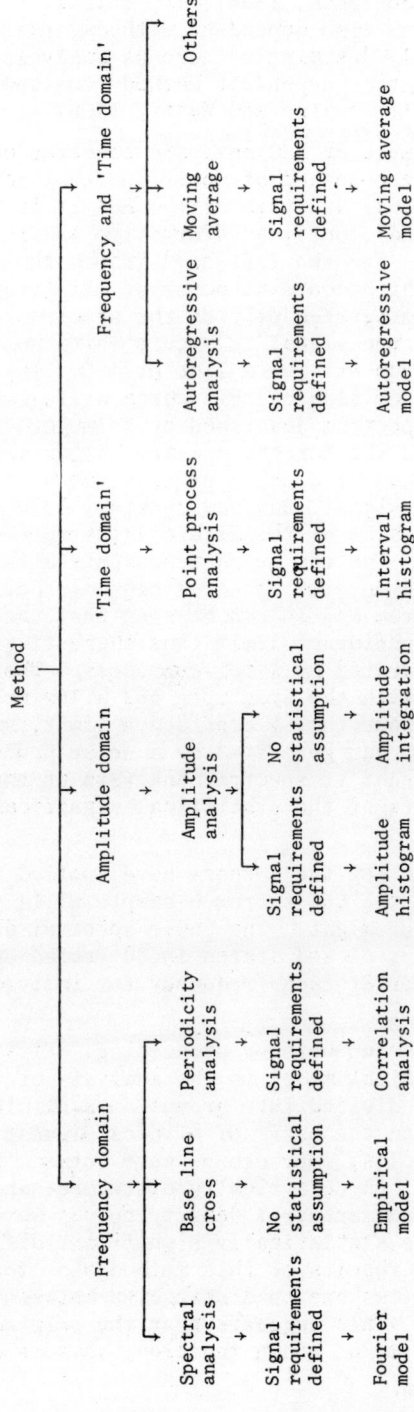

Figure 2 - This table shows those methods of EEG analysis which are now in common use and indicate whether or not precise statistical assumptions about each method are involved.

phenomena of the record (Drohocki, 1962; Sager and Herman, 1939; Saunders, 1963; Sugerman, 1964), and thirdly those methods which I have grouped under time dependent methods, realising that this is of course a purely descriptive term as analysis in the frequency domain is also a time dependent method (Cox and Lewis, 1966; Fenwick et al., 1971; Jenkins and Watts, 1968).

The first example of EEG analysis concerns only the frequency domain and uses the method of power spectral analysis. Before proceeding to frequency analysis of the EEG it is important to confirm that the EEG signal contains information and is not simply random noise, figure 3. The two left-hand graphs show the ideal spectrum of white noise which contains power at all frequencies, the bottom graph shows an integrated plot of the spectrum above. If the generator producing the signal is a pure white noise source then the integrated spectrum will be a line at 45°. It is possible to draw two lines on either side of this which will give the confidence limits for the spectrum described by Kolmogorov and Smirnov, so it can be calculated whether the spectrum being analysed is likely to have been generated by a noise process, or by a process which contains a definite signal (Box and Jenkins, 1970). The three graphs on the left-hand side of the figure illustrate this method applied to EEG analysis. The top graph represents a fairly typical spectrum of an EEG taken with the eyes closed, the second shows the integrated spectrum and it can be seen that the integrated curve crosses the 5% confidence limit thus suggesting that the spectrum has not been generated by a noise process. The third graph shows an EEG obtained with the eyes open and a low frequency filter; the graph does not cross the 5% confidence limit, suggesting that in this case the EEG was generated by a noise process. This indicates that it is important if spectral analysis of the EEG is to be meaningful, that tests of the statistical significance should always be included.

Figure 4 shows how the authors have applied the idea of frequency analysis to the EEG's from a sample of 14 year-old boys studied in the Isle of Wight. The power spectral densities for both eyes open and eyes closed states in 30 second epochs were estimated and the mean power at each frequency for individual groups was calculated.

Figure 5 shows two ways of proceeding. Firstly, we can apply the idea of a medical model to the analysis of the data. This means that the data is divided into groups on a clinical basis, and subjects are rated on the basis of clinical investigation and psychological test results; four groups were formed, that is; controls, backward readers, psychiatrically disturbed, and educationally subnormals. The power spectral density curves were then analysed to see if there were statistically significant differences between the groups. The results of this method show that simple power spectral analysis allows one to distinguish between the different clinical categories. This suggests that the original grouping was meaningful in terms of brain function, as some differences between

SIGNAL ANALYSIS

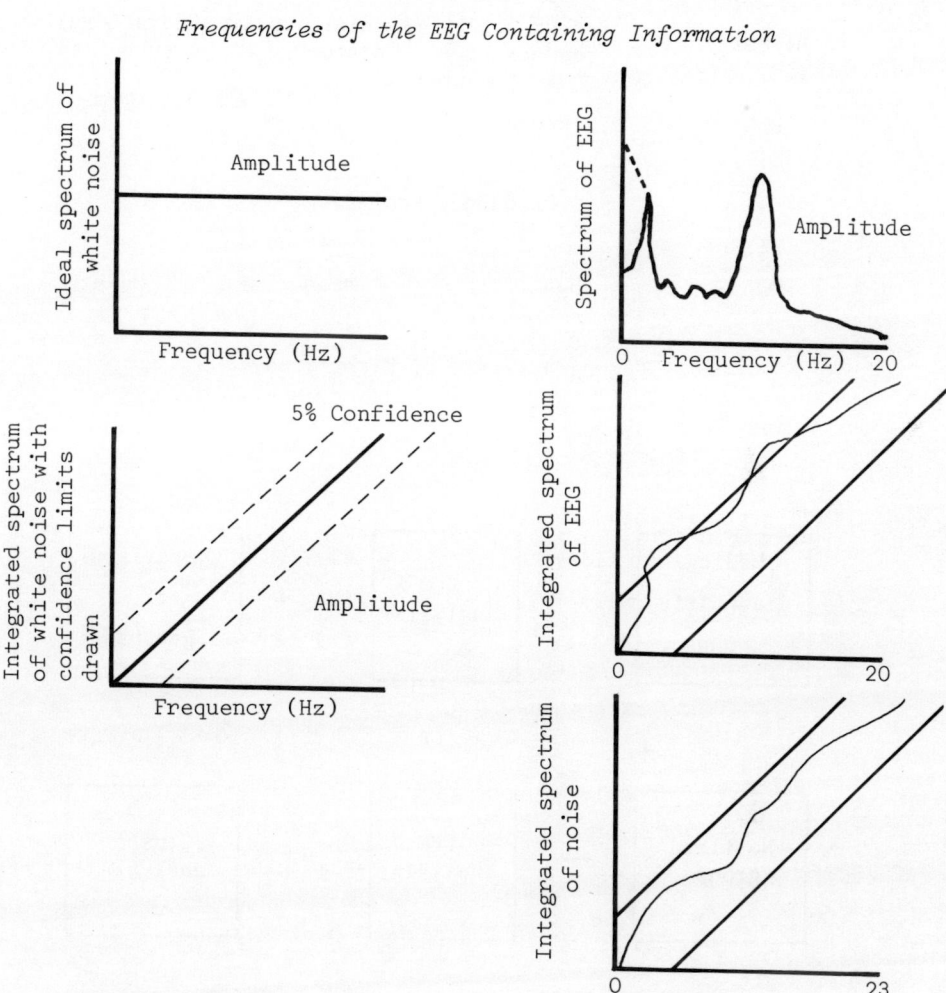

Figure 3 - The left-hand top graph shows the frequency spectrum of an ideal white noise source; the lower left-hand graph the integration of the spectrum and the 5% confidence limits defined by the Kolmorgorov and Smirnov method. The three right-hand graphs show the typical frequency profile of an EEG taken with the eyes closed. The middle graph shows this integrated and crossing the 5% line. The lower graph shows the integrated spec-spectrum of an EEG taken with the eyes open; this does not cross the 5% line, suggesting it could be generated by a noise process.

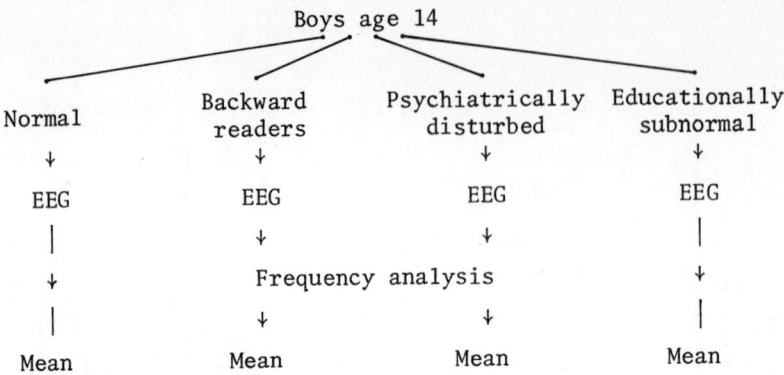

Figure 4 - Isle of Wight study.

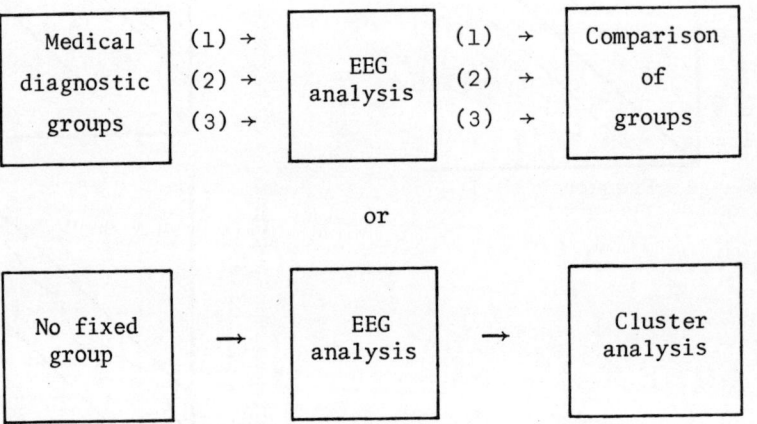

Figure 5 - EEG analysis.

the groups do exist (figure 6); the eyes open epochs were more successful at discriminating than the eyes closed epochs. Although power spectral density analysis has shown some differences which succeeded in separating the clinical groups, visual rating of the raw record was not so successful. In the Isle of Wight normal control group under 75% of the normal boys were classified by the EEG rater as having normal records while the other 25% were rated as abnormal. Power spectral density analysis of the normal group shows a prominent peak in the alpha band while the abnormal group shows some more theta activity in the temporal regions and very little

SIGNAL ANALYSIS

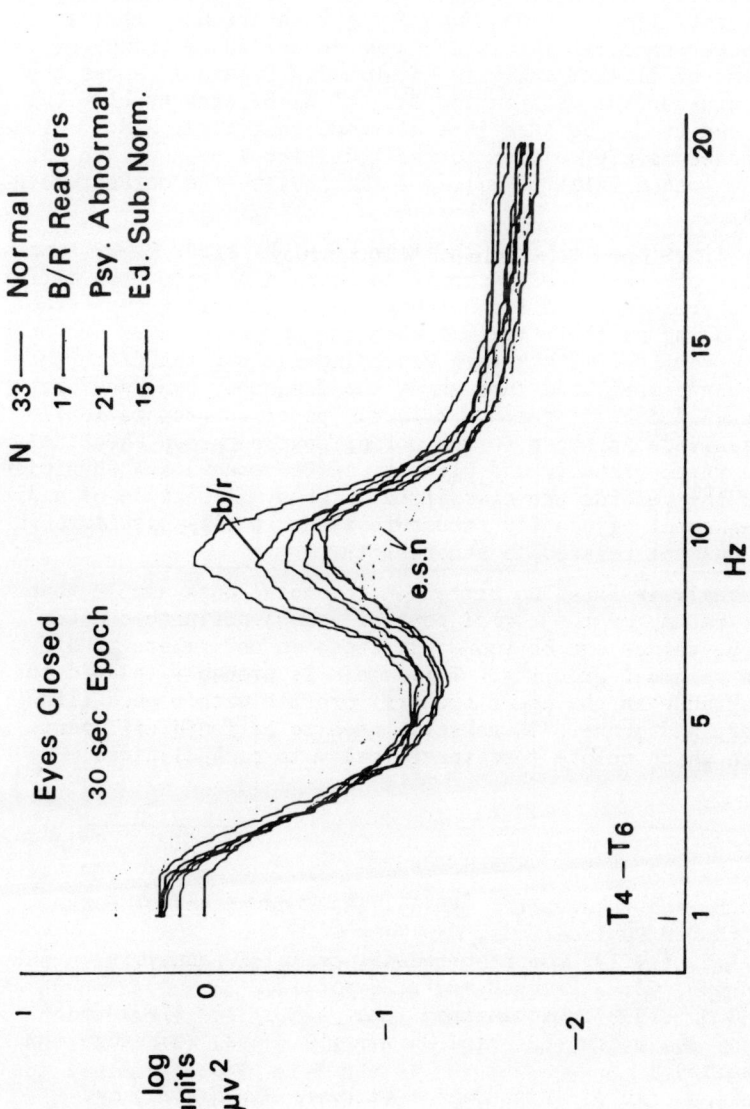

Figure 6 - Power spectral density curves derived from the Isle of Wight study of 14 year-old school children, 30 second epochs, eyes closed, electrode positions T4 - T6. Statistically significant differences exist between the groups.

power in the alpha band, figure 7. In the case of visual rating, however, power spectral analysis of the group with the eyes open shows very little difference, figure 8. This is consistent with clinical practice where more weight is given to a well formed dominant rhythm in the record than to the activity seen when the eyes are open.

An alternative method of proceeding where no a priori assumptions about the clinical grouping of the data are made is that in which the power spectral values are used to delineate groups of boys by means of cluster analysis, figure 9. Figure 10 shows the results of cluster analysis on the Isle of Wight data by clinical diagnosis, and it can be seen that although four clear P.S.D. clusters are formed mainly related to the total level of power in each cluster, the method fails to allocate the boys to the correct clinical groups.

These findings show that in the Isle of Wight study power spectral analysis of the EEG of 14 year-old boys is able to show differences in the frequency profile between the diagnostic groups, the differences being at their maximum when the subjects' eyes are open; however, the variance within each group is wide and the differences are not evenly distributed throughout the frequency band and are only just significant at the 0.05% level (paper in preparation). This wide variance is shown in the normal control group when the records are rated visually and blind by an EEG consultant physician. Over 25% of the records are classified as abnormal because of a different power spectral density structure although this structure in this study was not related to abnormality.

Cluster analysis fares no better on the total data sample than does visual rating on the normal control group; definite cluster of the P.S.D. values can be found but these do not relate to differences in clinical grouping. This again is probably related to the wide variance in the power spectral profile within each clinically determined group. There still need to be found different EEG criteria which relate more specifically to each clinical grouping.

REFERENCES

Blackman, R.B. and Tukey, J.W. (1958). *The Measurement of Power Spectra*, (Dover Publications, New York).

Brazier, M.A.B. (1961). Computer techniques in EEG analysis, *Electroenceph. Clin. Neurophysiol., Suppl. 20.*

Boldyrera, G.N. (1968). *Mathematical Analysis of the Electrical Activity of the Brain*, (Harvard University Press, Cambridge, Massachusetts).

Box and Jenkins. (1970). *Time Series Analysis Forecasting and Control*, (Holden Day, San Francisco).

Byford, G.H. (1965). Signal variance and its applications to continuous measurement of EEG activity, *Proc. Roy. Soc.*, **161**, 421.

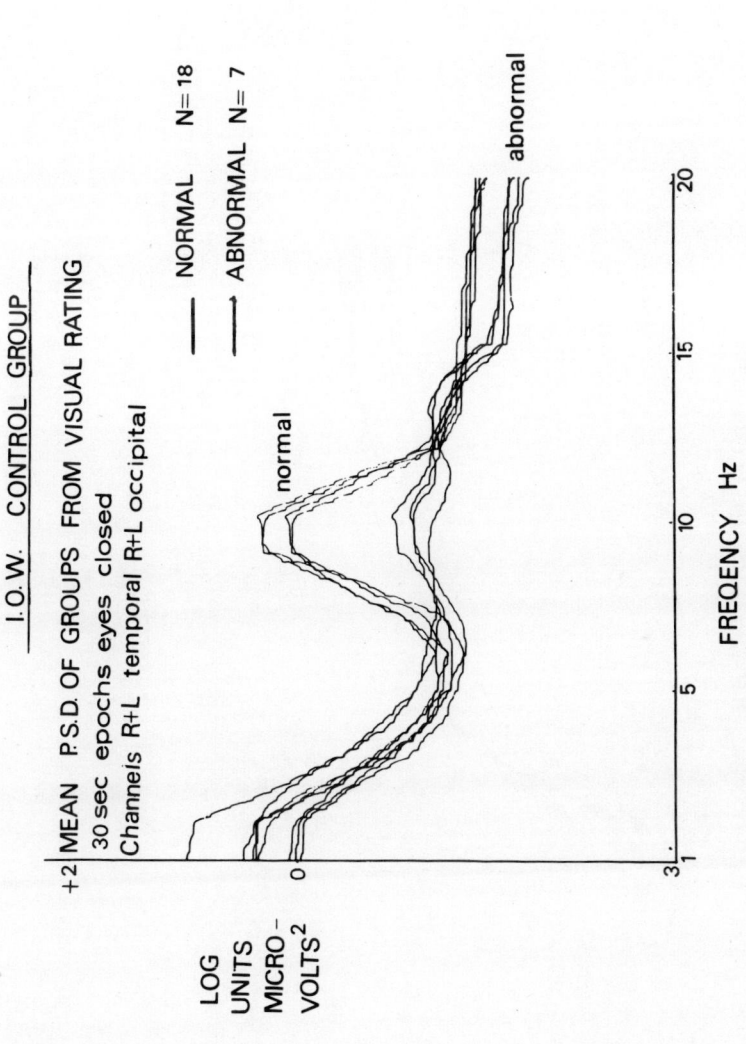

Figure 7 - Power spectral density curves derived from the Isle of Wight normal control group, eyes closed, 30 second epochs, rated visually by a 'blind' rater and classified as normal or abnormal. Over 25% of the records were allocated to the wrong group.

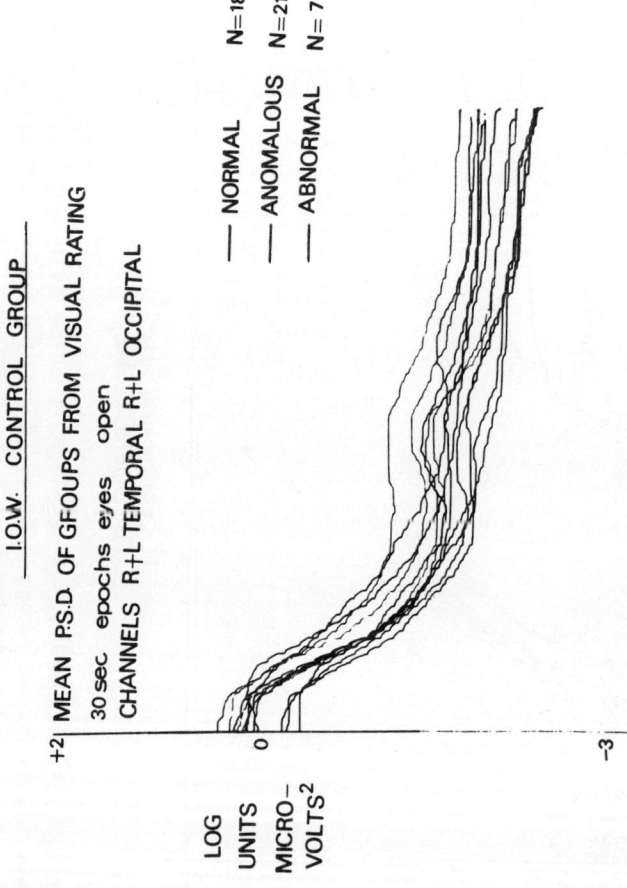

Figure 8 - P.S.D. curves taken from the same groups as figure 7, but this time with the eyes open. No differences exist between the groups, confirming that little importance is given to the E/O epochs by visual rater.

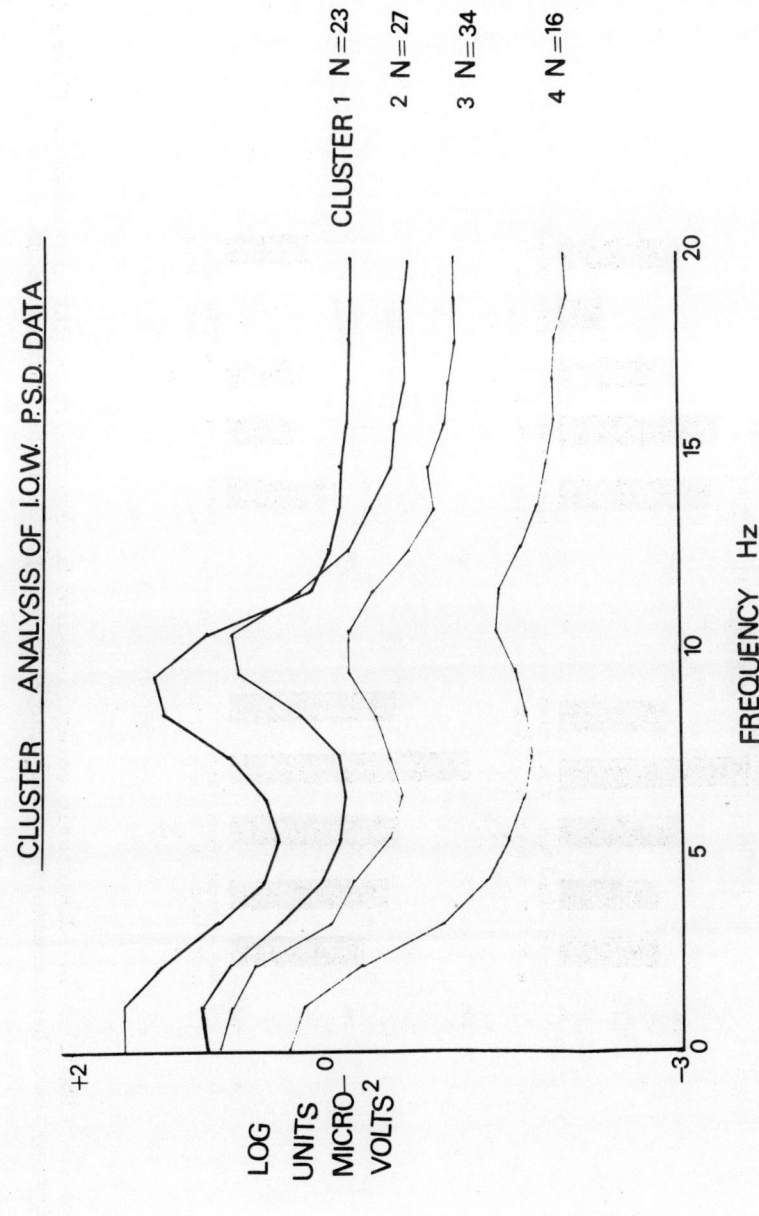

Figure 9 - Cluster analysis of 95 EEG records of all diagnostic categories from the Isle of Wight study. Four clusters are clearly found.

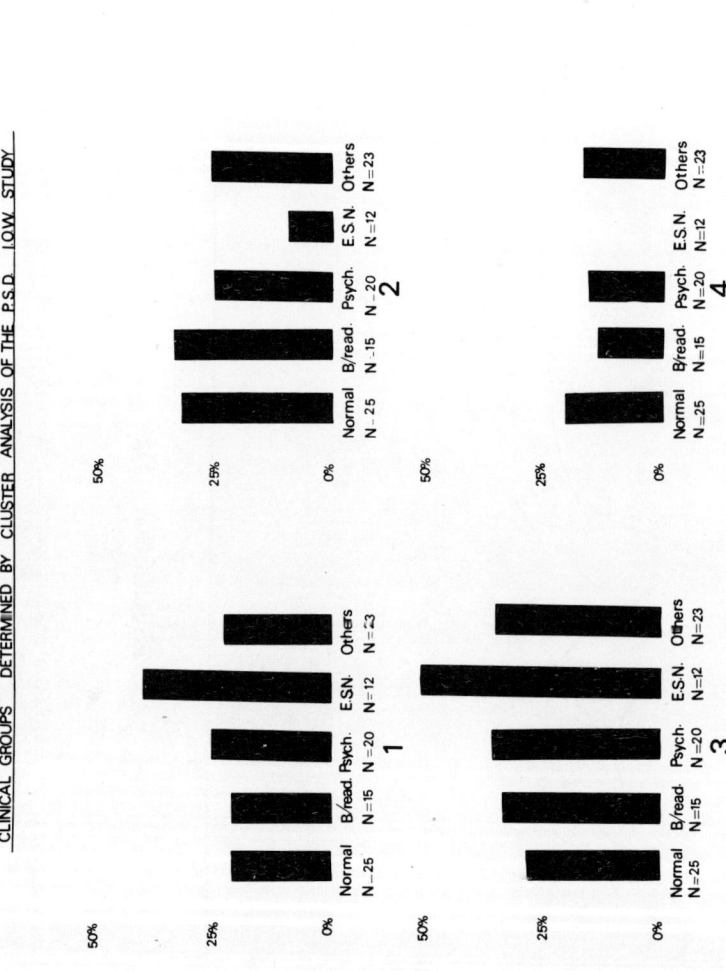

Figure 10 - The clinical diagnostic categories divide into the four clusters shown in figure 9, confirming that these clusters do not relate to any particular clinical group.

Cox and Lewis. (1966). *The Statistical Analysis of the Series of Events*, (Methuen).
Drohocki, Z. (1962). Quantitative electroencephalography. Objective detection of modification of the EEG produced by hyperpnoea, *Electroenceph. Clin. Neurophysiol.*, **23**, 223-240.
Elazar, Z. and Adey, W.R. (1967). Spectral analysis of low frequency components in the electrical activity of the hippocampus during learning, *Electroenceph. Clin. Neurophysiol.*, **14**, 959.
Fenwick, P.B.C., Michie, P., Dollimore, J. and Fenton, G.W. (1971). Mathematical simulation of the electroencephalogram using an autoregressive series, *Bio-Medical Computing*, **2**, 281-307.
Hannon, E.J. (1960). *Time Series Analysis*, (John Wiley and Sons, New York).
Jenkins, C.M. and Watts, D.G. (1968). *Spectral Analysis and Its Applications*, (Holden Day, San Francisco).
Kolmogorov and Smirnov. Sample distribution function, see Box and Jenkins, Chap. 8.
Liskie, E., Hughes, H.M. and Stone, D.F. (1967). Cross-correlation of human alpha activity: Normative data, *Electroenceph. Clin. Neurophysiol.*, **22**, 429-436.
Sager, O. and Herman, M. (1939). L'Analyse statistique de l'electroencephalogramme du point de vue des amplitudes, *Rev. Neurol.*, **71**, 625-633.
Saunders, M.G. (1963). Amplitude probability density studies on alpha and alpha-like patterns, *Electroenceph. Clin. Neurophysiol.*, **15**, 761-767.
Sugerman, A. Goldstein, L., Murphy, H., Pfeiffer, K. and Jenny, E. (1964). EEG and behavioural changes in schizophrenia, *Arch. Gen. Psychiat.*, **10**, 340.
Walter, D.O., Rhodes, J.M., Brown, D. and Adey, W.R. (1966). Comprehensive spectral analysis of human EEG generators in posterior cerebral regions, *Electroenceph. Clin. Neurophysiol.*, **20**, 224-237.

TOPOGRAPHIC ANALYSIS OF THE EEG

J.C. SHAW

MRC Clinical Psychiatry Unit, Graylingwell Hospital, Chichester, Sussex

The aim of this paper is to review the topographic analysis of the electroencephalogram (EEG). In the space available this can only be done briefly and reference will be made to the work of several investigators using this method to illustrate both techniques and applications. Only the analysis of ongoing, so-called "background", activity in man will be considered. For a more extensive account see Rémond (1960) and Petsche and Shaw (1972).

Electroencephalography has been likened to the problem of detecting what is being manufactured inside a factory building having no windows by listening to the sounds detected by a stethoscope placed on the outside wall. This apparently impossible task has caused the subject to be somewhat undervalued, if not overtly ridiculed, in some academic circles. The fact is that the EEG is of proven use as a diagnostic aid and indeed in some instances it may be vital. That it is of considerable value in studying the relationship between CNS activity and behaviour is evident from the wealth of information concerning normal and abnormal sleep patterns. It is true that in a large proportion of cases investigated by the EEG, the test has little influence on the case management but in judging the significance of this, one must not forget that lack of specificity and poor reliability is a common feature of very many medical diagnostic procedures (Cochrane, 1972).

The weight of evidence supports the hypothesis that the EEG is generated within the cerebral cortex, albeit under the influence of deeper structures in the brain. Its use for the study of the brain for diagnostic purposes is made difficult by the electrically diffusing nature of the tissues intervening between brain and recording electrodes, by the complex structure of EEG signals, and by the complex structure of the brain itself. Because of these limitations, the development of electroencephalography must be almost entirely empirical and must therefore rely on objective description of EEG signals. One way of doing this is to use well established methods for numerically describing signals, whilst taking into account the fact that EEG signals have random variable properties (Fenwick, 1972). It is being increasingly recognised, however, that what is required is objective information about the spatial distribution of these signals over the surface of the head. This spatial distribution is referred to as EEG topography, a term which is disliked or regarded as incorrect by some, but which has received official approval (Storm van Leeuwen et al., 1967). It is also used to describe the spatial distribution of EEG signals within the brain.

There are three main reasons for looking at the EEG from a topographic standpoint. Firstly, the clinical usefulness of the EEG depends on the recognition of particular patterns which have diagnostic significance and the detection of focal EEG phenomena in the hope that they reflect focal pathology. This detection of foci is made difficult because focal signs in the EEG are often masked by generalised EEG activity and because the model on which visual recognition of foci is based - the dipole model - only applies to a small proportion of practical cases. One application of topography then is to look for other localising features and other ways of detecting them.

Secondly, further advances in electroencephalography must come from a greater understanding of the relationship between the scalp electrical activity and function in the brain. Although this may depend largely on animal studies (Petsche, Rappelsberger and Trappl, 1970; De Mott, 1970), much can be learned from psycho-physiological experiments in man. Primary function in the cortex is spatially organized, so that it is reasonable to examine the association between the EEG and cortical function by topographic methods. A suitable model for such a study is that in cortical regions not involved in processing primary information, activity at the neuronal level comes under the influence of some synchronising mechanism resulting in detectable EEG waves in that region. Areas which are functionally active lose this synchronicity, with consequent reduction in EEG activity (Gastant et al., 1957; Cooper and Mundy-Castle, 1960). The largest proportion of cortex involved in the primary functions is used for vision. This may explain, on the basis of this model, why visual function appears to have such a large effect on the EEG.

The third aspect of electroencephalography where topographic methods are of value is the study of the relationship between the intra-cerebral electrical activity and scalp recording, or that between intra-cerebral activity recorded from different sites. The opportunity for such studies in man is rare, but it does occasionally occur (Cooper et al., 1965; Brazier, 1966, 1972).

It is convenient to classify methods for topographic analysis of the EEG as shown in figure 1. In the remainder of this paper, some examples of the four main members of this classification will be considered, with more emphasis on the first two of these. These are numbered in the figure.

The simplest way of looking at the EEG from the topographic point of view is to apply existing single channel analysis methods to each channel of a multichannel record, and to compare the results across channels. The latter step is done either by analysing the results statistically, or by displaying them in a two dimensional map in relative positions corresponding to their spatial derivation. This is called "within channel analysis" in figure 1.

This is an important method for relating the EEG to cortical function on the basis of the "synchronisation at rest" model described earlier. An example of this is the work in which the change in the EEG produced by a mental arithmetic task is compared with that resulting from vision. Consider the classical observation that the alpha rhythm in the EEG is most abundant when the subject

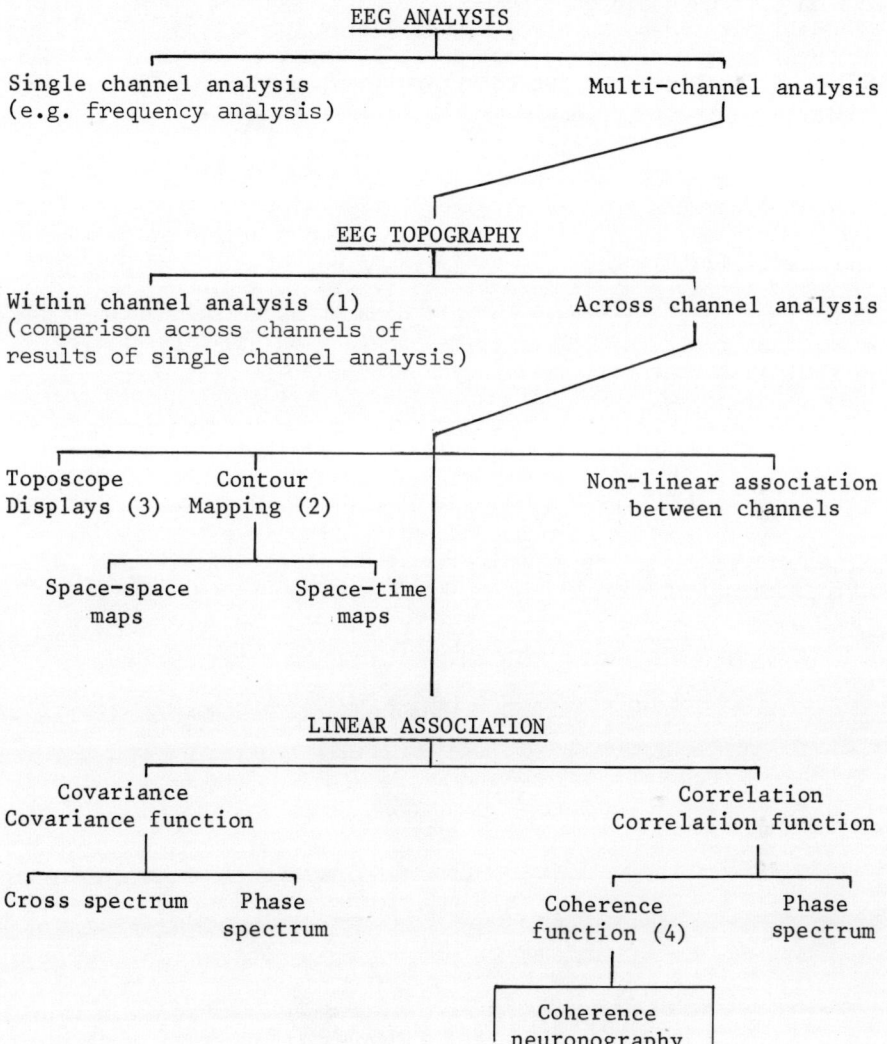

Figure 1 - Classification of methods for EEG topographic analysis showing some relationships between them.

is at rest with eyes closed. If the eyes are opened, the alpha rhythm abundance usually (but not always) decreases or blocks. If the eyes are kept closed, but the subject is asked to do mental arithmetic, the alpha rhythm abundance again decreases (but again this is not always the case, see Krietman and Shaw (1965)). The classical explanation is that both of these conditions involve an increase of arousal and it is this that blocks alpha activity (Whitteridge and Walsh, 1963). However, if there is a more specific relationship between cortical function and the EEG, regional (i.e. topographic) differences in the residual alpha abundance in these two conditions would be expected. Opening the eyes results in a visual input and so involves visual cortex. Mental arithmetic with the eyes shut does not produce a visual input (although there may be visual imagery) and probably involves the parietal cortex, particularly on the left (for example, lesions of the left parietal cortex result in acalculia, see Gerstmann, 1940).

Several workers have investigated this hypothesis. Dr. Glass in Birmingham has studied it with particular tenacity (Glass 1964, 1967; Glass and Kwiatowski, 1970) and was one of the first to examine the distribution of EEG activity as an indicator of differential cerebral involvement in a quantitative way (Glass, 1959, 1960). Glass found a significantly bigger drop in alpha abundance in parietal areas compared with occipital areas when subjects were doing mental arithmetic with eyes closed compared with the condition when subjects were mentally at rest with eyes open. The difference was greater on the left, in accord with what is known about function in this area (Gerstmann, 1940). These findings are illustrated in figure 2, which was kindly supplied by Dr. Glass. They were confirmed by Shaw (1971) and support the hypothesis that, as well as a generalised arousal effect on the alpha rhythm, tasks have more specific topographical effects in accord with the "synchronisation" model.

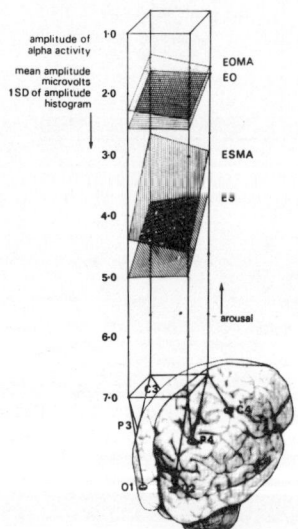

Figure 2 - The figure was derived from measurement of mean alpha amplitude recorded from four electrode pairs (C3-P3, P3-O1, C4-P4, P4-O2) in four conditions; eyes shut (ES), mental arithmetic with eyes shut (ESMA), eyes open (EO) and mental arithmetic with eyes open (EOMA). Note the amplitude scale increases from top down. (Kindly supplied by Dr. A. Glass).

TOPOGRAPHIC ANALYSIS OF THE EEG   137

A more complex implementation of the "within channel analysis" method is that used by D.O. Walter and his colleagues (Walter, Kado, Rhodes and Adey, 1967). Spectral estimates were computed for EEG signals derived from a number of bipolar electrode positions in each of fifty subjects and twelve recording conditions, some involving tasks. When averaged over all subjects and conditions, the spectra have the appearance shown in the top left corner of figure 3, which Walter calls a topo-spectrogram. The remaining topo-spectrograms in the figure show the difference between the spectra in each of five different recording conditions (averaged over the fifty subjects) and this overall average. Regional differences between the

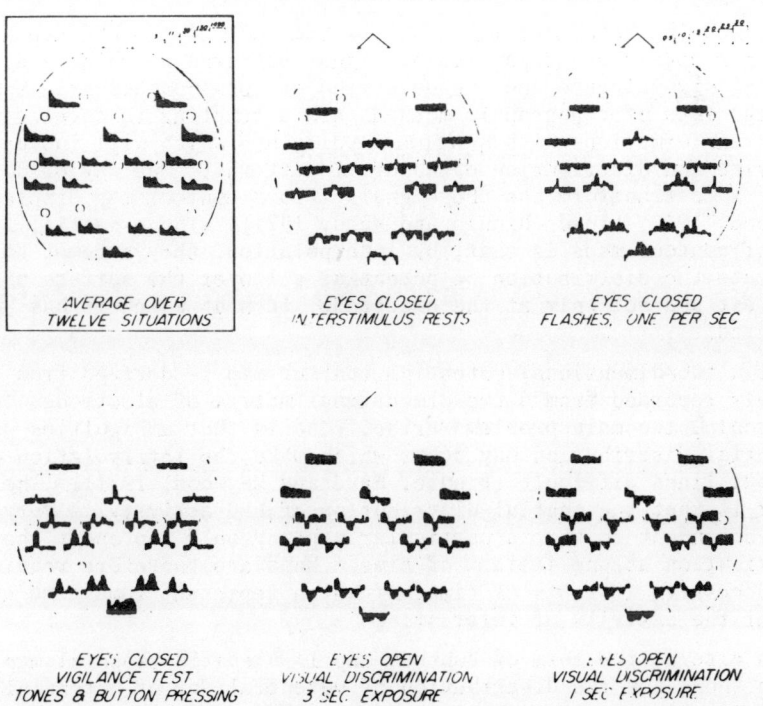

Figure 3 - Top left figure shows averaged spectral densities over the range 0 to 25 Hz for 50 subjects, 12 conditions, at the appropriate location on the scalp. Bipolar recording, circles show electrode positions. Remaining figures show deviation of spectra from average in each of 5 conditions (again averaged over the 50 subjects). From Walter, Kado, Rhodes and Adey 1967, by kind permission of the authors and Aerospace Medicine.

various conditions are seen. For example the three temporal derivations in each hemisphere show a notable difference between the three eyes closed conditions.

It is often pointed out that this particular work was carried out with the support of the considerable computing facilities of NASA. However, similar methods have been used by Giannitrapani (1970) with more modest facilities and with comparable results. There seems to be no reason why this technique should not be pursued with the currently available laboratory computer. While the signal analysis procedures are well formalised however, there is almost no agreement about the methods to be used for controlling cortical function by imposed task conditions. Experimental conditions vary greatly from laboratory to laboratory, making it difficult to integrate results into a meaningful model. Many questions remain unanswered about the particular stage of information processing in the brain which may influence the EEG, for example the relative importance of directing attention towards a task and the preparation for a motor response.

It was indicated earlier that clinical use of the EEG depends on the recognition of particular signal patterns which have diagnostic significance and the detection of focal pathology. Many protagonists of topographic methods are attempting to develop signal transformations with appropriate displays which will indicate the site and distribution of abnormal patterns. One way of doing this is to transform the EEG signals into a contour map display, (Rémond, 1960; Lloyd, Binnie and Ward, 1971). The essential feature of contour maps is that, by interpolation, they attempt to indicate the distribution of potential all over the surface of interest and not only at the electrode sites at which it has been measured.

If a two-dimensional potential contour map is derived from the signals recorded from a two-dimensional matrix of electrodes on the scalp, two main problems arise. One is that ambiguities of potential distribution may occur which make the interpolation of contour lines difficult (Binnie, Ward and Heywood, 1971). The other is that the spatial distribution of EEG activity is very time-dependent so that a particular map may only represent the distribution at one instant of time. Maps are therefore required at successive instants of time, or which represent some time average of the activity of interest.

An alternative form of contour map is a spatio-temporal map which shows how the distribution of potential, or of potential gradient, along a line of electrodes varies with time. This method was developed by Rémond (1960, 1964; Rémond, Lesèvre, Joseph, Rieger and Lairy, 1969) and the maps were originally referred to by him as chrono-topograms. They may be conveniently introduced in the following way.

The electrical activity generated in the cortex is diffused by the overlying tissues, skull and scalp into a continuous potential field over the scalp surface. This field is only sampled at discrete points by conventional recording methods. If signals are recorded from a line of electrodes and their amplitudes measured at discrete time instants, potential distribution graphs may be constructed as shown in figure 4. These may be simple graphs as shown, or may be derived by using interpolation formulae. Now these distributions will change with time so that to obtain a time picture of the changing topography, they must be measured at successive time instants

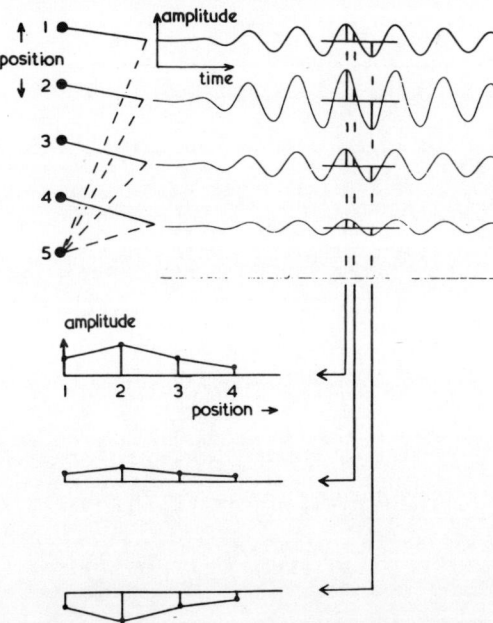

Figure 4 - Diagram to show how voltage/space distributions are derived from voltage/time signals.

throughout the record sample of interest (Rémond and Offner, 1952; Rémond, 1960). They can also be normalised to indicate the change in position of potential peaks (Shaw and Roth, 1955).

An alternative to presenting successive potential distributions is to transform them into a contour map. The resulting lines of constant potential will then show how particular potential values and potential peaks change position along the line of electrodes with time. The result is a spatio-temporal map or chrono-topogram. Rémond usually derived them from bipolar recordings so that they represent potential gradients rather than potential.

To describe the chrono-topogram transformation more specifically, they are constructed by the following steps. (1) All channels of the multichannel record are amplitude sampled at successive time instants. (2) For each time instant, a potential distribution curve is computed by interpolation to fit the measured amplitudes for that instant. (3) This interpolated curve is used to find the position along the space dimension (the electrode line) of selected

amplitude levels (with for example 2 micro-volt increments). (4)
When this has been done for successive instants of time, points
corresponding to the same amplitude levels can be joined up (by
interpolated curves if required) to form a contour map.

Considerable research on these contour mapping methods is being
carried out by Dr. Binnie and his colleagues at St. Bartholomews
Hospital (personal communication). Figure 5 is an example of the

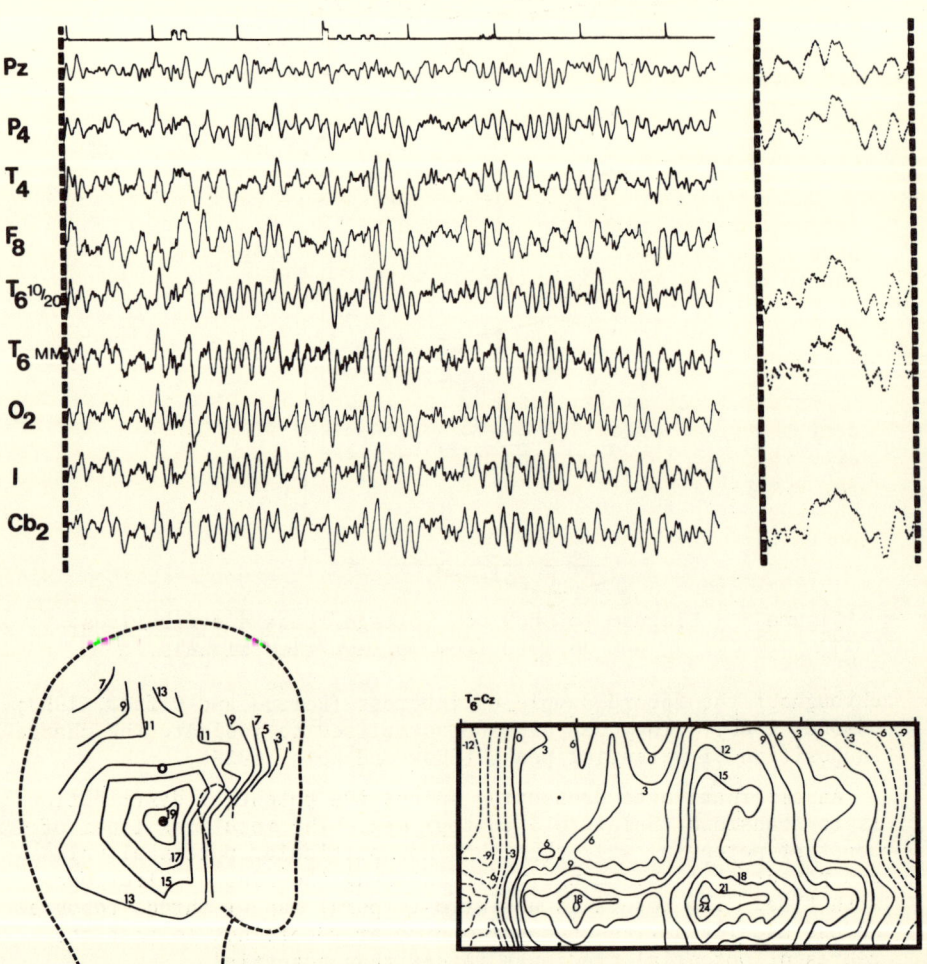

Figure 5 - (a) Multichannel EEG record from common references
recording to vertex (CZ). 10-20 system with T6 MM 3 cm T6
10-20. The signals at the right are averages of the wave
complexes. (b) Contour map derived from the averages in (a).
(c) Chrono-topogram derived from the same averages. (Reproduced by kind permission of Dr. C. Binnie).

application of these methods, kindly supplied by Dr. Binnie. In (a) is shown a multichannel record using common references recording to a vertex electrode (CZ on the 10-20 system). The electrodes are over the right scalp and the record shows alpha rhythm and a slow component more obvious at the posterior temporal electrodes. At the right of this record, averages of the wave-complexes are shown for these electrodes which run in a transverse right posterior temporal line. Figure 5 (b) shows a contour map constructed from the average signals indicating that the activity is focal around the posterior temporal electrode (T6). In 5 (c) the same data is shown in topogram form. Here the contours corresponding to the alpha peaks are seen in the lower half of the picture. The lack of negativity (dotted line) between these peaks indicates that the alpha waves are superimposed on the slower component which again appears to be centred around T6.

One criticism of the chrono-topogram approach has been the not inconsiderable computing requirements. Dr. Binnie and his colleagues have recently shown that it is possible to compute these maps on-line and to display them concurrently with the EEG being recorded. The display is recorded on the same paper record as the EEG by using high speed ink jet writers to produce the write out (personal communication).

Chrono-topograms are usually derived to indicate the time-dependent change of potential distribution along a particular line of electrodes on the head. However, similar maps may be derived for any electrode matrix and may be useful as another means of studying the way in which EEG topography is related to cortical function as controlled by behavioural tasks.

The third method of topographic analysis to be described is classified as toposcope analysis in figure 1. In its simplest form it consists of a visual display in which a number of light sources are arranged in a matrix corresponding to a matrix of electrodes from which EEG signals are derived. The amplitude variations of the signals are made to modulate the light intensity of the sources. The display may be viewed by eye or photographed. This was one of the earliest methods for looking at the topography of the EEG and more complex forms have developed (Walter and Shipton, 1951; Marko and Petsche, 1960; Shipton, 1963; De Mott, 1970).

One interesting feature of EEG topography which is not seen by visual inspection of the record is the small time difference that occurs between similar EEG waves recorded from different parts of the head. Toposcopic displays have been used to study this phenomena, both normal rhythms (Cooper and Mundy-Castle, 1960) and pathological activity, for example the spike and wave activity of Petit Mal Epilepsy (Petsche, 1962). The functional significance of this property remains obscure, although there is some indication that it is associated with arousal (Cooper and Mundy-Castle, 1960; Shaw and McLachlan, 1968) and with hemisphere dominance (Giannitrapani, 1965).

Toposcopes are currently rather out of fashion. However, one problem with the current vogue for digital computation of EEG signals is the vast amount of output data this often produces. One way of dealing with this may be via suitable transformation and a toposcope display.

The methods described so far have the common property that they give information about the actual distribution of potential over the area covered by the recording electrodes. In order to relate this distribution to function within the brain, it may be more useful to measure the degree of dependence of activity recorded from different sites. In this way it may be possible to separate activities arising from independent sources which are selectively influenced by differing behavioural conditions. The amount of dependence between signals recorded from different areas may be measured by correlation analysis. There are several techniques for doing this (Petsche and Shaw, 1972; Shaw and Ongley, 1972).

One method of interest is the coherence function. This is really a correlation spectrum, it expresses the correlation between two signals as a function of frequency. One interesting application of this is the study of the degree of association between signals recorded from different parts of the brain. This method has been actively pursued by Dr. Brazier in a study of epileptic patients with onplanted electrodes. The epilepsy in these patients was uncontrolled by drug therapy and they were candidates for therapeutic surgery. The electrodes were inplanted to assist in finding the primary epileptic focus (Brazier, 1966, 1968, 1972). In one study, Dr. Brazier (1966) has shown that in the absence of seizures, the coherence between EEG activity from different brain centres and between these centres and the cortex is low and usually not significant. During an epileptic seizure the coherence between some regions, amygdala and ipsilateral hippocampus for example, becomes significantly high over a wide frequency band. In other regions the coherence may not change or may become coherent in restricted frequency bands.

In another study (Brazier 1972), records were obtained from psychotic (non-epileptic) patients who also had implanted electrodes. Records were obtained with the patients awake and asleep, the latter both natural and thiopentone induced. In the waking state, high coherence was found at theta frquencies between the dorsal medial nucleus of the thalamus and the amygdala and between the amygdala and septum. High coherences were also found between amygdala and hippocampus, but restricted to ipsilateral hemispheres.

Previously, functional relationships between different parts of the brain have been studied by histological examination of degeneration pathways following destruction of nuclei and by oscillographic detection of responses to electrical stimulation of different centres. The investigation of relationships between brain centres by coherence measurements of the spontaneous electrical activity arising from these centres has the advantage that interference with normal function is reduced to a minimum. Of course it is restricted to the few patients in whom intra-cerebral recording is justified for therapeutic reasons. This techniques has been named coherence neuronography.

It has already been said that if the same waveform occurs in two different brain areas or scalp regions, there is almost invariably a small time difference between their time of occurrence. This means that the frequency components of the waveforms in the two regions have a definite phase relationship. For a waveform arising in one location to be reproduced in a different place with a time delay, it is necessary for the phase log of the components to be proportional to frequency. When making measurements of coherence functions and related correlation measures, it is usual to also measure the phase spectra relating the two signals. In fact the interpretation of the significance of a frequency correlation may depend on this (Perronet, Laviron and Sindou, 1972). The requirement that phase be proportional to frequency makes the interpretation of phase spectra difficult. Dr. Ackroyd of the University of Loughborough has suggested that interpretation would be made easier by the use of group delay spectra in place of phase spectra (personal communication). The components of two correlated waveforms would all have the same delay value. This method also reduces the complexity of computation. It is being used by the author to study the functional significance of the small time displacements in scalp recordings.

This brief review of topographic methods of EEG analysis has attempted to draw attention to this approach, and to emphasize some particular methods and their applications. It may be argued that this is an unnecessary emphasis, that topographic analysis is implicit in all EEG interpretation. Nevertheless, the explicitly topographic approach suggests a number of analysis techniques not normally used, and these may find some important significance in EEG features not usually detectable by visual inspection of the record. In addition, ignoring the topographic approach may lead to gross errors. As an example of this, many investigations have been carried out attempting to find a relationship between the EEG and personality variables assessed by standard psychological tests. There is almost no agreement between the various studies that have been done (Gale, Coles and Blaydon, 1969; Gale, Coles, Kline and Penfold, 1971). One reason for this may be that in these studies only one EEG channel may be analysed and the electrode derivation may differ between studies. It is well known that schizophrenic and psycopathic patients have EEG's which differ from "normal" population in terms of the topography of activity, although they do not contain specific EEG abnormalities (Hill, 1952; Kennard and Schwartsman, 1957; Bruck, 1964). It seems likely therefore that the differences in personality measures of a non-patient group may have more subtle EEG differences very dependent on topography and electrode placement.

One final comment - the interpretation of topographic EEG data is completly dependent on the mode of electrode derivation used (see for example, Cooper, 1959) and no amount of signal transformation will compensate for inadequate recording techniques.

REFERENCES

Binnie, C.D., Ward, P.A. and Heywood, J. (1971). EEG contour mapping: I Theory and practice. *Proc. E.P.T.A.*, **18**, 12-21.

Brazier, M.A.B. (1966). An application of computer analysis to a problem in epilepsy, in *Comparative and Cellular Pathophysiology of Epilepsy*, (eds. Servit, Z and Black, R.), (Excerpta Medica, Amsterdam), pp. 112-128.

Brazier, M.A.B. (1968). Electrical activity recorded simultaneously from the scalp and deep structures of the human brain, *J. Nerv. and Ment. Dis.*, **147**, 31-39.

Brazier, M.A.B. (1972). Interactions of deep structures during seizures in man, in *Synchronisation of EEG activities in Epilepsies*, (eds. Petsche, H and Brazier, M.A.B.), (Springer-Verlag, Vienna), (in press).

Bruck, M.A. (1964). Synchrony and voltage in the EEG of schizophrenics, *Arch. Gen. Psychiat.*, **10**, 454-468.

Cochrane, A.L. (1972). *Effectiveness and Efficiency: Random Reflections on Health Services*, (Nuffield Provincial Hospitals Trust, Oxford).

Cooper, R. (1950). An ambiguity of bipolar recording, *Electroenceph. clin. Neurophysiol.*, **11**, 819-820.

Cooper, R. and Mundy-Castle, A.C. (1960). Spatial and temporal characteristics of the alpha rhythm: a toposcopic analysis, *Electroenceph. clin. Neurophyiol.*, **12**, 153-165.

Cooper, R., Winter, A.L., Crow, H.J. and Walter, W.G. (1965). Comparison of subcortical, cortical and scalp activity using chronically indwelling electrodes in man, *Electroenceph. clin. Neurophyiol.*, **18**, 217-228.

DeMott, D.W. (1970). *Toposcopic Studies of Learning*, (Charles C. Thomas, Springfield, Illinois), p. 262.

Fenwick, P. (1972). *Signal Analysis, Proceedings of the S.A.M.B. Congress on Interdisciplinary Investigation of the Brain*, (Oxford).

Gale, A., Coles, M. and Blaydon, J. (1969). Extraversion-intraversion and the EEG, *Br. J. Psychol.*, **60**, 209-223.

Gale, A., Coles, M., Kline, P. and Penfold, V. (1971). Extraversion-intraversion, neuroticism and the EEG: basal and response measures during habituation of the orienting response, *Br. J. Psychol.*, **62**, 533-543.

Gastaut, H., Storm van Leeuwen, W., Jus, A.C., Morrell, F., Dongier, S., Naquet, H., Regis, H., Roger, A., Bekkering, D.H., Kamp, A., Werre, J. (1957). Étude topographique des réactions électroencephalographiques conditionnées chez l'home, *Electroenceph. clin. Neurophysiol.*, **9**, 1-34.

Gerstmann, J. (1940). Syndrome of finger agnosia, disorientation for right and left, agraphia and acalculia. *Arch. Neurol. Psychiat. (Chicago)*, **44**, 398.

Giannitrapani, D. (1965). EEG phase symmetries and laterality preference, in *Proc. 6th Int. Congr. Electroenceph. clin. Neurophysiol., Vienna Academy of Medicine, Communications EEG-EMG*, (Vienna), 301-305.

Glass, A. (1959). Blocking of the occipital alpha rhythm and problem solving effeciency, *Electroenceph. clin. Neurophysiol.*, **11**, 605.
Glass, A. (1960). A hypothesis concerning the epistemological problem in neurology, *Anat. Rec.*, **136**, 198.
Glass, A. (1964). Mental arithmetic and the occipital alpha rhythm, *Electroenceph. clin. Neurophysiol.*, **16**, 595-603.
Glass, A. (1967). Changes in the prevalance of alpha activity associated with the repetition, performance and magnitude of arithmetical calculations, *Psych. Forsch.*, **30**, 250- 272.
Glass, A., and Kwiatowski, A.W. (1970). Power spectral density changes in the EEG during mental arithmetic and eye-opening, *Psych. Forsch.*, **33**, 85-99.
Hill, D. (1952). EEG in episodic psychotic and psychopathic behaviour. A classification of data, *Electroenceph. clin. Neurophysiol.* **4**, 319-442.
Kennard, M.A. and Schwartzman, A.E. (1957). A longitudinal study of electroencephalographic frequency patterns in mental hospital patients and normal controls, *Electroenceph. clin. Neurophysiol.* **9**, 263-274.
Kreitman, N. and Shaw, J.C. (1965). Experimental enhancement of alpha activity, *Electroenceph. clin. Neurophysiol.*, **18**, 147-155.
Lloyd, D.S.L., Binnie, C.D. and Ward, P.A. (1971). EEG contour mapping: II. Automation, *Proc. E.P.T.A.* **18**, 21-24.
Marko, A. and Petsche, H. (1960). The multivibrator toposcope: an electronic polygraph, *Electroenceph. clin. Neurophysiol.*, **12**, 209-211.
Peronnet, F., Sindou, M., Laviron, A., Quoex, F. and Gerin, P. (1972). Human cortical electrogenesis through stratigraphy and spectral analysis, *Synchronisation of EEG activity in Epilepsies*, (eds. Petsche, H. and Brazier, M.A.B.), (Springer-Verlag, Vienna). (in press).
Petsche, H. (1962). Pathophysiologie und Klinik des Petit Mal. Toposkopische Untersuchungen zur Phanomenologie des Spike-Wave-Musters, *Wiener Z. Nervenheilk*, **19**, 345-422.
Petsche, H. Rappelsberger, P., and Trappl, R. (1970). Properties of cortical seizure potential fields, *Electroenceph. clin. Neurophysiol.*, **29**, 567-578.
Petsche, H. and Shaw, J.C. (1972). EEG Topography, in *EEG Handbook*, Vol. 5B (Theme 10), (Elsevier, Amsterdam), (in press).
Rémond, A. (1960). Recherche des renseignements significatifs dans les enregistrements éléctrophysiologiques et mécanisation possible, *Actualités neurophysiologiques*, (Masson, Paris), 167-210.
Rémond, A. (1964). Level of organisation of evoked responses in man, *Ann. N.Y. Acad. Sci.*, **112**, 143-159.
Rémond, A. and Offner, F. (1952). Études topographiques de l'activité EEG de la region occipitale, *Rev. Neurol.*, **87**, 182-189.
Rémond, A., Lesèvre, N. Joseph, P., Rieger, H., and Lairy, G. (1969). The alpha average. I. Methodology and description, *Electroenceph. clin. Neurophysiol.*, **26**, 245-265.
Shaw, J.C. (1971). A method for measuring characteristics of EEG topography for the study of psycho-physiological correlates of the EEG, (Ph.D. Thesis), (University of Southampton, England).

Shaw, J.C., and Ongley, C. (1972). The measurement of synchronisation, in *Synchronisation of EEG Activity in Epilepsies*, (eds. Petsche, H. and Brazier, M.A.B.), (Springer-Verlag, Vienna), (in press).

Shaw, J.C. and McLachlan, K.R. (1968). The association between alpha rhythm propagation time and level of arousal, *Psychophysiology*, **4**, 307-410.

Shaw, J.C. and Roth, M. (1955). Potential distribution analysis. I. A new technique for the analysis of electrophysiological phenomena, *Electroenceph. clin. Neurophysiol.*, **7**, 273-284.

Shipton, H.W. (1963). A new frequency-selective toposcope for electroencephalography, *Med. and Biol. Eng.*, **1**, 403-495.

Storm van Leeuwen, W., and the Terminology Committee (1966). Proposal for an EEG terminology, *Electroenceph. clin. Neurophysiol.*, **20**, 306-310.

Walter, D.O., Kado, R.T., Rhodes, J.M. and Adey, W.R. (1967). EEG baselines in astronaut candidates estimated by computation and pattern recognition techniques, *Aerospace Medicine*, **38**, 371-379.

Walter, W.G. and Shipton, H.W. (1951). A new toposcopic display system, *Electroenceph. clin. Neurophysiol.*, **11**, 374-375.

Whitteridge, D. and Walsh, E.G. (1963). The physiological basis of the EEG, in *Electroencephalography: a Symposium on its Various Aspects*, (eds. Hill, D. and Parr, G.), (Macdonald, London), pp. 99-146.

ELECTRIC RESPONSE AUDIOMETRY

M.L. HYDE

Audiology Group, Institute of Sound and Vibration Research, University of Southampton

The behavioural threshold intensity for a continuous pure-tone and the pattern of its change with frequency are important in the diagnosis of dysfunctions of the auditory system. Classical techniques for the estimation of pure-tone thresholds involve serial presentation of stimuli at intensity levels ordered in accordance with any of several psychophysical designs, together with recording of the behavioural responses. The threshold level is a statistical concept, normally defined as the intensity at which the subject achieves a 50% detection score.

These techniques make several demands of the patient, who must have a general understanding of the nature and aims of the test, must cooperate and must give a precise voluntary response. Many patients give inadequate or incorrect threshold data as a result of failure on one or more of these counts. There are two important categories of such patient. The first category includes patients with any disorder describable as 'non-organic' hearing loss, which term covers those cases in which there is apparent loss of hearing but no evidence of organic dysfunction of the auditory system. Included here are several psychological disorders, as well as deliberate falsification of test results, and often a mixture of the two is encountered. It is also common to find a non-organic component superimposed upon a real loss of hearing. The second category of patient for whom classical testing is unsatisfactory includes several classes of child. Following Davis (1971), these types are infants, active and uncooperative young children, hyperactive or retarded older children, and those with multiple neurological handicaps. Although special behavioural techniques exist to deal with some of these cases, their practice requires considerable skill and may be inordinately time-consuming. Rarely are sufficiently quantitative data obtained. In addition, there is an increasing requirement for detailed audiological assessment in connection with legal actions by persons allegedly sustaining auditory impairment as a result of noise hazard in their work environment. In some of these cases there is a need for threshold estimations independent of voluntary response from the patient.

There is a number of methods of pure-tone audiometry which do not depend on understanding or voluntary response on the part of the patient. Electric Response Audiometry or ERA is the most successful of these methods, and has been developed in the last five years into a valuable clinical test for the types of patient mentioned above.

The method is dependent upon the properties of what may be called the evoked vertex response, or EVR. This response is one of a complex set of electrical events occurring in response to auditory stimulation and measurable on the head using gross surface electrodes. The auditory EVR is a slow fluctuation in potential occurring shortly after any change in the auditory environment constituting transition from a state of sensory rest to a state of sensory motion (Clynes, 1968). Sensory motion is a state of continuous change of any subjective variable associated with the stimulus, for example in the loudness or pitch of a continuous pure tone, although physical descriptors of the auditory environment such as intensity or frequency may be used in analyses of EVR dynamics. Sensory rest is absence of sensory motion. Silence, for example, may be considered a degenerate case of sensory rest, with zero values on all sensory dimensions. If a pure tone of constant intensity is then initiated, an EVR develops shortly after tone onset, namely after the transition from silence to a state of changing intensity. If the tone is sufficiently long, say of several seconds duration, then a somewhat smaller EVR appears shortly after the start of the tone offset envelope. No complete theory of EVR dynamics exists, nor has functional significance of the response been established.

Now the EVR is a diphasic potential of some 300 msec duration, and starts to develop approximately 80 msec after the tone onset crosses some threshold intensity. The response is a representation of a spatiotemporal sum of numerous cortical electrical events. Presumably these events are related to post-synaptic potentials on radially oriented pyramidal cells, though the details of the electrophysiology of response generation are not clear, and conflicting viewpoints exist. The EVR can be detected over a large area of the scalp, and usually develops maximum amplitude at or near the vertex. This result is a consequence of brain geometry rather than of special significance of the cortex underlying the vertex. The response is normally recorded using a bipolar derivation, with the active electrode on the vertex and the reference on a mastoid process. Even with this optimal derivation however, the EVR is usually an order of magnitude smaller than the typical spontaneous EEG activity. Before the response can be reliably detected or measured, therefore, some means of improving the signal-to-noise ratio is needed. This enhancement is commonly achieved by time-domain averaging techniques. Using as stimuli shaped pure-tone bursts of ~200 msec duration, presented periodically at a typical rate of approximately one per 2 sec, the amplified and band-pass filtered EEG is fed to an online averager or more commonly a summing device. This device stores the sum of short segments of EEG following stimulus onset for each and every stimulus presentation. Typically 50 stimuli may be used, the length of each stored EEG segment is ~1 sec. Each segment can be simply modelled as a superposition of an invariant signal, namely the EVR, and an independent random process, namely the spontaneous EEG. If the random process has zero mean value, then the improvement in signal-to-noise ratio as a result of summing or averaging N segments is $N^{\frac{1}{2}}$. The statistics resulting from this simple model are not very appropriate, however, because not only is the EEG often appreciably non-random, but also the EVR itself is subject to both random and systematic variation over the stimulus set. These changes are at the present time not well understood, thus the properties of EVR's to single stimuli are poorly defined. However, these difficulties are usually ignored, and the averaged EVR considered in terms of the simple model outlined above.

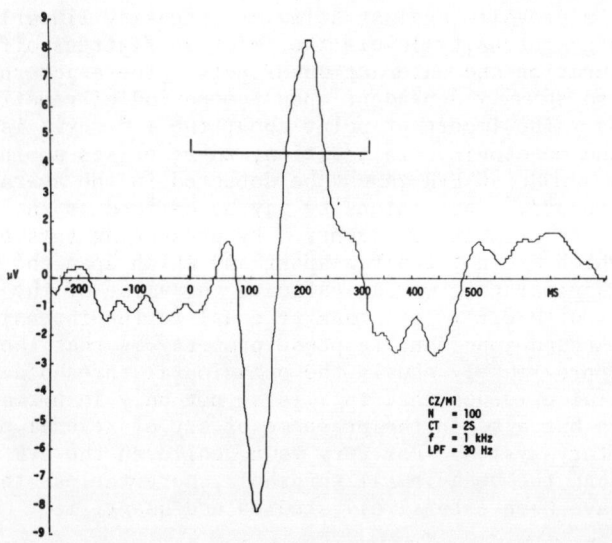

Typical averaged auditory evoked vertex response (EVR). Response to 100 1 kHz pure-tone bursts at 60 dB Sensation Level. EEG low-pass filtered at 30 Hz. Duration of stimulus marked by horizontal bar.

The figure shows a typical averaged auditory EVR to 100 moderately loud 1 kHz tone bursts presented regularly at one per 2 sec. The total response time history shows at least four peaks, though the prominent negative-positive complex starting approximately 100 msec after stimulus onset constitutes the auditory EVR. The various peaks may relate to activity in distinct physiological systems, however, there is some basis for regarding the EVR as a separable entity, since this complex shows some homology of topography and morphology regardless of the modality of stimulation (Goff, 1969).

The response time histories show considerable variation between individuals, and to a lesser extent between occasions in the same individual. Fairly systematic changes in response size and morphology occur as a function of age and of stimulus conditions.

Two properties of the EVR are of particular importance with respect to its use as an audiometric measure. The first is the form of the functional dependence of response amplitude, normally a peak-to-peak measure, upon stimulus intensity. Due to the considerable variability of the EVR from test to test, the form of this so called input-output or I-O function is difficult to determine in any single individual. Nevertheless it appears that EVR amplitude is a monotonic increasing function of stimulus intensity, other conditions being equal. The I-O function is approximately linear up to moderate intensity levels, plotting response amplitude linearly in microvolts against stimulus intensity linearly in decibels. At high intensity levels the function flattens off as a result of saturation and interaction effects. The exact shape of the curve is also strongly dependent upon the period of repetition of the stimulus. The important point about the I-O curve is that it is smooth and monotonic. In addition, there exists an intensity level below which an EVR cannot be detected in the averaged or summed EEG record. This intensity may be defined as the EVR threshold for a given stimulus frequency. By presenting sets of stimuli at levels which are not too far apart and which span the point of response disappearance, we can estimate the value of the EVR threshold, ideally with error less than or equal to the intensity step size. The second important response property.is that the EVR threshold approximately equals the behavioural threshold. There is substantial evidence that this is so not only in normal adults and children but also in the presence of any of several pathologies of the auditory system. For very young children the EVR threshold is higher than the behavioural threshold, nevertheless these relationships have been extensively studied and quantified.

In fact the estimate of EVR threshold obtained in any particular case depends upon many variables, notably upon several facets of stimulation, recording and analysis technique, as well as upon stimulus frequency. However, on the basis of the two properties just outlined it is reasonable to assume that if an EVR is detectable in the summed response record to a given stimulus intensity, then that intensity is above behavioural threshold. The converse assumption, namely that if no EVR is obtained the level is below threshold, is by no means as reliable.

The basis for a clinical test is now apparent. We can estimate the EVR threshold for any stimulus frequency. In the light of our knowledge of the empirical relationships between EVR and behavioural thresholds expected to obtain under the conditions of interest, we can derive an estimate of the behavioural threshold for that stimulus frequency. We have therefore a method of estimating the behavioural pure-tone threshold without any voluntary response from the patient.

A clinical ERA test is simply a set of EVR threshold estimations. As far as the test environment is concerned, the patient should sit quietly or lie in an acoustically-treated test room. The acoustic treatment is necessary not primarily to exclude environmental noise, which rarely interferes with the test other than by possible masking effects, but to ensure some degree of uniformity of incident sound field at the patient's head when stimuli are delivered by loudspeaker. It is often necessary to resort to this technique, since stimulus delivery by headphone is not appropriate for the majority of infants and active very young children. During the test the patient is encouraged to read or, in the case of a child, to play quietly. Specific stimulus-oriented attention is not required. The sets of stimuli are presented according to a predetermined strategy of ear-frequency combinations. There is usually a considerable pressure of time during the test, a reasonable maximum test duration being one and a half hours. Since it may take 15 min or longer to estimate a single EVR threshold with acceptable accuracy, the number of testable conditions is severely limited. The amount of data required varies greatly from patient to patient, though it is common to use ERA in a limited fashion, to confirm or contradict the results of prior behavioural tests, where these are possible.

The details of EEG processing and response judgement vary greatly from centre to centre, and a detailed account is out of place here. It is emphasised, however, that the ultimate success of any ERA test is strongly dependent upon these matters of technique. In addition the test is complex, time-consuming and expensive both in terms of instrumentation and manpower. With regard to the latter, for example, the effective testing of a difficult child demands knowledge ranging from child psychology to random process analysis.

Certainly the most important application of the test is the evaluation of the hearing of infants or young children who cannot be tested by behavioural methods. But one of the most serious difficulties with the test is that it is in precisely these patients that problems of summed record interpretation arise. The main source of difficulty is that an excessive amount of movement on the part of the patient can contaminate the summed record with large transient voltage artefacts. These artefacts are due both to summated myogenic activity and to physical movement of the electrode leads, and can obviate reliable judgement of response presence or absence, particularly if narrow-band EEG filtering is used. The artefact problem can be attacked in many ways. It is possible, for example, to perform ERA during sleep, or under sedation or light general anaesthesia. Each of these methods has attendant problems. ERA during sleep necessitates skilled continuous monitoring of the spontaneous EEG, since the size and morphology of the EVR have been shown to vary considerably with sleep stage. It is difficult under these conditions to reliably relate summed records obtained during different sleep stages or combinations of stages. Both sedation and general anaesthesia are under intensive study and in some centres sedation has been incorporated into clinical procedure. However, neither has been satisfactorily fully evaluated, particularly with respect to the effects of the available drugs upon the EEG and EVR.

Without resorting to such methods, some progress can be made by means of instrumentation and technique. Continuous monitoring of the summed response as the stimuli are delivered is essential in artefact-ridden cases, as are a number of other interpretational and instrumentational techniques. One of the most promising is limiting of the EEG amplitude before input to the band pass filter and subsequent summing device. Studies on normal adults have shown that amplitude limitation to 0 ± 2 standard deviations, say to ± 20 μV in an adult EEG, causes negligible change in the averaged response time history, which result is predictable from the properties of the typical EEG amplitude density function. Clearly such limiting would reduce the effect of an isolated 200 μV movement artefact. However, some caution is necessary in choosing appropriate limits for use with very young children, the EEG's of whom have amplitude distributions which are often far from Gaussian.

There is also the possibility of performing the entire test under the control of a digital computer. This would allow the limiting process, automatic editing of contaminated EEG sections, stimulus timing to occur in periods of low-level EEG activity, selection of stimulus conditions, display of results and possibly the application of automatic statistical response detection criteria. Furthermore time domain averaging is not the only process which can be used to detect periodic transients such as the EVR, and most of the alternatives require quite extensive computer facilities. However, at the present time the majority of ERA is performed using small special purpose machines.

A final point is emphasis of the empirical nature of ERA. Not enough is known about the physiology of EVR mediation to permit detailed diagnostic evaluation of responses per se. Under these circumstances, ERA is certainly carried out to best effect in advanced audiology centres, wherein the test results can be evaluated in conjunction with those of all other available assessment procedures.

REFERENCES

Clynes, M. (1968). Dynamics of vertex evoked potentials: the R-M brain function, in *Average Evoked Potentials. Methods, Results, and Evaluations*, (eds. Donchin, E. and Lindsley, D.B.), NASA Symposium Report SP 191, pp. 363-374.

Davis, H. (1971). Is ERA ready for routine clinical use? *Arch. klin. exp. Ohr.-, Nas.-, Kehlk. Heilk.*, **198**, 1, pp. 2-8.

Goff, W.R. (1969). Evoked potential correlates of perceptual organisation in man, in *Attention in Neurophysiology*, (eds. Evans, C.R. and Mulholland, T.B.), (Butterworth, London), pp. 169-193.

PATTERN RECOGNITION IN EEG

D.S.L. LLOYD, C.D. BINNIE

Department of Clinical Neurophysiology,
St. Bartholomew's Hospital, London

and

B.G. BATCHELOR

Department of Electronics, University of Southampton

INTRODUCTION

A *Classification of Patterns*

The term 'pattern recognition' requires definition as a variety of meanings is currently in use. Even within a single discipline there may exist several kinds of processes to which the name 'pattern recognition' is applied. As the term suggests, there are two concepts to be considered. Firstly, the definition of a pattern and, secondly the manner of its recognition or detection. Three alternative definitions are now presented, as a basis for discussion, but it is recognised that further kinds of pattern exist.

The first, and possibly most easily appreciated type of pattern, is a primary physical phenomenon and may usually be observed by Man using his primary senses. Examples include a particular distribution of optical density on an X-ray plate, a musical chord, or an arrangement of dots in relief as in the Braille character recognised by touch. There is room for slight variation in the exact shape or nature of such a pattern which is reflected in the degree of certainty associated with its detection. In most practical situations the pattern may be partially obscured by other information and the recognition will involve some process akin to filtering to increase the contrast between the pattern and the background. This form of pattern recognition is sometimes called 'Template Matching'.

The second type of pattern is defined as some logical combination of characteristics, a familiar medical example being a syndrome. The physical characteristics are measured in whatever units are appropriate and each may have a single value or a range of values associated with it. In logically combining the measured characteristics, no marginal cases are allowed. Thus the statement that quantity A lies inside a given range of values can only be either true or false. All the usual logical operators, e.g. AND, NOT, OR etc. may be used to construct a decision tree which itself defines, and can be used to identify, the pattern.

The third type of pattern and its recognition uses concepts of a statistical nature. As in the second type, some physical characteristics are measured in appropriate units. Here it should be noted that certain non-numeric information must be converted into

into a suitable numerical form, preferably forming a continuum. For
example - TRUE and FALSE can be represented as 1 or 2, or as 1 and
0; SMALL, MEDIUM, LARGE may be 1,2,3; but GREEN, MAUVE, BROWN cannot be represented by interval or ordinal measurements and will not
usually have a meaningful numerical equivalent. This measurement
or coding process is common to the recognition of all type 2 and 3
patterns and is generally called 'feature extraction'. The remainder of the definition of a type 3 pattern involves a classification or discrimination process to distinguish different patterns
within the same class. One such method known as 'linear discriminant analysis' defines a number as some weighted combination of
the original measurements. The weighting function used will be
specific to a class of patterns and the value of the derived number allocates the pattern to a particular group of the class when
its value falls within the range associated with that group.

The process is alternatively called 'Statistical Pattern Recognition' or 'the hyperspace approach'. It has a formal resemblance
to the subjective process of medical diagnosis, which involves
making observations on many variables and attaching to them different weights determined by past experience of their predictive value.

The discrimination process may alternatively be realised using
a system of coordinate axes in n-dimensional space, one axis being
assigned to each of the n measured characteristics. A pattern is
now defined by a region or regions of n-space in which the end of
a vector, constructed from the set of measurements, will lie. The
boundaries of these regions may be plane or non-linear, but, in
either case, recognition of the pattern is based on a statistical
statement of the probability that the pattern belongs to a particular group.

Figure 1 shows a set of hypothetical observations on two groups
(open and solid circles) which are obviously separable, but with a
surface which is neither continuous nor linear. One of the techniques now available for defining such non-linear decision surfaces
involves automatic adaptive learning processes. Briefly the procedure is as follows: In order to separate two groups A and B in a two-dimensional space, a circle is found which most nearly enclosed all
examples in group A and excludes group B. In most cases this will
produce an incomplete separation. A further circle is then defined
and the radii and centre positions of the circles are systematically
changed until the optimum separation of groups A and B is achieved.
The number of circles (each being a subclassifier) is increased
until either an acceptable degree of separation is achieved or a
previously defined limiting number of subclassifiers is reached.
The coordinates of the centres of the circles together with their
radii now completely specify a compound classifier. These values
constitute a full and numerical definition of a type 3 pattern and
provide an adequate means of communication between all users of
the technique.

The method readily extends to 3 dimensions, using spheres, and
beyond, using hyperspheres. A common variant employs cubes and

hypercubes instead of spherical shapes, and in some special cases, the distribution of the data may justify the use of more complex shapes.

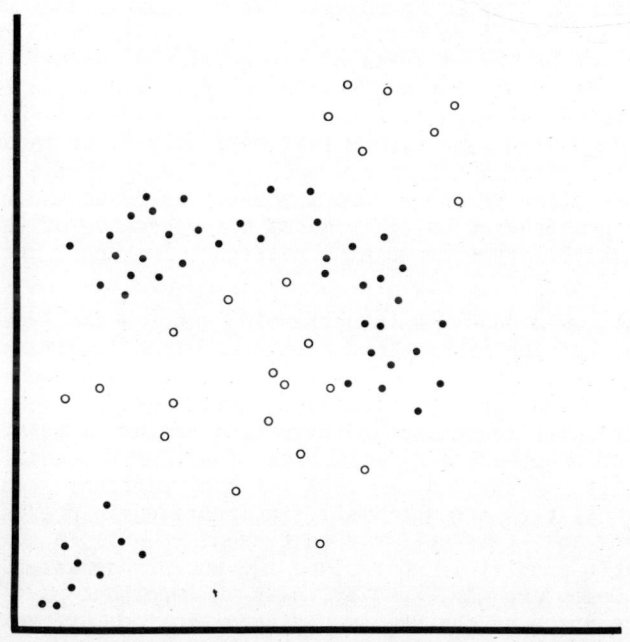

Figure 1 - Distribution of a hypothetical set of observations on two groups (solid and open circles) which are separable only by a discontinuous, non-linear surface.

For the purposes of the present account these kinds of patterns will be referred to simply as types 1, 2 and 3. There is an inherent hierarchy in these three definitions of patterns which has implications for the choice of recognition technique. In general it is possible to regard type 1 patterns in terms of types 2 and 3 definitions and similarly type 2 patterns in type 3 terms, but the reverse is not usually true and, indeed, the boundaries between the types are sometimes rather vague.

PROBLEMS OF EEG PATTERN RECOGNITION

Pattern recognition in electroencephalography has, until fairly recently, been restricted to visual detection of EEG phenomena by trained observers. Over the past forty years a considerable body of expertise has been built up in hospitals and laboratories all over the world and the trained human observer can clearly become extremely skilled at recognising patterns of type 1. Indeed the whole range of EEG phenomenology so far described in the literature is largely the result of visual observations of type 1 patterns in EEG charts. There is, however, an obstacle to the efficient transfer of skills between the observers and therefore further to progress in the accurate assessment of EEG tracings in a wide range of clinical conditions. To describe type 1 patterns verbally, it is first necessary to convert them to type 2 or 3. This is a very difficult task for the human observer as he usually does not know exactly how he identifies a particular EEG phenomenon and cannot therefore describe the criteria of recognition in words. Consequently, it is difficult for one specialist to communicate EEG observations to another or even to ensure that one observer's performance does not change with time either systematically or at random. Moreover, once the primary EEG phenomena have been identified, the clinical interpretation of the record involves assessing the various features in combination and this makes heavy demands of the very limited human ability to recognise patterns of types 2 and 3.

The use of computers has already overcome some of the inadequacies of the human observer in performing types 2 and 3 pattern recognition, but the automatic detection of type 1 patterns is usually much more difficult. Despite the problems of consistency of performance mentioned previously, practising electroencephalographers currently recognise EEG phenomena against a relatively high level of other EEG activity which itself may be changing greatly; they do it rapidly and can look for many patterns simultaneously. These abilities are not easily incorporated in present computer systems and it is unlikely that machines will in the near future be able completely to replace the human observer to type 1 patterns. Computers may, however, play an important part in increasing the power of the EEG as a diagnostic tool by their ability to extract features not visible to the naked eye and by implementing techniques for the detection of type 2 and 3 patterns using these features.

EXPERIENCE OF EEG PATTERN RECOGNITION

Extensive use of computer assisted pattern recognition in EEG has been made by Adey and his co-workers in the University of California, using frequency domain techniques for feature extraction.

Figure 2 is redrawn from Walter et al. (1967) and indicates the reliability achieved in distinguishing 5 test conditions in pooled EEG data from 4 subjects. Only four features were used here, relating to the amount and frequency of alpha activity in four derivations. The reliability with which each of the 5 test conditions could be identified was 49%. If individual rather than pooled data were used for each subject, the reliability rose to between 60 and 70%, and when 15 features were employed, it increased further to between 90 and 95%.

Adey and his colleagues extracted a large number of features based on mathematical properties of the EEG and used step-wise discriminant analysis to identify those features which were of most importance and which made up the patterns characteristic of the various test conditions. Such an empirical method may well prove eventually to be the best available, particularly for recognising

very small changes. However, this approach makes no use of the
existing body of knowledge concerning the clinical significance
of particular waveforms. Rather than using the methods of time
series analysis for feature extraction, much might be gained by
first using EEG phenomena of known clinical predictive value. These
phenomena are, of course, type 1 patterns and readily identified by
eye, but less easily by computer. At this stage of technological
development, it may be necessary to use a human observer to identify type 1 patterns as features for a subsequent discriminant
analysis.

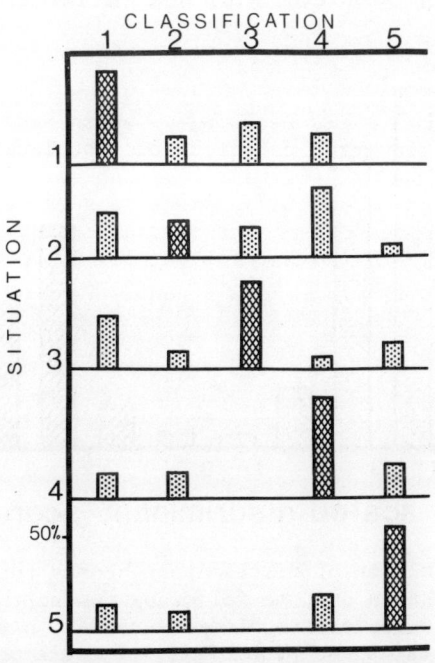

Figure 2 - Adapted from Walter et al. (1967). Automatic
classification of samples of EEG from five test situations.
Cross-hatched columns indicate percentage of samples correctly classified.

Such a method was employed by Binnie et al. (1970) in an investigation of the prediction of outcome following presentation from
Cardiac Arrest. Previous authors had established a relationship
between the degree of EEG abnormality and the probability of survival. Using very simple criteria based on the amplitude and dominant frequency of the EEG and the presence of the burst suppression phenomenon, outcome could be predicted with a limited reliability (of the order of 80%). In an effort to increase the predictive value of the EEG, a visual analysis was made of 93 records
obtained from patients in whom the eventual outcome of cardiac
arrest had been reliably established either as recovery of normal

cerebral function or as death from anoxic brain damage demonstrated at autopsy. Some 50 EEG features were extracted by conventional visual rating methods. The data which comprised 93 sets of observations on 50 variables were subjected to linear discriminant analysis in the hope of detecting characteristic patterns (type 3 in the classification suggested earlier) for distinguishing the EEG's of patients who died from those of the survivors. Figure 3 shows the results of the linear discriminant analysis, in which the discriminant score represents the distance from the decision surface, which separates two groups as completely as possible, of a point in n-dimensional space representing the observations on each subject. A large absolute value of discriminant score denotes

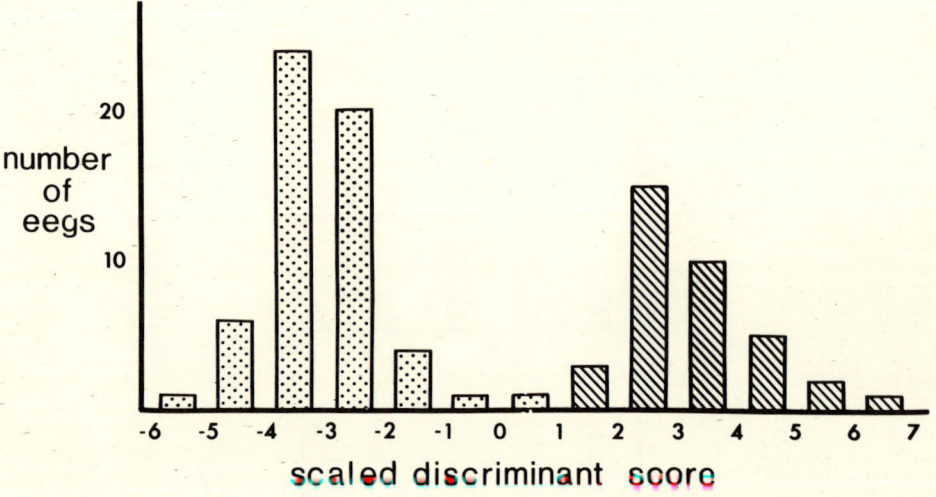

Figure 3 - Distribution of discriminant scores from 93 EEG's of patients with known outcome following resuscitation from cardiac arrest. Outcome: stippled = survival, hatched = died. A score of 0 indicates equiprobability of death or survival.

a high level of confidence for allocating the patient to one or other group. In this instance it was possible to set up a decision surface which separated the EEG's of those who survived and those who died with only one error in a sample of 93. This suggests a substantial improvement over the reliability of previous methods and this has been confirmed with further records assessed in the same way.

So far as the practical application of pattern recognition techniques to electroencephalography is concerned, it must be admitted that methods for the recognition and description of type 3 patterns have out-stripped the methods for feature extraction. For example - a fundamental flaw of the work on the quantitative prediction of outcome following cardiac arrest is the reliance upon a human observer to fill in a proforma in the first place. The criteria employed cannot be communicated verbally, but only by practical demonstration and cannot therefore be widely disseminated. Equally, when a criterion is a purely operational one based on the behaviour of a particular human observer, it is impossible to ensure the stability of performance of the observer himself, particularly over a period of years. Automatic feature extraction is therefore essential for the practical application of the already highly developed techniques available for recognising type 3 patterns. Further, if EEG waveforms of known pathological significance are considered likely to be the appropriate features for clinical prediction, it is necessary to develop means of identifying these type 1 patterns automatically.

All three methods of pattern recognition may be used to detect primary EEG phenomena. Waveforms of fairly constant outline may be treated as type 1 patterns and can be identified by continuously comparing the EEG with some previously defined model. This can, for example, be achieved by means of a matched filter. This may be implemented in hardware or by a computer program, and has the properties of a network whose impulse response is the time-inverse of the waveform to be identified. Figure 4 shows the result of passing a sample of EEG containing spike activity (top trace) through such a filter. The filter output (second trace) shows a peak, delayed by the length of the complex, each time that a spike-wave discharge occurs. In this case, the matched filter is not very selective, as the spectrum of the ongoing EEG is neither uniform nor constant and often contains components in common with the complex being detected. One solution is to modify the impulse response of the filter to compensate for the non-uniform spectrum of the ongoing activity, but this is time consuming, and not usually feasible in real time. A second solution, less than perfect but useable in real time, is to measure the sharpness of the peaks of the filter output. The third trace of figure 4 displays the second derivative as a measure of sharpness of the peaks of the filter output. The fourth trace shows the second derivative only when it exceeded a specified threshold value, and this occurrence was taken to signify the presence of a spike-wave complex. The threshold can be adjusted to give close agreement with the decisions of a human observer, or lowered to recognise complexes buried under ongoing activity which often escape detection by eye. Figure 5 shows some examples of the detection of complexes of differing prominence.

We are using this technique to quantify spike-wave activity in patients with epilepsy as an aid to assessing responses to medication. Another possible application lies in the immediate detection of evoked responses without the use of averaging. The complex waveform made up on a CNV and its associated evoked potentials is particularly suitable for recognition by a matched filter, owing to its wide bandwidth. Such a technique is being used by Dr. Cooper and his colleagues at the Burden Neurological Institute at Bristol. The detection of simple auditory or visual evoked responses is more difficult, as their spectrum is narrow and similar to that of the alpha rhythm. One solution is to base the criteria of recognition on the outputs of multiple filters linked to channels recording from several different regions of the head. Another approach is

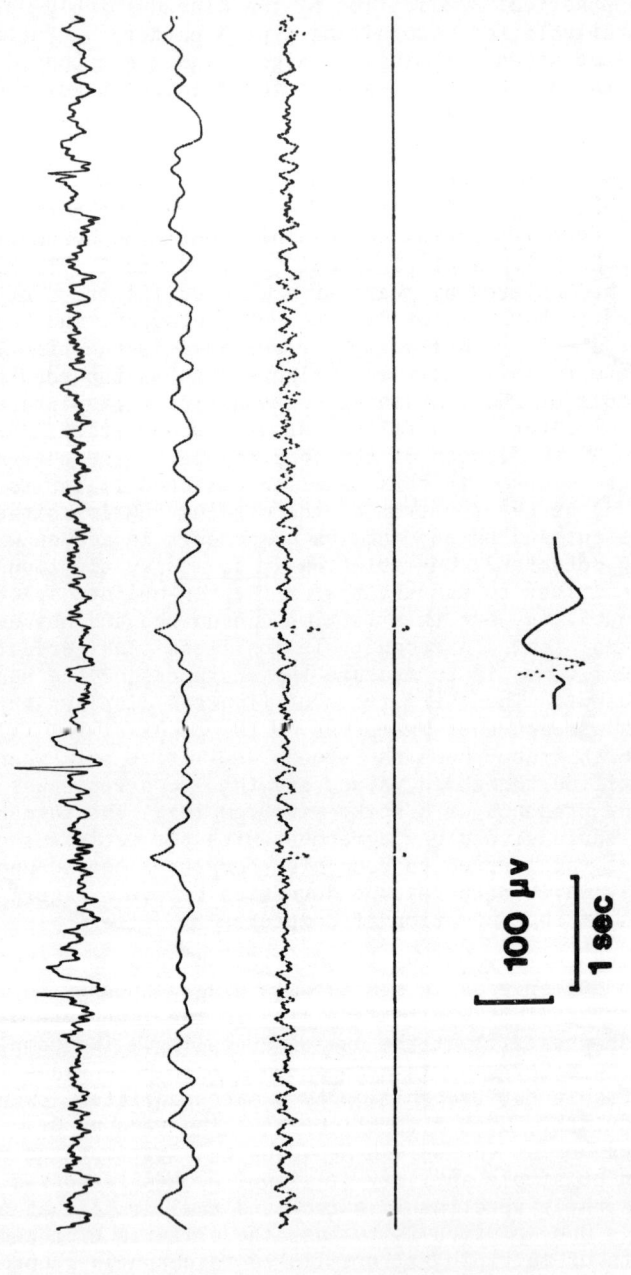

Figure 4 - Matched filter performance on one channel of EEG containing spike and wave complexes. Trace 1) (top) raw analogue signal; 2) filter output; 3) second derivative of trace 2; 4) threshold version of 3; 5) time inverse of the filter impulse response.

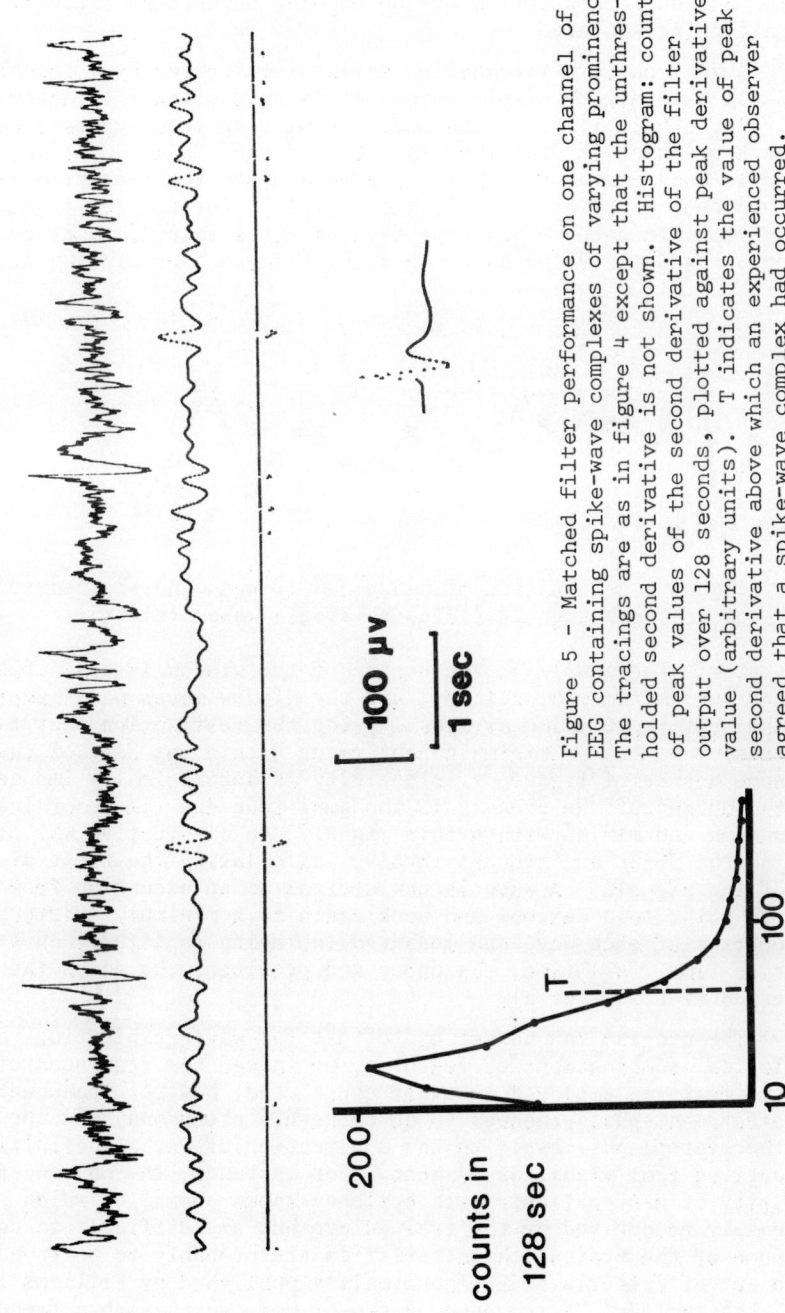

Figure 5 - Matched filter performance on one channel of EEG containing spike-wave complexes of varying prominence. The tracings are as in figure 4 except that the unthresholded second derivative is not shown. Histogram: counts of peak values of the second derivative of the filter output over 128 seconds, plotted against peak derivative value (arbitrary units). T indicates the value of peak second derivative above which an experienced observer agreed that a spike-wave complex had occurred.

to adapt the impulse response of the filter so as to correct for the non-uniform spectrum of the ongoing background activity in a particular subject.

Type 2 pattern recognition may be illustrated by a technique which uses a very simple method of feature extraction described by Leader et al. (1967). The EEG is split up into separate waves each of which is described in terms of amplitude, duration, peak angle and related features. Figure 6 shows the operations required to detect each wave. Following digitising of the raw signal at an appropriate rate, n adjacent samples are examined. n is an odd number and its value determines the frequency resolution of the

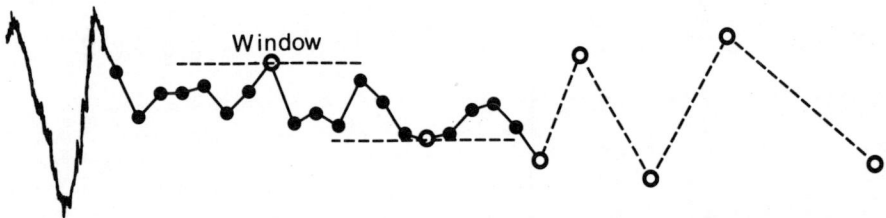

Figure 6 - Detection of peaks and troughs and the reduction of analogue signals (left) to single waves (right).

system. The sample at the centre of the window is classified as a maximum, minimum or neither, and the window moves on 1 sample as the next input value arrives. Using the restriction that two successive maxima or minima cannot recur within one half of the window, some degree of frequency selectivity is automatically imposed, and the output of the process is the amplitude and time coordinates of maxima and minima within this signal. An alternative way of detecting the peaks and troughs involves calculating the first directions of the signals. A wave is now defined as an excursion from a minimum point to a maximum and back again to a minimum. Various properties of each wave are measured including amplitude, duration, rise time, fall time, sharpness and prominence based on the K criterion of Leader et al..

The program can be set up to test for waves exhibiting various logical combinations of features, or indeed for sequences of waves. The features employed resemble those used, however inadequately, by electroencephalographers to describe EEG phenomena, and the method therefore lends itself to the application of verbal definitions derived from visual assessment. For instance, the ongoing EEG activity of many patients with epilepsy shows anomalies which are easily recognised by the trained eye but are difficult to define. Some of the typical characteristics are probably to be found among a set of criteria of EEG abnormality published by Williams in 1941. These include: "A sequence of two or more waves with a frequency of less than 8 a second and an amplitude of more than half that of the dominant frequency ...". Such patterns can easily be detected by the procedure just described, but not, incidentally, by more elaborate techniques based on power spectra.

Type 3 methods have the advantage that they do not require the human observer to give a verbal or numeric description of the phenomenon to be identified but only to present some examples of it, and further that they can recognise classes of waveforms having some general properties in common but differing totally in detail. The features employed can be selected automatically from among a larger number without guidance from the operator, and some indeed may relate to mathematical properties of the signals which cannot be detected by eye.

Figure 7 shows the extraction of 3 features from a section of EEG. Their nature is not relevant to the present account; suffice it that they are three spectral descriptors described by Hjörth (1970) and relate to the mean square amplitude, root mean square frequency and complexity of the power spectrum. Here they are being computed in real time and written out on the chart immediately following the 1.28 second samples of EEG to which they relate. this record contains paroxysmal activity of complex and inconstant waveform which could not be identified by either of the two previous methods described. There are also artefacts due to eye movement and finally there is some more or less normal ongoing EEG activity.

Figure 8 shows the values of these variables for a few minutes of EEG plotted in a 3-dimensional discriminant space, and it is found that the observations on the different types of EEG activity occupy separate regions. The values for ongoing EEG activity lie within this larger region. The overlap between the two (shown as a shaded cuboid) is very small. Observations on artefacts have been omitted for the sake of clarity but occupied a separate region in the lower right part of the figure.

CONCLUSION

Automatic pattern recognition is already finding some limited but practical applications for identifying particular transients in the EEG, notably paroxysmal activity and evoked potentials. Discriminant analysis of spectral properties has been used for some years to characterise the EEG in various test situations and such studies may eventually show how mental function affects different features of the EEG. Various recent studies as, for instance, that of Martin and others (1972) on identification of different stages of sleep, have used a hierarchy of pattern recognition procedures. This last approach, involving feature extraction by identification of EEG phenomena and subsequent clinical prediction based on discriminant analysis, offers the possibility of automating many of the skills of the electroencephalographer and its effects could be more far reaching than almost any other recent technical development in this discipline.

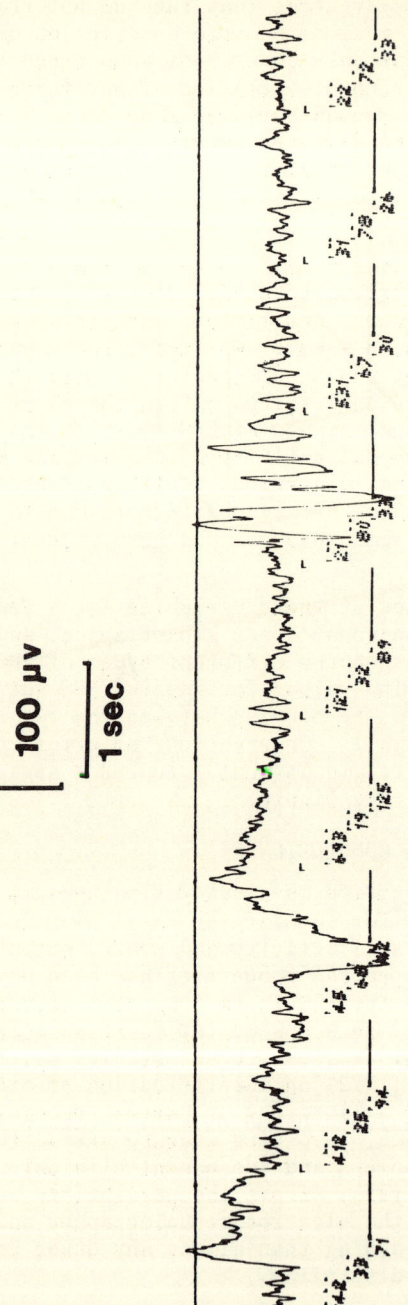

Figure 7 - The derivation of 3 spectral parameters from successive 1.28 second epochs of EEG. The values (read from top to bottom) denote mean square voltage, RMS frequency and spread of the power spectrum (complexity). Scales: µV2/10; Hz×10; Hz×10.

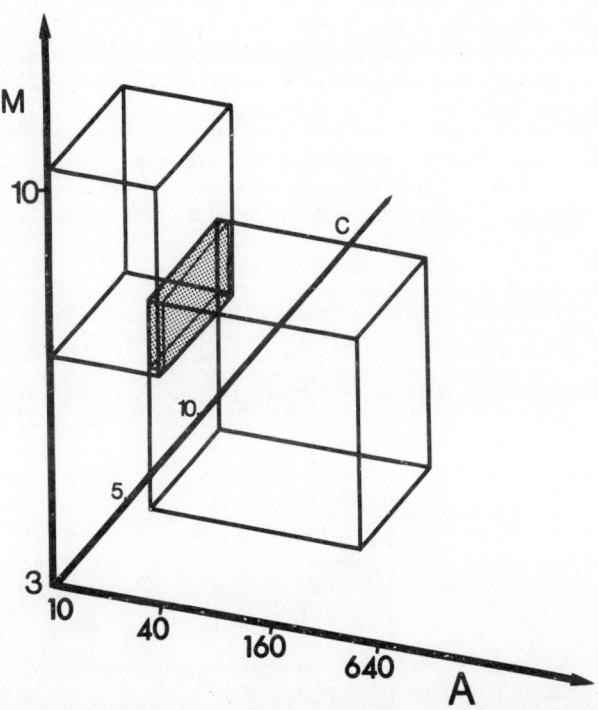

Figure 8 - Regions of 3 dimensional space occupied by epochs of EEG as in figure 7. Axes: A) activity (mean square voltage) $\mu V^2/10$; M) mobility (RMS frequency) Hz×10; C) complexity (power spectrum spread) Hz×10. Regions: Top Left - normal background activity; Centre - paroxysmal activity; Bottom Right Back (not shown) - eye movements.

REFERENCES

Binnie, C.D., Prior, P.F., Lloyd, D.S.L., Scott, D.F. and Margerison, J.H. (1970). Electroencephalographic prediction of fatal anoxic brain damage after resuscitation from cardiac arrest, *Brit. Med. J.*, **4**, 265-268.

Hjörth, B. (1970). EEG analysis based on time domain properties, *Electroenceph. Clin. Neurophysiol.*, **29**, 306-310.

Leader, H.S., Cohn, R., Weihrer, A.L. and Caceres, C.A. (1967). Pattern reading of the clinical electroencephalogram with a digital computer, *Electroenceph. Clin. Neurophysiol.*, **23**, 566-570.

Martin, W.B., Johnson, L.C., Viglione, S.S., Naitoh, P., Joseph, R.D. and Moses, J.D. (1972). Pattern recognition of EEG-EOG as a technique for all-night sleep stage scoring, *Electroenceph. Clin. Neurophysiol.*, **32**, 417-427.

Nilsson, N.J. (1965). *Learning Machines: Foundations of Trainable Pattern Classifying Systems*, (McGraw Hill, New York).

Walter, D.O., Rhodes, J.M. and Adey, W.R. (1967). Discriminating among states of consciousness by EEG measurements. A study of four subjects, *Electroenceph. Clin. Neurophysiol.*, **22**, 22-29.

Williams, D. (1941). The significance of an abnormal electroencephalogram, *J. Neurol. Psychiat.*, **4**, 257-268.

A NOTE ON THE VISUAL NEUROSENSORIUM

HERBERT G. VAUGHAN, Jr.

Department of Neurology,
Albert Einstein College of Medicine,
Bronx, New York 10461

There is a striking discrepancy between the stable and continuous impression of the visual world we experience when contrasted with the spatially and temporally discontinuous series of retinal images which occur in the ordinary course of vision. The information about the environment gained through the eye is defined at each instant by the character of the image sensed by the photoreceptors, which in turn is defined by the position of the eye with respect to the external scene. During normal vision the position of the eyes ordinarily shifts abruptly at an average rate of from two to four times per second, so that there is a corresponding change in the neural input to the brain associated with each shift of the visual image. Although there has been considerable theoretical speculation on the nature of the central mechanisms which might stabilize the visual percept in the face of the discontinuity induced by the saccadic eye movements (Sperry, 1950; von Holst and Mittelstaedt, 1950; Teuber, 1960; MacKay, 1966) neurophsyiological studies of the visual system have largely ignored the implications of these frequency shifts of the retinal image for the processing of afferent information. It seems likely that a substantial portion of the cerebral structures which have been implicated in vision, largely on the basis of lesion and stimulation studies, must in some way be involved in the conscious representation of the visual scene. This neural substrate of visual experience, which we call the 'visual neurosensorium', must display physiological characteristics quite distinct from the visual mechanisms which process the saccade linked afferent inflow and which control the shifts in fixation. For brevity, the latter mechanisms will be designated the 'visuomotor apparatus'.

An experimental differentiation of the visual neurosensorium from the visuomotor apparatus can be made on the basis of a simple functional distinction. Neural activity in the visuomotor system must be temporally linked to the occurrence of saccades, whereas the visual neurosensorium should display a continuous flow of neural activity corresponding to the continuity of visual experience. Thus, when recording brain activity during normal viewing we would expect to observe time locked activity preceding each eye movement, associated with the commands which produce each saccade. Following the eye movements a surge of afferent activity should occur, reflecting the inflow of visual information with each fixational pause. We should not, however, detect phasic changes in the neurosensorium under active conditions of viewing. By contrast with the situation which obtains in normal viewing, a discrete visual stimulus, as obtained by tachistoscopic exposure, would generate a transient neural response within the neurosensorium corresponding to the brief visual percept it engendered (Efron, 1970).

In our studies of the human brain potentials associated with vision, we have used the averaging method for extracting time locked signals from the ongoing EEG activity, and have recorded visually evoked responses under the two experimental conditions outlined above. By means of a topographic analysis of these potentials, we have obtained an estimate of the location and extent of their cortical generators (Vaughan, 1969; Kurtzberg and Vaughan, 1970). Thus it has been possible to approach experimentally the problem of identifying some physiological concomitant of the cerebral processes associated with conscious experience.

In presenting our evidence for the cortical representation of the visual neurosensorium, we shall first describe the configuration and distribution of the evoked responses to brief photic stimuli and then contrast them with the potentials recorded when the eyes are moved across a patterned visual scene.

THE VISUAL EVOKED RESPONSE (VER) TO DISCRETE STIMULI

When a patterned flash of light is briefly (e.g. 10 msec) presented to the central portion of the retina, a characteristic sequence of waves is observed (figure 1). In most individuals this VER

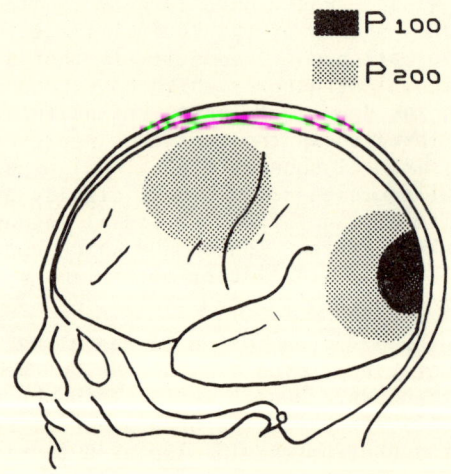

Figure 1 - Sources of the VER.

is triphasic, with an initial positive peak at about 100 msec, followed by a negative and a positive deflection, the latter peaking around 200 msec. The total duration of the response is approximately 250 msec. When the topographic distribution of each component is mapped, it is found that the initial positivity is maximal in amplitude over the occipital pole of the cerebrum and its extent is compatible with a cortical origin within the confines of the striate cortex (area 17) and its immediate surroundings (area 18). The later positive component has a somewhat more widespread distribution over the posterior portion of the head, indicating a cortical generator which includes area 19 and the adjacent posterior parietal region. It is often possible to identify subcomponents of this late peak, one of which arises from a region coextensive with the source of the early positivity (areas 17 and 18) and the other from a more anterior site overlying area 19. In addition to these posterior foci of activity, a secondary maximum in the VER distribution is observed over the central and posterior frontal regions, corresponding to a distinct generator which encompasses the motor and premotor cortex. The latter source includes the region of the classic frontal eye field (area 8). Thus we see that the VER to a discrete visual stimulus invades the cortical regions which have previously been implicated in some aspect of the visual process.

CORTICAL POTENTIALS (EMP) ASSOCIATED WITH SACCADIC EYE MOVEMENTS

When the eyes are moved across a patterned field between fixation points, a characteristic sequence of cortical potentials is observed (Kurtzberg and Vaughan, 1970). These consist of activity which precedes each saccade, as well as a deflection called the 'lambda wave' (Evans, 1952). The antecedent EMP (figure 2) consist of a slow positive ramp-like wave typically beginning about 200 msec

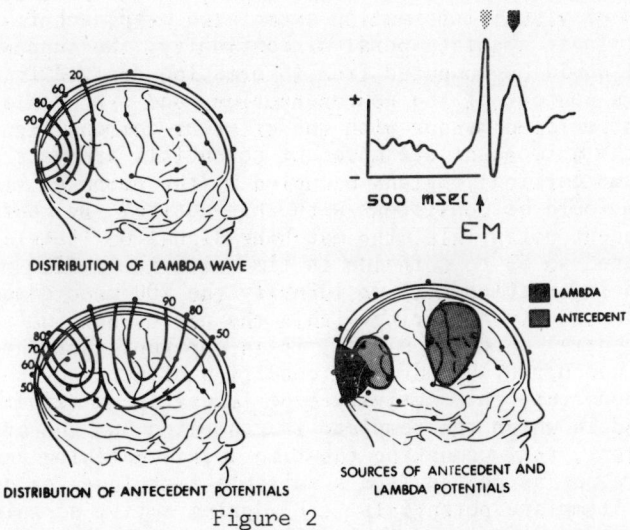

Figure 2

before the saccade, and culminating in a positive sharp wave which precedes the eye movement by 20-40 msec. Both components of the antecedent activity have essentially the same topographic distribution, with a posterior maximum overlying area 19 and an anterior focus overlying the motor and premotor regions. The succeeding lambda wave possesses a single positive peak at about 100 msec after onset of the eye movement. Its distribution is similar to that of the comparable early positive component of the VER. That the lambda wave reflects input from the visual scene is shown both by its change in latency with alteration in field illumination similar to those shown by the VER and its disappearance when saccadic movements are performed in darkness (Kurtzberg, 1972).

Thus, the lambda wave differs from the VER primarily in the absence of the late components emanating from the posterior parietal and posterior frontal cortex. According to our postulate, the VER components arising from prestriate area 19 and from the frontocentral region may represent activity in the neurosensorium, since there is no time-locked activity in these areas following the eye movements under the active viewing condition. However, the antecedent potentials, presumably related to the initiation of the saccades, arise from the same cortical regions which we implicate as a part of the neural substrate of visual experience. We cannot, therefore, consider the visuomotor apparatus and the neurosensorium to be anatomically distinct mechanisms, but rather as systems which share to some extent coextensive cortical regions.

Previous theoretical considerations of the mechanisms for stabilizing the visual scene have not specified the location of the postulated operations, but have been concerned with the formal analysis of an hypothetical visuomotor system (e.g. MacKay, 1966). The suggested mechanisms require a centrally generated signal, linked in time with each eye movement, which interacts with the inflow of visual information associated with each fixational pause to eliminate spatiotemporal discontinuity. We suppose that this signal would be computed from information derived from the instantaneous content of the neurosensorium, and synchronized in some as yet unspecified manner with the efferent command signal. The fact that the antecedent eye movement potentials are generated within the same cortical regions occupied by the proposed visual neurosensorium would be consistent with this notion. By contrast with the antecedent potentials, the matching signal or 'template' must be generated so as to coincide in time with the inflow of saccade linked information. If we identify the 200 msec components of the VER as activity appearing within the neurosensorium in the absence of a central matching signal, it is apparent that the template must occur concurrently under the condition of active viewing. In order to demonstrate this activity experimentally, a situation must be devised in which the template is generated but the afferent signal is absent, thus unmasking the time locked matching central activity. We have not as yet devised a suitable technique for demonstrating these 'template potentials' (TP) during active scanning of a visual scene, but an equivalent situation can be readily created by a tachistoscopic simulation of the discontinuous input produced by saccadic eye movements. In this experiment, a visual pattern is abruptly changed at frequent, regular intervals. Under these circumstances, the brain is able to predict the occurrence of each change in visual input in a manner analogous to that which obtains with active saccadic shifts in gaze. The main difference is that a passive but predictable change in input is occurring rather than an actively induced one. If a stimulus in the regular sequence is occasionally omitted in unpredictable fashion, the average of brain activity time locked to the 'missing' stimuli should provide us with an indication of central activity generated in the expectation of a change in visual input but in the absence of an objective change in stimulation. Several investigators have now shown that time locked brain potentials may be present in response to the deletion of an expected stimulus (e.g. Barlow, 1969; Klinke et al., 1968). In our experiments with unexpected deletion of a stimulus within a train of visual stimulation, we observe an initial negative deflection beginning about 100 msec after the anticipated change which reaches a peak at about 250 msec. Topographic analysis of this negative potential indicates a major source in the region of cortical area 19 and adjacent parietotemporal cortex (figure 3), with a small focus of activity also centred on the premotor region. Thus the sources of this TP are coextensive with the previously delineated cortical confines of the visual neurosensorium.

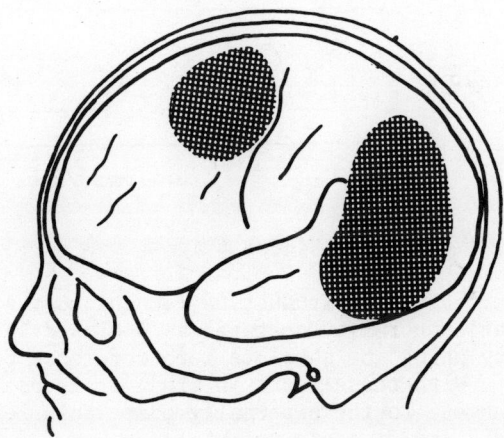

Figure 3 - Sources of the template potential.

Figure 4 provides a schematic representation of the temporal relationships among the various potentials we have previously discussed. In the upper section two saccades are depicted at their average spacing of about 300 msec, with the lambda wave and the antecedent EMP separately displayed for clarity. The center section illustrates the TP, and the lower portion the typical VER to a discrete visual stimulus. The latter potentials have been aligned so that the stimulus (or missing stimulus) coincides with the onset of the saccade. By reference to these traces we can compare the timing of the postulated neural processes within the visual neurosensorium. It must be kept in mind that the processes represented by these gross potential waveforms are occurring in different structures which are connected by pathways which entail various conduction delays. Furthermore, the processes are not sequential but overlapping in time, so that a precise separation of the neural events

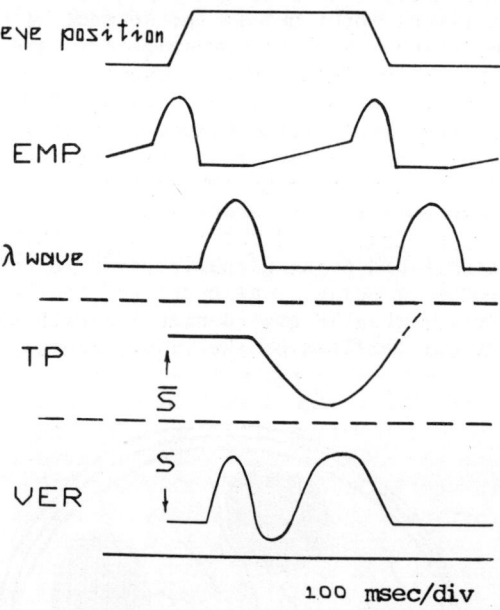

Figure 4

is not possible. Finally, it must be recognized that the system under consideration normally operates as a closed loop, so that there is no 'beginning' or absolute zero reference point of a visuomotor sequence. With these facts in mind, it is useful to relate the neural phenomena to the externally observable reference events, i.e. the saccades and discrete stimuli.

We note again that the lambda potential and initial VER component arise at the same latency from their reference events - saccade and stimulus, respectively - within the confines of the striate and immediate prestriate cortex. We and others have shown (Gross, Vaughan and Valenstein, 1967) that there is a sharp reduction in the capacity to process any change in patterned input to the visual system during a saccade. This suppression is highly dependent upon the pattern characteristics of the visual stimuli and is essentially identical regardless of whether the pattern shift is active, due to eye movement, or passive, due to field displacement (Vaughan, 1970; MacKay, 1970). We have interpreted the presaccade suppression as a form of backward masking. In view of the close relationship between saccadic suppression and the lambda wave, it is still a moot point whether the neural activity represented by that potential reach the neurosensorium as information concerning the stimulus field, or whether this activity serves an inhibitory function which prevents the rapidly moving retinal image during the saccade from serving as an effective stimulus. The latter interpretation seems to us to be more plausible and in accord with most of the existing experimental evidence. If this interpretation is accepted, it is necessary to suppose that information from the retinal image is almost totally ineffective for a period of approximately 50 msec. Due to retinal processing and transmission delays, this would correspond to suppression of input to visual cortex of about 50 msec after the beginning of each eye movement and continuing for a comparable period. According to our psychophysical and physiological evidence, changes in visual stimulation achieve two-thirds of their maximum effectiveness by the end of each saccade, but some degree of reduced sensitivity persists for about 200 msec. Thus we would hypothesize that the effective visual input begins at the end of each eye movement and continues until the blanking associated with the next saccade. We note that both the antecedent potential and the template potential display a gradual increase in amplitude during the period which would be associated with active input from the visual scene. In the case of EMP the gradual increment terminates in a sharp deflection which precedes the saccade by an interval appropriate for an oculomotor command signal. The TP, which coincides both spatially and temporally with the EMP, might be viewed as a manifestation of the 'corollary discharge' (Sperry, 1950). This hypothetical process has invariably been linked to the mechanisms which generate eye movements, serving primarily a corrective function. It is of interest, however, that the experiment by which the TP is disclosed does not involve oculomotor activity, so that a more general predictive mechanism underlying the perceptual process may well be involved. In our current view of this process, we suppose that the neurosensorium must be in continuous interaction with the substrate of memory storage, as well as with the visual input and with the oculomotor control apparatus. Thus, we would envisage the likelihood of several interleaved processes, occupying a common processing zone within the neurosensorium, one of which would lead to production of successive saccadic vectors and another achieving the shift in coordinates of the incoming visual signals required to match the existing content of the neurosensorium. It is very likely that these processes would be highly integrated with one another and operate in coextensive areas of brain.

Two aspects of our present suggestion require brief comment. First, we are proposing a role of posterior frontal cortex in the neural substrate of visual experience. This may seem a novel idea but it is not without complementary experimental support. Several observations in the older literature noted a neglect of contralateral visual space following lesions of the arcuate cortex (or frontal eye field) in the monkey (Kennard and Ectors, 1938). It was never clear whether this disorder could properly be considered a 'sensory' defect until the recent work by Latto and Cowey (1971) which has established the presence of a specific ambylopia following ablation of the prearcuate region in the rhesus macaque. This finding makes it impossible to uphold for vision the long-held distinction between sensory and motor cortical regions. The common cortical origin of the evoked activity we have suggested as representing a manifestation of visual experience and the potentials which precede saccades further underlines this point.

The significance of the antecedent EMP represents the second matter of concern. As yet, it has not been possible to identify unitary neural activity preceding eye movements in either the frontal or the posterior eye fields of monkeys (Bizzi, 1968; Bizzi and Schiller, 1970; Bizzi, personal communication). These negative results are especially puzzling in view of the extensive body of lesion and stimulation evidence which implicates these frontal and parietal regions in oculomotor control, as well as the close anatomical linkage between the cortical eye fields and the superior colliculi in which antecedent unitary activity has recently been identified (Wurtz and Goldberg, 1970; Schiller and Koerner, 1970). The probable explanation for this discrepancy is to be found in the experiment of Robinson and Fuchs (1969) who found that microstimulation within the frontal eye fields generated saccades of specific size and direction. Thus, it might be difficult to find the cells appropriate to a given saccade unless special methods to determine the movement generated by a particular neurone were employed. This has been done in the superior colliculus but not yet in the cortex.

In future studies of the cerebral mechanisms of vision, it will be essential to take into consideration the active role of the oculomotor system in the processing of afferent input. It is likely that we are approaching the point at which the classic approaches to understanding the visual process which involve the analysis of receptive field properties of single neurones will fail to meet the analytic demands of the mechanisms under study. It is clear that further studies of the spatial and temporal pattern of activity within the brain, under experimentally controlled conditions of normal vision, are required to identify the extent of the mechanisms which must be dissected by more analytic techniques.

ACKNOWLEDGMENTS

The research reported here was supported in part by NIMH Grants MH 06723 and 17442. I thank Diane Kurtzberg, Richard Simson and Walter Ritter for collaboration in these studies.

REFERENCES

Barlow, J.S. (1969). Some observations on the electrophysiology of timing in the nervous system, *Electroenceph. clin. Neurophysiol.*, **27**, 545.

Bizzi, E. (1968). Discharge of frontal eye field neurons during saccadic and following eye movements in unanaesthetized monkeys, *Exp. Brain Res.*, **6**, 69-80.

Bizzi, E. and Schiller, P.H. (1970). Single unit activity in the frontal eye fields of unanaesthetized monkeys during eye and head movement, *Exp. Brain Res.*, **10**, 151-158.

Efron, R. (1970). The minimum duration of a perception, *Neuropsychologia*, **8**, 57-63.

Evans, C.C. (1952). Some further observations on occipital sharp waves (λ waves), *Electroenceph. clin. Neurophysiol.*, **4**, 371.

Gross, E.G., Vaughan, H.G., Jr. and Valenstein, E. (1967). Inhibition of visual evoked responses to patterned stimuli during voluntary eye movements, *Electroenceph. clin. Neurophysiol.*, **22**, 204-209.

Kennard, Margaret A. and Ectors, L. (1938). Forced circling in monkeys following lesions of the frontal lobes, *J. Neurophysiol.*, **1**, 45-54.

Klinke, R., Fruhstorfer, H. and Finkenzeller, P. (1968). Evoked responses as a function of external and stored information, *Electroenceph. clin. Neurophysiol.*, **25**, 119-122.

Kurtzberg, Diane and Vaughan, H.G., Jr. (1970). Electrocortical potentials associated with eye movement, in *The Oculomotor System and Brain Functions*, (Proceedings of the International Colloquium, Smolenice).

Kurtzberg, Diane (1972). Electrocortical potentials associated with eye movement, (Doctoral dissertation, City University of New York), (unpublished).

Latto, R. and Cowey, A. (1971). Visual field defects after frontal eye-field lesions in monkeys, *Brain Res.*, **30**, 1-24.

MacKay, D.M. (1966). Cerebral organization and the conscious control of action, in *Brain and Conscious Experience*, (ed. Eccles, J.C.), (Springer-Verlag, New York), pp. 422-445.

MacKay, D.M. (1970). Elevation of visual threshold by displacement of retinal image, *Nature*, **225**, 90-92.

Robinson, D.A. and Fuchs, A.F. (1969). Eye movements evoked by stimulation of frontal eye fields, *J. Neurophysiol.*, **32** (5), 637-648.

Schiller, P.H. and Koerner, F. (1971). Discharge characteristics of single units in superior colliculus of the alert rhesus monkey, *J. Neurophysiol.*, **34**, 920-936.

Sperry, R.W. (1950). Neural basis of the spontaneous optokinetic response produced by visual inversion, *J. comp. physiol. Psychol.*, **43**, 482-489.

Teuber, H.-L. (1960). Perception, in *Handbook of Physiology; Section 1: Neurophysiology, Vol. 3*, (eds. Field, J., Magoun, H.W. and Hall, V.E.), (American Physiological Society, Washington, D.C.), pp. 1595-1668.

Vaughan, H.G., Jr. (1969). The relationship of brain activity to scalp recordings of event-related potentials, in *Average Evoked Potentials: Methods, Results, Evaluations*, (eds. Donchin, E. and Lindsley, D.B.), (NASA #SP-191), (National Aeronautics and Space Administration, Washington, D.C.), pp. 45-94.

Vaughan, H.G., Jr. (1970). The role of stimulus pattern in suppression of vision during eye movements, in *The Oculomotor System and Brain Functions*, (Proceedings of the International Colloquium, Smolenice).

von Holst, E. and Mittelstaedt, H. (1950). Das Reafferenzprinzip (Wechselwirkungen zwischen Zentralnervensystem und Peripherie), *Naturwiss.*, **37**, 464-476.

Wurtz, R.H. and Goldberg, M.E. (1971). Superior colliculus cell responses related to eye movements in awake monkeys, *Science*, **171**, 82-84.

CORTICAL EVOKED POTENTIALS

D. REGAN

Department of Communication,
University of Keele

Buttressed by some undeniably sloppy evoked potential research there are some who would dismiss out of hand the recording of electrical signals from the human scalp as being comparable to "holding an oscilloscope probe six feet in diameter up to a computer and pronouncing from the resultant waveform on the underlying structure and function". Such extreme views are often associated with an implication that the method of recording electrical activities of individual nerve cells is the only electrophysiological technique which merits serious scientific consideration. This view has more than a grain of truth in it. Although a fair case can be made for the clinical possibilities of scalp recording, it is certainly true that the contribution made by the scalp recording method to our present day understanding of brain function are very much less than the contributions made by single-cell recording. It could be argued that although a deal of taxpayers' money has been absorbed by evoked potential research, the scientific returns have been many articles, much equivocal data, but little additional understanding of brain function. Very well, but is our present day understanding of brain function so profound that it can support a judgement that the single-unit technique is, in itself, an adequate electrophysiological tool for unravelling the problem of brain function? Unless this is the case, then there must be a need for other and complementary electrophysiological methods. I will argue that the methods of recording electrical responses from the human scalp offers promise as such a method.

The title of this paper is "Cortical Evoked Potentials" although the title of Dr. Spekreijse's paper, "System Analysis Approach to the Problem of Vision" would be more accurate. The evidence that most of the generators of scalp-recorded potentials are located in the cortex is strong, but confusing [24]. On the other hand I am quite sure that scalp electrodes are indeed stuck onto the scalp, so that I would prefer to use the term 'scalp evoked potentials'.

One way of using scalp evoked potentials has been to study the waveform of the electrical responses elicited by a sensory stimulus. This approach would be undermined if either of the following proved to be true:- (a) scalp potentials were some mere concomitant of the activities which correlate with the processing of sensory information; (b) scalp potentials contained substantial contributions from glial cells such that their waveforms were not in general similar to the waveforms generated by neurons [3].

One counter to these problems is to adopt approaches analogous to the methods long used by classical psychophysicists who have to content themselves with the responses "yes, stimuli S1 and S2 produce the same sensation under condition X" or "no, stimuli S1 and S2 produce different sensations under condition X (i.e. Brindley's Class A observations). This approach is to ask only whether a particular signal has reached a particular response generator. There is evidence (much of which has been provided by Spekreijse and van der Tweel), that this method can be used to investigate activities at sites as peripheral as the retina. The rationale here is that, although scalp responses may be *generated by* cortical cells, some features of these responses can be *determined by* activities at sites peripheral to those cortical cells.

There is growing evidence of an aspect of scalp potential research which can be a pitfall, but can alternatively be used as a tool. This evidence is that some constraints are common both to perception and to scalp recordings. Other constraints are not common. The result is that if an experiment confounds constraints which are common to scalp recordings and to perception with constraints which are not common, then any resulting correlations between perception and scalp responses will be difficult to interpret. Examples of constraints which seem to be common to perception and to scalp responses are suppression of pattern vision [*2, 31*], the visual acuity threshold [*1,24*] and orientation selectivity [*1*]. Examples of constraints which are not common to perception and scalp responses are whether the subject can or cannot see flicker, [*8,13,35,34*], saturation [*13,32,35*], nonanalytic distortion [*29,32,34,35*], phase [*15*], changes in apparent size due to ocular convergence [*22*], apparent brightness versus check size [*23*], the subject's psychophysical criterion [*33*], electrode position [*24*], bipolar versus referential recording [*5,26*], location of reference electrode [*10*], upper versus lower visual field [*6, 7,37*] and foveal versus extrafoveal location of the stimulus [*9, 27,38*].

Anyone who studies physiological tissue by comparing an input (stimulus) with an output (response) is engaged in systems analysis. The 'classical' stimuli such as pulses (e.g. flashes), or square waves fall under this heading. Yet the terms 'systems analysis' can sometimes seem to carry implications of the occult. To explicitly invoke 'nonlinear systems analysis' sometimes seems to risk exorcism to some dark engineering department. Yet the behaviour of physiological tissue abounds with nonlinearities, a number of which seem inherent to normal function. One may ask, "what's in a name?" One answer to this question is, "a row of bookshelves in a library". They might be in the electrical engineering section, the mechanical engineering section or the mathematical section. They hold a body of knowledge which has been developed in trying to slove problems in fields other than brain research. A number of these problems are analogous to problems encountered in brain research. A further point is that mathematical treatments may have been developed which could both sharpen one's physiological experiments and expose limitations and pitfalls inherent in one's current experimental techniques.

There is a point which can lead to misunderstanding when presenting the results of experiments on sensory information processing. Such results could be summarised in the form of a series of mathematical equations which describe the processing of the signals generated by some sensory stimulus. It is easier to visualise such a summary by representing each mathematical equation in the form of a graph or even as an object with analogous mathematical properties. Such a visual aid may contain graphs and terms such as 'rectifier', 'integrator' and 'capacitor'. I have often been asked whether I, and others, believe that there really are resistors, capacitors and rectifiers in the visual system. Before electronics became fashionable, it was common to cast physiological models in mechanical terms. This is quite straightforward, since mechanical equations are quite analogous to electrical equations. In mechanical terms, the visual system would appear to be filled with springs, masses, gearwheels, governers and water cisterns containing ballcocks. Such models throw a sharper light on the distinction between the real brain and one's hypotheses. Some nonlinearities can be illustrated more easily by mechanical than by electrical analogies. Now might well be an appropriate time to re-introduce water cisterns into the visual system.

TIME DOMAIN AND FREQUENCY DOMAIN ANALYSIS

Among the ways of studying the behaviour of a system are the methods of time-domain and frequency-domain analysis. The majority of scalp evoked potential studies have been time-domain studies. These have been reviewed elsewhere. The studies described in this paper are mainly frequency-domain studies.

The transient response to a sensory stimulus can be illustrated by the notional, extreme situation in which the sensory stimulus is repeated at intervals which are sufficiently long that the response to one stimulus has died away before the arrival of the next stimulus (e.g. the system is given a 'kick'). One way of displaying transient evoked potential is as a voltage versus time plot. This is the form of display familiar to users of averaging devices. The 'steady-state'response to a sensory stimulus can be illustrated, again by the extreme case, this time when the responses to an infinitely long train of repetitive stimuli overlap to such an extent that in general no single response cycle can be associated with any individual stimulus (i.e. the system is 'gently shaken'). Steady-state data can be presented as plots of voltage versus frequency (figure 1).

There are a number of distinctions between transient and steady-state scalp responses. Among these are:-

(1) In a linear system, the time-domain and frequency-domain (figure 1) descriptions are equivalent. In a nonlinear system, however, the two descriptions are to some extent complementary. Now the behaviour of the visual system can be very nonlinear indeed [12,13,29,32,35] (for example, see figure 2). In principle, therefore, transient and steady-state investigations offer different insights into brain function. (This point applies with equal

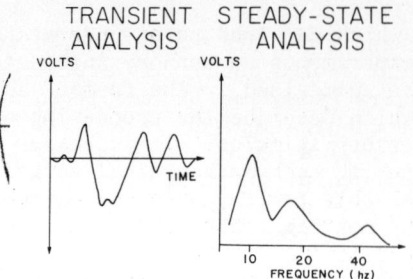

Figure 1 - Left Side: The response of a system to infrequently repeated transient stimuli presented as a time-domain plot of volts versus time. Right Side: The steady state response of a system to reptitive stimulation presented as a frequency domain plot of volts versus the repetition frequency of the stimulus. Here it is assumed that a sinewave output results from a sinewave input and that both sinewaves have the same frequency. In such a linear system either the time domain or the frequency domain description is adequate. One indication that a system is nonlinear is that a sinewave input does *not* produce a sinewave output which has the same frequency as the input. Such nonlinear behaviour is illustrated in figure 2.

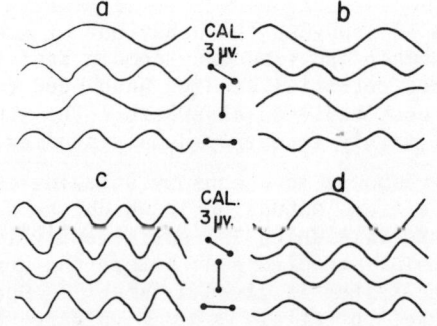

Figure 2 - (a) and (b) Averaged scalp potentials evoked in two different subjects by a spatially-unstructured stimulus field of 60° subtense sinusoidally modulated to a depth of 33% at 24.4 Hz. The top channel was recorded from a photocell which sampled the stimulus light. Note the second harmonic responses in the second and third traces. These are high frequency components of frequency 48.8 Hz. The third trace is predominantly a fundamental component. This is a medium frequency component of frequency 24.4 Hz. (c) Fundamental components of the high frequency type evoked by a stimulus modulation frequency of 55.5 Hz. The dots and lines indicate that the second trace was recorded between electrodes 2 and 4, the third trace between electrodes 2 and 1 and the fourth trace between electrodes 2 and 3. Electrode 1 was located 1 cm above the inion, electrode 2 was 7 cm in front of electrode 1 along the midline, electrode 3 was 5 cm from 1, perpendicular to the midline and electrode 4 was 7 cms from 1 and 2. (From [12]).

force to single-unit and slow wave studies). An example of this point is that transient evoked potentials are markedly affected by 'psychophysical' factors, sometimes difficult to define in other than operational terms, which include 'attention', 'signal detection', and 'cognitive evaluation of stimulus significance'. In contrast, steady-state scalp responses seem unaffected by such 'psychological' factors as attention (except for components at frequencies near the alpha frequency).

(2) A complete time-domain description of a system is compressed into a single transient evoked potential (figure 1). However, individual items of information may be imprecise and difficult to disentangle. On the other hand, a single steady-state recording may be described by as little as four or even two numbers. A full frequency-domain description of the system must be built up of many individual recordings of the responses to stimuli of different frequencies. Each response gives only a little information, but this is precise and unequivocal. In this sense the transient response resembles a telescope while the steady-state response resembles a microscope.

(3) A device which is appropriate for recording transient responses is not necessarily the most appropriate device for recording steady-state responses. By the use of devices which reject all redundant information, steady-state response analysis can provide certain items of information (e.g. visual acuity) very much more rapidly than when transient responses are averaged. Increases in speed exceeding 100 times are quite possible.

Figure 3a shows the running average of the amplitudes of steady-state scalp responses elicited by a patterned stimulus and recorded by an averaging device. Figure 3b shows the running average of steady-state scalp responses elicited by an identical stimulus, but recorded by an analogue Fourier analyser. It is clear that the moment-to-moment variability is much less when the Fourier analyser was used. The most likely reason is that much of the variability of the averaging device's output was due, not to signal variability, but to noise which passed through the device. The bandwidth of the Fourier analyser was much less than the bandwidth of the averaging device. When analysing steady-state responses this is no disadvantage, since just as much signal passes through the Fourier analyser as through the averager (if N harmonics are present, N analysers are needed). However, much less noise passes through the Fourier analyser than through the averaging device. This advantage can be traded either for increased speed or for the capacity to measure smaller signals.

Figure 4 shows a calibration of a simple Fourier analyser in typical use [24]. The half-power bandwidth can be some 0.001 Hz, with a 100-fold attenuation within 0.05 Hz. In comparison with an averaging device with a bandwidth of (say) 50 Hz, this represents a bandwidth compression of some 50,000:1 without loss of signal.

Much faster devices than the simple analyser described here can be designed for specific applications.

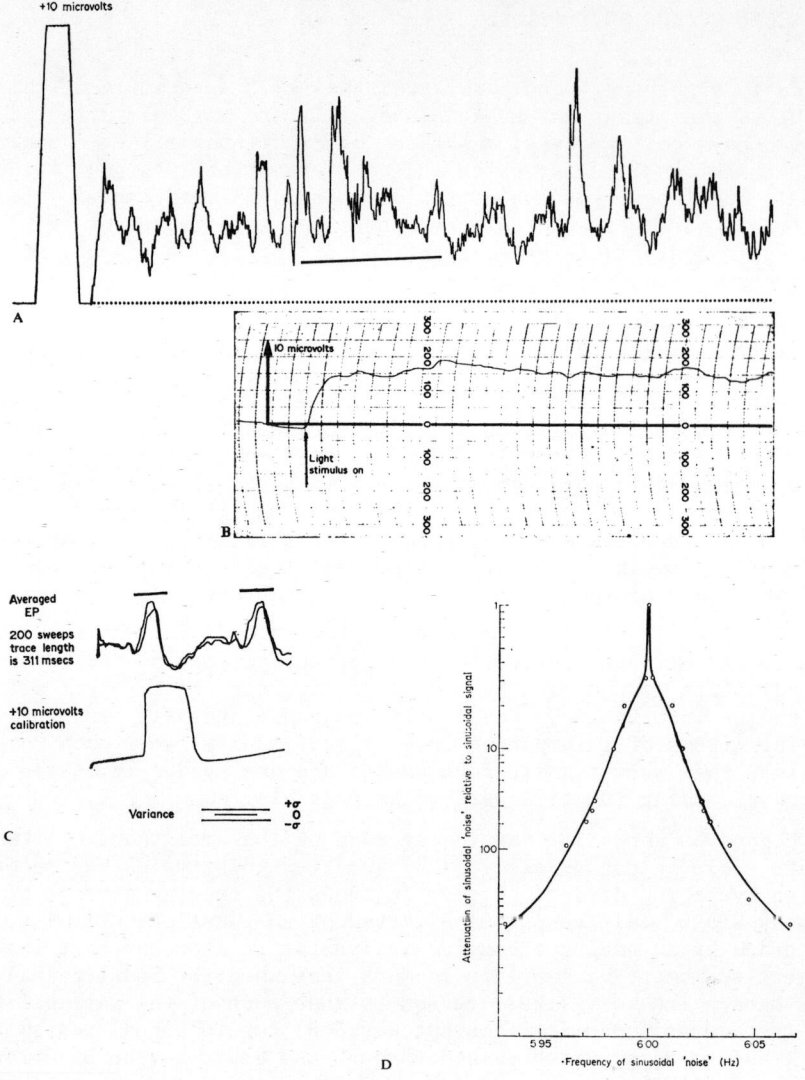

Figure 3 - This figure illustrates the way in which the variability of scalp responses is influenced by the bandwidth of the recording device. (a) and (b) compare the moment-to-moment variability of scalp responses evoked in the same subject by similar stimuli. An averaging device computed trace (a); an analogue Fourier analyser computed trace (b). The stimulus was a foveally-viewed 4 deg. pattern of 13 min checks whose spatial contrast reversed 6 times per second. The recording period in (a) was 320 secs and in (b) 420 secs. A digital computer integrated the EEG for a 50 msec period centred on a latency of 90 msec after each stimulus. Two 50 sec periods are shown by the black bars in (c). A running average was formed of a block of 16 successive responses. The horizontal dotted line in (a) is zero amplitude. (d) shows an experimental calibration of the Fourier analyser as a frequency filter showing its extremely narrow effective bandwidth (1 minute analysis period). The half power bandwidths of this analyser was 0.002 Hz. The analyser attenuated sinusoidal 'noise' by a factor of 100 when the noise fequency differed form the signal frequency by only 0.05 Hz. (From [24]).

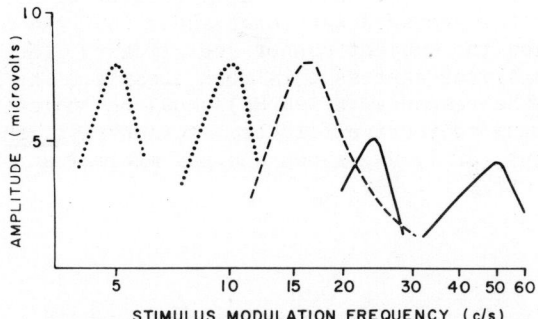

Figure 4 - Steady-state scalp responses are composed of three (at least) types of frequency component. Dotted lines: low frequency region (fundamental and second harmonic components). Chain line: medium frequency components. Full lines: high frequency components (fundamental and second harmonic). Note: The relative amplitudes of these types of component vary considerably with the subject, electrode position, stimulus intensity, field size and colour. Components other than fundamental and second harmonic are omitted for clarity. (From: [15]).

FREQUENCY-DOMAIN ANALYSIS OF STEADY-STATE SCALP RESPONSES

A steady-state scalp response can be analysed into a number of frequency (Fourier) components. The characteristic of a particular frequency component depends both on its frequency and on the type of stimulus which elicited the response.

Steady state responses to flickering, spatially-unstructured patches of light often have complex waveshapes. The picture is simpler when the steady-state responses are split into frequency components. The characteristics of a particular component seems to depend on which of three frequency regions it falls into (figure 4). These regions are roughly: (a) 45-60 Hz ('high-frequency' components), (b) 13-25 Hz ('medium frequency' components) and (c) near the alpha frequency ('low frequency' components).

Components in different frequency regions can relate quite differently to perception and to stimulus variables. Figure 5 shows the steady-state scalp responses elicited by alternating the colour of a patch of light twenty times per second. When the two colours were made equally bright, the patch of light appeared to be steady, with no flicker. (0 on abscissa, "b" in centre of figure 5). Nevertheless, an averaging computer recorded a clear response ("b" on right lower part of figure 5). When one coloured light was made brighter or dimmer than the other, the subject was clear flicker ("a" and "c", centre of figure 5). The averaged responses were, however, little different in amplitude from when the stimulus appeared steady (compare "a", "b" and "c" right lower figure 5). The averaged potentials elicited by flicker, then, seem to be little different when the subject sees flicker or not. A closer inspection of the averaged waveforms shows that the waveform is 'smoother' when the subject cannot see flicker. The outputs of the Fourier analyser express this more clearly. The fundamental component of the response (at 20 Hz) shows no indication of the point of minimum subjective flicker. In contrast, the second harmonic component (at 40 Hz) shows a clear minimum at the point of minimum subjective flicker.

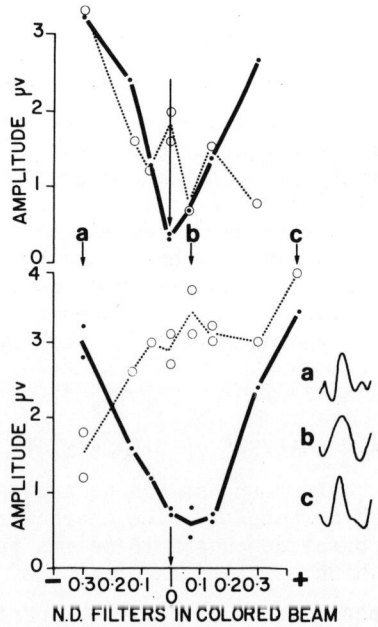

Figure 5 - Comparison of subjective and objective measures of the stimulus 'strength' of different colours. A standard white light was alternated 24 times per sec with a coloured light whose intensity was adjusted by the subject to a point where the stimulus flicker was a minimum. At this point the white and coloured lights are defined to be equally bright. The second harmonic component of the scalp response (48 Hz high frequency component) had a sharp minimum at the point of brightness equality. The fundamental component (24 Hz medium frequency component) showed no consistent indication of the point of brightness equality, and might even be largest when flicker was zero and smallest when flicker was maximal. The amplitudes of averaged scalp potentials (a,b,c) showed no indication of the point of minimum flicker since they were compounded of 24 Hz plus 48 Hz components. (From [14]).

The spectral sensitivity of components in the high frequency region agrees very closely (within 0.05 log unit) with the subjective spectral sensitivity of vision. Oddly enough the notion of spectral sensitivity seems to have little meaning for components in the medium frequency range (e.g. the dotted lines in figure 5).

A curious property of these medium frequency components is that they show large relative phase shifts between different colours. These phase shifts can reach 180° and are much larger than phase shifts measured psychophysically. The most obvious explanation would be relative time delays between the responses to stimuli of different colours. If this were so, then the relative phase shift would vary with stimulus flicker frequency. Figure 6 shows that this is not so. The phase shift shown in figure 6 is frequency-

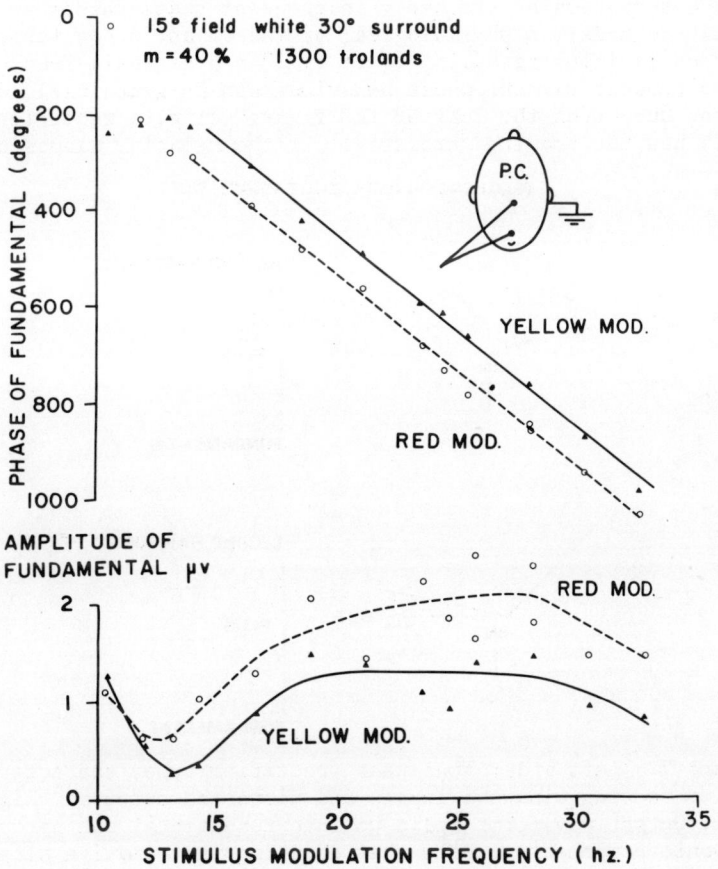

Figure 6 - Top Half: Plots of phase versus stimulus modulation frequency for modulation of a red stimulus and modulation of a yellow stimulus. Lower Half: Plots of corresponding response amplitudes. The stimulus was composed of a yellow patch of light superposed on a red patch of light of the same brightness. The intensity of the red light was modulated while the yellow was constant or vice versa.

invariant. The phase difference between the responses to red and yellow stimuli remains constant at 60° to within ±10° while the absolute phase of each response changes by some 800°. This means that the 'apparent latencies' of the responses to red and yellow stimuli are constant to within roughly 1.5 msec (in 100 msec). The frequency-independent phase shift depended markedly on the wavelengths of the stimuli, but changing the relative intensities of the stimuli merely tilted the lines. The plots in the lower half of figure 6 show that the phase shift could not easily be attributed to differences between the shapes of the amplitude versus frequency curves.

This observation of frequency-independent phase shifts proved difficult to model in physiological or indeed any other terms. One suggestion is illustrated in figure 7. "An hysteresis-free, frequency-independent element whose behaviour can be graphically described by the curves on the left of the figure" (i.e. a rectifier-type element) has the required property. If the relative slopes of the

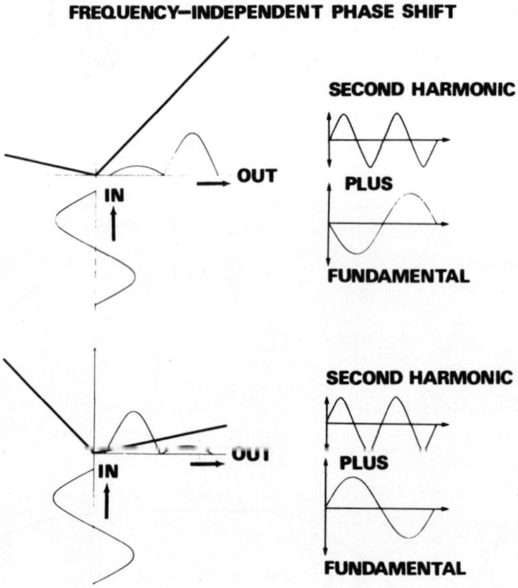

Figure 7 - Left Side: Nonlinear (rectifier-type) characteristics showing sinewave inputs and distorted outputs. Right Side: Output waveforms split up into fundamental and second harmonic components. Note that changing the relative slopes of the branches of the rectifier shifts the phase of the fundamental component of the output by 180°, while leaving the phase of the second harmonic unchanged.

two branches is changed as shown in figure 7, then the phase of the fundamental component of the output shifts through 180°. The shift will be frequency-invariant. The interesting point is that Spekreijse has experimentally found phenomena which resemble rectification both in human, and animal visual systems [28,30,32]. Furthermore, Spekreijse's physiological 'rectifiers' are frequency-independent - exactly the property which is required to explain why the phase shifts of figure 6 are independent of frequency.

Information processing which has the property described in figure 7 can only explain frequency-invariant phase shifts of 0° or 180°. If, however, a frequency-independent differentiation stage were located before the stage of figure 7, then frequency-invariant phase shifts of 90° and 270° could also be modelled. By adding the outputs of direct-coupled and differentiating stages any phase shift could be produced.

This tentative mathematical model points to a physiological speculation. Dr. Spekreijse's paper presents evidence that the outputs of his hypothetical 'rectifier' elements can be associated with the frequencies of spike firing of ganglion cells leading from the retina. There is evidence for both retinal neurons which respond to the absolute level of illumination ('tonic units') and also for retinal neurons whose firing is determined by changes in the level of illumination ('phasic units'). The response of these neurons would differ in phase by 90° when the retina was stimulated by sinusoidally modulated light.

De Valois has shown that the firing characteristics of some cells in the lateral geniculate body of rhesus monkey are suggestive of opponent colour processing [4]. For example an increase in the brightness of a red light might increase the firing rate of such a cell while an increase in the brightness of a green light would have the opposite effect of decreasing the firing rate of the cell. (Figure 7 can easily be modified to include decreases in mean firing rate). Speculatively, then, the colour-dependent, frequency-independent phase shifts of figure 6 might reflect opponent colour processing either at the level of retinal ganglion cells or peripheral to this site.

Spekreijse has described experimental evidence that the hypothetical 'high frequency' channel separates from the 'low frequency' channel at a level peripheral to the rectifier stage. In physiological terms this suggests that the separation lies peripheral to ganglion cell level. More speculatively, the 'high frequency' components (which correlate with the subjective brightness of the stimulus) might reflect activities which are functionally separate from the activities which underlie 'medium frequency' components (which may correlate with opponent colour processing), and the separation occurs at or peripheral to the level of retinal ganglion cells.

It seems necessary to postulate parallel channels to account for all the properties of scalp responses elicited by spatially-unstructured (blank) stimulus fields. Further parallel channels are required when spatially-structured stimuli are used. If the brightness contrast across the borders of a white checkerboard or strip pattern is increased, decreased or reversed, then scalp responses may be evoked which are quite different from the responses elicited by spatially-unstructured stimulus fields [32,2,6,7,24]. This also holds for coloured stimuli.

Scalp responses which are specific to sharply-accommodated chromatic contrast borders can be elicited by a foveally-viewed stimulus pattern or small (less than some 12 mins subtense) checks or stripes. Steady-state scalp responses can be elicited by rhythmically exchanging the colours of adjacent checks or stripes [21,23a]. Similarly, transient scalp responses can be elicited by causing a pattern of coloured checks or stripes to appear from a previously uniform, monochromatic stimulus field. Although the brightness of adjacent squares may be maintained *subjectively* equal, the effective intensities of the different colours are quite unequal when measured by means of contrast-specific scalp responses. Our working hypothesis is that the signals which underlie contrast-specific scalp responses are segregated into broad-band colour channels at least until the stage at which lateral interactions elicit neural signals which are specific to changes in spatial brightness contrast [23a]. The colour characteristics of responses to changes in chromatic contrast are, therefore, quite different from 'low frequency', 'medium frequency' or 'high frequency' responses to changes in the brightness of spatially-unstructured fields.

Spekreijse and I have evidence that in a deuteranopic subject the red and green channels which underlie contrast-specific responses are fused before the site at which contrast-specific signals are first elicited.

The amplitudes of steady-state scalp responses elicited by changes in chromatic contrast can, in specific experimental situations, provide a measure of visual acuity. There is, however, evidence against the notion that the same organization of retinal receptive fields underlies all subjective and objective responses to spatial contrast. One item of evidence is that the check size which elicits the largest scalp response is dissociated from the check size which produces the maximum subjective brightness contrast in a checkerboard pattern [23,29] (figure 8). For the subject shown in figure 8 a 2° foveal check pattern elicited scalp responses of maximum amplitude when individual checks subtended some 12 mins of arc. This held whether the angle of convergence of the subject's eyes was high or low, even though the change in convergence produced marked alterations in the apparent size of the external world. On the other hand, figure 8 shows that the apparent brightness of checks had a weak maximum for checks of 6 mins of arc when the convergence of the eyes was small, and a broader maximum near 14 mins of arc when the convergence of the eyes was increased. A second way of dissociating apparent brightness from the amplitude of the scalp response was to blur the stimulus pattern.

In an attempt to record scalp potentials which were minimally influenced by retinal events we stimulated the eyes with a random pattern (Julesz pattern) which appeared to oscillate in depth although the stimulus to either eye alone hardly varied. Our notion was that these responses would reflect neural activities which occurred after the signals from the two eyes came together. We were able to record scalp responses which correlated with changes in the perceived depth of the stimulus [21]. However, the amount of perceived depth exerted little influence on the amplitude of the scalp response. This seems to be due to a saturation of the amplitude of the stereoscopic scalp response which takes place for retinal disparities considerably less than 10 mins of arc; this saturation does not occur for perceived depth.

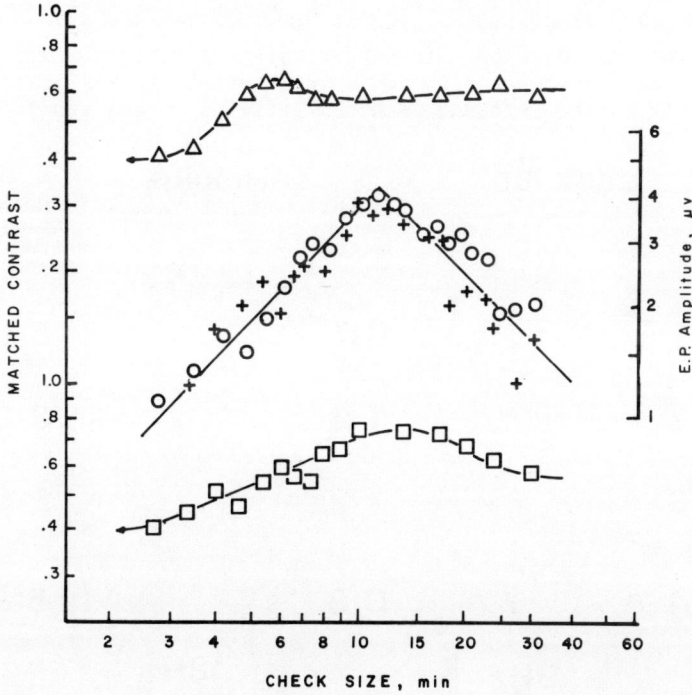

Figure 8 - Relation between check size and EP amplitude (circles and pulses), subjective brightness at 175 cm (triangles) and subjective brightness at 24 cm (squares). The fixation distance was changed from 175 cm to 24 cm by means of prisms and appropriate lenses, so that the retinal images remained approximately identical while the subject was forced to converge his eyes. (From [23]).

CLINICAL APPLICATIONS OF STEADY-STATE SCALP RESPONSES

Summarising then, there is evidence that suggests that scalp responses can be used to investigate: (a) activities at sites which may be as peripheral as the retina; (b) activities in parallel functional channels. These possibilities suggest that scalp responses could be used as a tool for detailed objective exploration of the different functions of the visual pathway. One example of this is that by comparing scalp responses to patterned and unpatterned stimuli, hemianopia with and without macular sparing can be detected. Changes of visual acuity which are restricted to a foveal quadrant subtending some 2° by 2° can easily be detected by simultaneous stimulation with several almost identical stimuli. There is evidence which suggests that this technique can detect lesions which are not detected by angiography or brain scan [8].

Normal subjects show quite different topographical distributions of the 'high frequency', 'medium frequency' and 'low frequency' scalp responses. This suggests that the generators of these responses are differently-located or differently-oriented, even though they may overlap. In support of this notion figure 9 shows steady-state responses elicited by flickering patches of light which fell on the left and right half-fields of one eye [8]. The

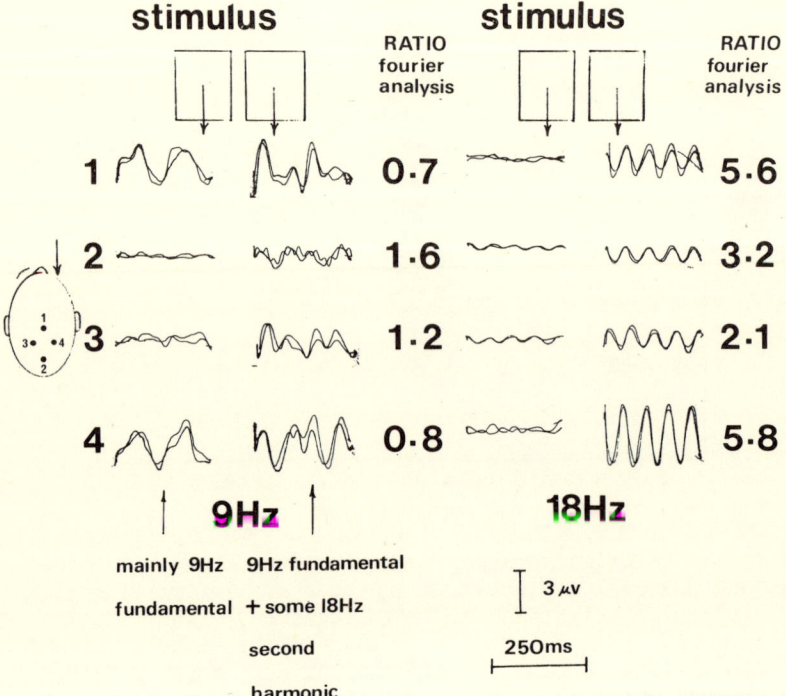

Figure 9 - Pairs of steady-state scalp responses recorded simultaneously from each of 4 electrodes. The responses were elicited by simultaneous stimulation of the left and right halffields of one eye by weakly flickering patches of light whose flicker frequencies were almost identical (0.3 Hz difference). The subject's right occipital pole had been removed surgically. Medium frequency (18 Hz) components elicited by stimulation of nasal and temporal half-fields were very different in amplitude, whereas low frequency components were not. (From [8]).

right occipital pole of this patient had been surgically removed so that she was blind in her left visual fields. The two light stimuli flickered at slightly different rates (0.3 Hz difference) so that two Fourier analysers could simultaneously record the responses elicited by the left and right stimuli respectively [*18*]. Figure 9 shows that stimulation of the blind half-field produced much smaller medium frequency (18 Hz) responses than stimulation of the 'good' half field. On the other hand, the differences between the low frequency (9 Hz) responses to stimulation of the 'good' and blind half-fields hardly fell outside normal limits. This suggests that medium frequency response components can be abolished by occipital pole lesions while low frequency components are spared. Conversely, patients whose clinical indications suggested anterior cortical lesions which did not affect vision showed marked changes in low frequency responses, but little change in medium frequency responses.

Such findings suggest that by comparing the relative effects of brain lesions on 'low frequency', 'medium frequency', 'high frequency' and contrast-specific scalp responses, an estimate of the location of destructive brain lesions can be made.

By combining such empirical findings with the powerful method described by Halliday of using prior knowledge of 'quirks' in retino-cortical projections [*6*] it is not too much to hope that some future development of scalp response methods will find a place alongside present objective methods used for detecting and locating neurological and neuro-opthalmological lesions.

ACKNOWLEDGMENTS

I wish to thank the Medical Research Council, the Migraine Trust and Sandoz Pharmaceuticals for their support. Robert F. Cartwright's technical expertise has been invaluable in this work. I thank Dr. H. Spekreijse for critical comments and for correcting the English.

REFERENCES

1. Campbell, F.W. and Maffei, L. (1970). *J. Physiol.*, **207**, 635.
2. Cobb, W.A., Morton, H.B. and Ettlinger, G. (1967). *Nature*, **216**, 1123.
3. Cohen, M.W. (1970). *J. Physiol.*, **210**, 565-580.
4. De Valois, R.L., Abramov, I. and Jacobs, G.H. (1966). *J. Opt. Soc. Amer.*, **56**, 966.
5. Haider, M., Spong, P. and Lindsley, D.B. (1964). *Science*, **145**, 180.
6. Halliday, A.M. and Michael, W.F.J. (1970). *J. Physiol.*, **208**, 409.
7. Jeffreys, D.A. (1971). *Nature*, **229**, 502.
8. Milner, B.A., Regan, D. and Heron, J.R. (1972). *Proceedings of the 9th ICSERG Symposium*, (Plenum Press, New York).
9. MacKay, D.M. (1968). *Nature*, **217**, 81.
10. Michael, W.F. and Halliday, A.M. (1971). *Brain Res.*, **32**, 311.
11. Regan, D. (1966). *Electroenceph. clin. Neurophysiol.*, **20**, 238.
12. Regan, D. (1968). *Electroenceph. clin. Neurophysiol.*, **25**, 231.

13. Regan, D. (1968). *Psychophys.*, **4**, 347.
14. Regan, D. (1970). *J. Opt. Soc. Amer.*, **60**, 856.
15. Regan, D. (1970). *Vison Res.*, **10**, 163-178.
16. Regan, D. and Heron, J.R. (1969). *J. Neurol. Neurosurg. Psychiat.*, **32**, 479.
18. Regan, D. and Cartwright, R.F. (1970). *Electroenceph. clin. Neurophysiol.*, **28**, 314.
19. Regan, D. and Heron, J.R. (1970). In *Background to Migraine*, (Heinemann), 67.
20. Regan, D. and Spekreijse, H. (1970). *Nature*, **225**, 92.
21. Regan, D. and Sperling, H.G. (1971). *Vision Res.*, **11**, 173.
22. Regan, D. and Richards, W. (1971). *Vision Res.*, **11**, 679.
23. Regan, D. and Richards, W. (1972). *J. Opt. Soc. Amer.*, (in press).
23a. Regan, D. (1972). *Advances in Medicine and Biology, Vol. 24.*
24. Regan, D. (1972). *Evoked Potentials in Psychology, Sensory Physiology and Clinical Medicine*, (Chapman and Hall, London; J. Wiley, New York).
26. Ritter, W. and Vaughan, H.G. Jr. (1969). *Science*, **164**, 326.
27. Schiller, P.H. and Chorover, S.L. (1966). *Science*, **153**, 1398.
28. Spekreijse, H. (1969). *Vision Res.*, **9**, 1461.
29. Spekreijse, H. and Tweel, L.H. van der, (1965). *Nature*, **205**, 913.
30. Spekreijse, H., Norren, D. van, and Berg, T.J.T.P. van den, (1971). *Proc. Nat. Acad. Sci.*, p.1.
31. Spekreijse, H., Tweel, L.H. van der, and Regan, D. (1972). *Vision Res.*, **12**, 52.
32. Spekreijse, H. (1966). *Analysis of EEG Responses in Man Evoked by Sine Wave Modulated Light*, (Junk, The Hague).
33. Sutton, S. (1969). In *Average Evoked Potentials*, (eds. Donchin, E and Lindsley, D.B.), NASA SP-191.
34. Tweel, L.H. van der, (1961). *Ann. N.Y. Acad. Sci.*, **89**, 829.
35. Tweel, L.H. van der, and Verduyn Lunel, H.F.E. (1965). *Electroenceph. clin. Neurophysiol.*, **18**, 587.
36. Tweel, L.H. van der, and Spekreijse, H. (1969). *Ann. N.Y. Acad. Sci.*, **156**, 678.
37. Tweel, L.H. van der, Regan, D. and Spekreijse, H. (1969). *Proceedings of the 7th International ICSERG Symposium*, (University of Istanbul).
38. Vaughan, H.G. and Silverstein, L. (1968). *Science*, **160**, 207.
39. Westheimer, G. (1967). *J. Physiol.*, **190**, 139-154.

SYSTEM ANALYSIS APPROACH TO THE PROBLEMS OF VISION

HENK SPEKREIJSE

*Laboratory of Medical Physics, University of Amsterdam,
Herengracht 196, Amsterdam*

Investigations of the dynamic properties of the visual system date from as early as the 18th century. At first the choice of stimulus was based on simplicity. But this simplicity was for the designer of equipment rather than for the system analysist. Perhaps this technical simplicity accounts for the almost exclusive use of square wave flashes of variable durations. Such stimuli, however, do not allow the effects of luminance change and mean luminance to be separated with any facility. The resulting chaos in writings on the subject of flicker perception rapidly becomes clear to any determined reader who peruses the (roughly) 1350 papers listed in 1953 by Landis. It could be claimed that de Lange (who was by the way a Dutchman) introduced some measure of order into this chaos.

de LANGE CURVES; FLICKER FUSION IN MAN

Although Ives in 1922 introduced the harmonic analysis approach that underlies present day understanding of flicker perception, the full potential of Fourier analysis only became evident after de Lange's (1954, 1958) extensive study at photopic levels of illumination. De Lange, who perhaps significantly was an engineer, used mainly sine wave modulated light, a signal which had proved to be so useful in the analysis of linear systems. The two important parameters of a sinusoidal stimulus are the average luminance L_0, and the amplitude of the luminance modulation A, which can be controlled independently of L_0 (insert of figure 1). For a given average luminance, L_0, de Lange plotted the threshold modulation m ($m = A/L$) as a function of frequency. For historical reasons he used logarithmic scales. Examples of such curves of flicker sensitivity versus frequency (de Lange curves) are given in figure 1 (left side). De Lange demonstrated that for conventional waveforms the high frequency (> 10 Hz) flicker threshold depends only on the amplitude of the fundamental Fourier component. This suggested that the system behaved linearly near threshold. In order to account for the extremely sharp attenuation in the high frequency region models were proposed that are made up of as many as ten cascaded temporal integrations or RC-elements (DeVoe, 1964; Sperling, 1964; Marimont, 1965). One should, however, be cautious with such a linear description based on a constant response criterion since it only holds if the threshold detector is the last and *only* nonlinear element in the chain of transformations. Suppose, for example, that the chain consists of the following three subsequent stages: (1) a static square-root saturating element, (2) a single RC-element and (3) a threshold detector (figure 2). With

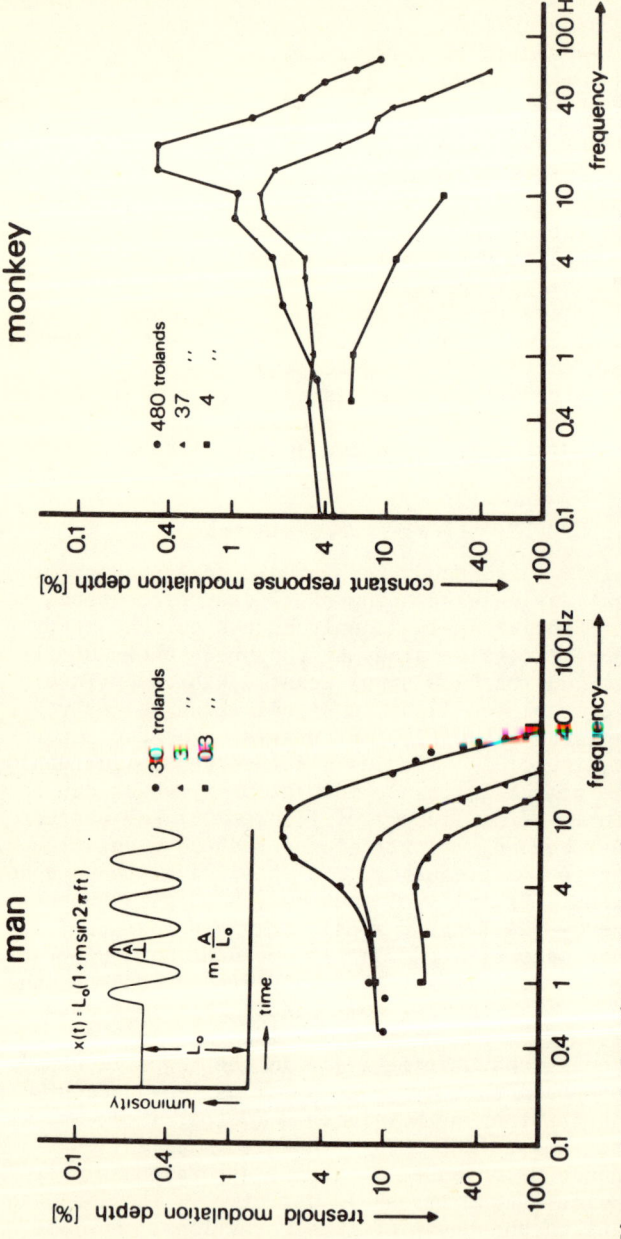

Figure 1 - Left Side: Modulation depth for flicker fusion in man as a function of frequency. White, sinusoidally modulated light is used at three different average retinal illuminations. The Maxwellian field subtended 15° of visual angle. Insert: The unmodualted stimulus, of intensity L_0, changes at a given moment into a sinusoidal modulated light with amplitude A. The depth of modulation is conveniently expressed by the parameter $m = A/L_0$. The stimulus frequency is f (Hz).
Right Side: Amplitude characteristics of a yellow⁻ blue⁺ monkey LGN cell determined with blue, sinusoidally modulated light at three different retinal illuminations. The amplitude characteristics (de Lange curves) are obtained by plotting the modulation depth required for each stimulus frequency to reach a constant response of 8.6 spikes/sec.

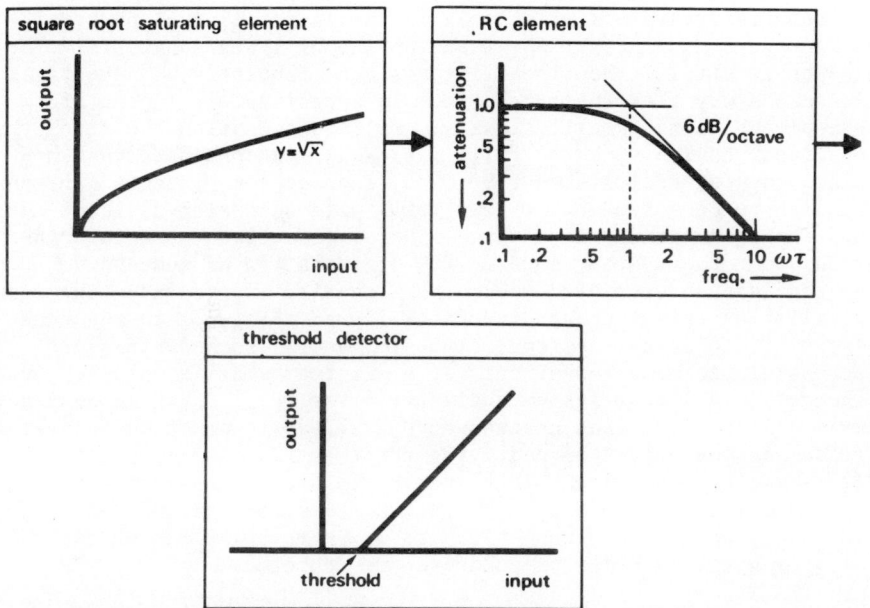

Figure 2 - Example of a nonlinear system for which the constant response method will give erroneously a two-stage integrator (2 RC-elements) description.

this model the compression caused by the saturation element has the result that the amplitude of the luminance modulation must increase more than proportional to frequency in order to maintain a constant output. This results in a steeper high frequency fall-off than could be attributed to a single RC-element, so that a linear description would erroneously consist of a two-stage integrator model! However, Talbot's Law may still provide a criterion (van der Tweel, 1961).

FLICKER RESPONSES IN MONKEY LATERAL GENICULATE NUCLEUS

In order to determine whether an N-stage integrator model holds for human flicker sensitivity, we studied the spike discharge patterns evoked by sinusoidal luminance modulation in single lateral geniculate cells of macaque monkey (Spekreijse et al., 1971). We plotted the modulation depths required to reach an arbitrary threshold criterion as a function of stimulus frequency (right side of figure 1). Since the psychophysical data in the left side of figure 1 were obtained for a human subject under the same stimulus conditions as those of the animal experiment, both sets of data may be compared directly. The overall similarity is evident. The only difference is the steepness of the high frequency fall-off. Although this fall-off in psychophysical data may reach values as high as 60 dB/octave (10 RC-elements), we never observed such high values in our LGN-data. In the case shown, the attenuation amounts only to 12 dB/octave (2 RC-elements). All this suggests that an N-stage linear integrator model for flicker fusion seems valid.

Yet linear systems exist only in the mind; all real physical systems are nonlinear. Why then the use of linear analysis? The answer is simple. Nonlinear systems can frequently be investigated in such a way that their behaviour is approximately linear, for example by using 'small' signals. In this situation the strengths of linear analysis can be fully deployed. In contrast, when nonlinear system analysis must be used, each system presents a fresh problem to be solved on its own terms with a 'custom-designed' approach. Yet there is a paradox here. Sometimes more information about the system, such as the organization of successive stages, can be extracted when a nonlinearity is present. The possibility of this approach is especially advantageous in the analysis of biological systems, since in general such systems are accessible to measurement only at a limited number of sites. Furthermore, in linear system analysis, noise (e.g. 'spontaneous' activity) is no more than an annoyance, whereas in a nonlinear system noise has the effect of modifying the transfer characteristics. It is worth pointing out that 'noise' is one of the most striking characteristics of biological systems. A direct demonstration of the above points is given at figure 3, where spike responses of retinal ganglion cells of goldfish are depicted.

NONLINEAR GOLDFISH GANGLION CELL RESPONSES

If a goldfish retina is stimulated with sine wave modulated light a burst of action potentials occurs only once during each stimulus cycle (left column of figure 3). The mid column of figure 3 gives period averaged spike responses as a function of modulation depth. For half the stimulus period the density distribution of the nerve impulses has roughly the same shape as the sinusoidal stimulus but during the other half of the stimulus cycle no spike discharge is observed at all. Since the 'amplitude' of the average response is approximately proportional to the amplitude (modulation depth) of the sinewave stimulus, the waveform distortions in the discharge pattern of goldfish ganglion cells can be modelled by a half-wave linear rectifier (Spekreijse, 1969). This rectifier dominates the response for modulation depths as small as 5% but for a still lower modulation depth (2%) we find an almost pure sinusoidal response. This demonstration that even an essential nonlinear system may behave linearly near threshold, provides a further example of the wide applicability of the 'small' signal approach. The data in the right column of figure 3 show that it is the internal noise of spontaneous activity which is responsible for such a seemingly linear behaviour. If the 'amplitude' of the noise sufficiently exceeds the stimulus amplitude, the input-output relation may suggest that the system is linear, although it contains nonlinear or even essential nonlinear elements. During the experiment depicted in the right column of figure 3 the spontaneous discharge rate increased up till a frequency of 30 spikes/sec. When this level was reached we observed an almost linear response even for a modulation as high as 60%! Our conclusion is that if you get a linear output from a biological system, don't be too certain that the system is linear, since it is quite possible that

SYSTEM ANALYSIS APPROACH TO THE PROBLEM OF VISION

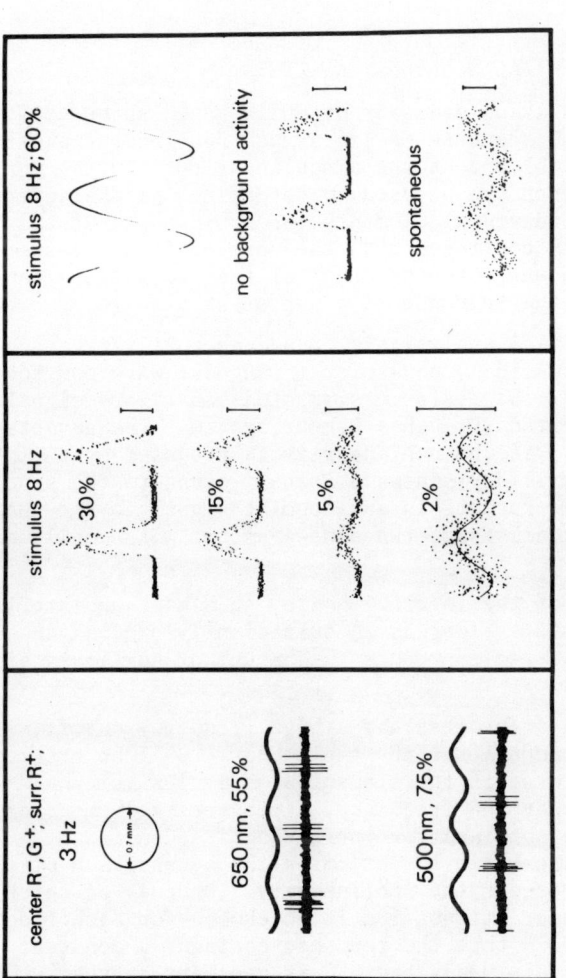

Figure 3 - First Column: Ganglion cell responses to sine wave modulated light. The parameter m varies between 0 (0%) for unmodulated and 1 (100%) for fully modulated light. The mean intensity of the stimulus is approximately 6 µW/cm2 for the red and 20 µW/cm2 for the green stimulus.

Middle Column: Average spike response of a red-off centre process as a function of the modulation depth. The mean intensity of the red stimulus is approximately 1 µW/cm². The number of summations with the CAT computer amounts to 300. The calibration bars are 20 spikes/bin. The bin duration is 625 µsec.

Right Column: After an increase in spontaneous activity the highly distorted ganglion cell response (middle figure) becomes undistorted (bottom figure), even at a modulation depth of 60%. The number of summations with the CAT computer is 400; the mean intensity of the red sinusoidal modulated light is approximately 1 µW/cm2.

noise has masked the nonlinearities. Such noise can arise within
the system or can be quantal noise inherent to the stimulus (van
der Tweel and Spekreijse, 1969). On the other hand, if strongly
nonlinear responses occur in the presence of neural noise, then
this means that there is no interaction between the system noise
and the responses. One example of this possibility is the visually
evoked responses in man. These responses are highly distorted,
although the spontaneous cortical activity is many times larger
than the responses.

SEQUENTIAL NONLINEAR ANALYSIS

The masking or linearizing property of noise can also be used to
determine the functional sequence of linear and nonlinear transformations in a system which contains a nonlinearity. Furthermore,
the linearizing phenomenon can be used to determine the characteristics of the various individual elements (Spekreijse and Oosting,
1970). This possibility contrasts with the case of linear systems
or of a linear approach where the sequence of transformations can
never be detected from the response of a system as-a-whole.

The method of sequential analysis is to add an auxiliary signal
such as noise, or a sinusoidal, square or triangular waveform to
the sinusoidal stimulus. We prefer a sinusoidal auxiliary signal
since it passes undistorted through a linear system. The advantage
of this feature is that, if the nonlinearity is preceded by a linear process, then an auxiliary sinewave $B\sin \omega t$ added to the sinusoidal stimulus $A\sin \omega t$, results in an incoming signal to the non-
linearity which still consists of two sinewaves but with amplitudes
A^* and B^*.

Just as in the case of the internal noise, an almost undistorted
response will be obtained as long as B^* sufficiently exceeds A^*.
Period averaging is required to reduce the amount of auxiliary signal in the final record.

Suppose that the linear process has a high frequency cutoff,
then for increasing frequencies β the amplitude B^* will be progressively reduced. Therefore, if the sinusoidal stimulus $A\sin \omega t$
retains the same amplitude and frequency, a progressively more distorted response will be obtained for increasing frequencies β.
With this method it is possible to determine the attenuation of a
linear process which precedes the nonlinearity. One way of determining this initial linear attenuation is to choose for each frequency β such an amplitude B that the response contains a constant
amount of distortion. This means that B^* is constant at the input
of the nonlinearity. By plotting B against β on logarithmic scales
(just as in the case of the de Lange curves), the amplitude characteristic of the first linear process can be obtained.

This method is illustrated in figure 4 where the linearizing
effect of high frequency auxiliary signals upon the visually evoked
potentials in man (left column) and the spike-discharges in goldfish
(right column) is shown. Both sets of data show high frequency attenuation since for increasing auxiliary frequencies the response

becomes progressively more distorted. This type of data suggested that both in man and goldfish the elements preceding the nonlinearity have a high frequency attenuation of the order of 18 dB/octave (Spekreijse, 1966).

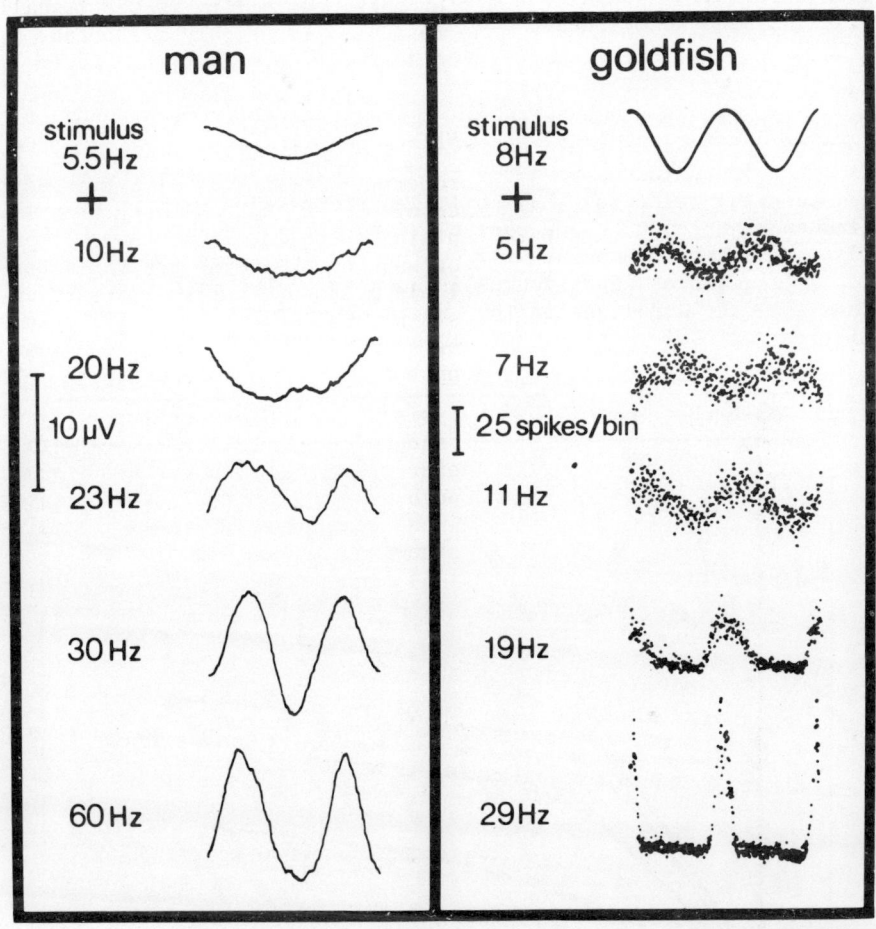

Figure 4 - Linearizing of visually evoked potentials in man (left column) and the spike discharges in goldfish (right column) as a function of the frequency of the sinusoidal auxiliary signal. In man the responses are to a 10% sinusoidally modulated light with a frequency of 5.5 Hz and a mean luminance of 200 asb. The sinusoidal auxiliary signal has the same modulation depth. In goldfish the period averaged spike responses are to a sinusoidal stimulus of 8 Hz with a modulation depth of 5%. The sinusoidal auxiliary signal is 50% modulated. The intensity of the red stimulus is 1 µW/cm^2. The bin duration is 625 µsec.

The similarity between these two sets of data, and the correspondence with the lateral geniculate data in monkey has an implication which I would like to stress. This implication is that the sequential method provides information about retinal processing in man from signals recorded at electrodes attached to his scalp. Such information would have been impossible to obtain if the human visual system were linear.

The same kind of information about the human visual system which can be deduced from linearizing experiments can also be obtained more directly from the saturation characteristics. If the amplitude of a sinewave modulated light is progressively increased, it is often found that a point is reached above which the visual evoked occipital response (VER) no longer increases. Suppose that high frequency attenuation precedes the saturating element. In that case the saturation point will be reached at higher modulation depths for increasing stimulus frequencies. The data in figure 5 show that the amplitude of the VER in man saturates at higher modulation depths for stimulus frequencies below and above 30 Hz.

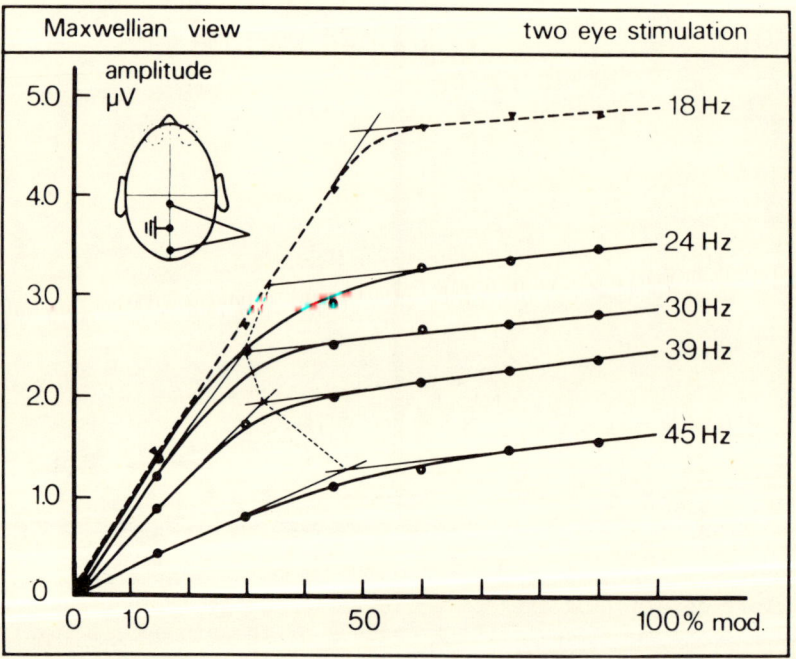

Figure 5 - Saturation of the occipital responses in man as a function of the frequency of the sinusoidal light stimulus. The mean luminance is 20,000 asb, the Maxwellian field extended 20°. For clarity the saturation curve to the 18 Hz stimulus has been doubled in amplitude.

These shifts in saturation with frequency suggest a high frequency attentuation of some 18 dB/octave, indicating also that the rectifying and saturating element probably coincide. Therefore all the electrophysiological data in man, monkey and goldfish described above point to the notion that the human high frequency flicker sensitivity can be modelled with an N-stage integrator model, distributed along the visual pathway probably up to the cortex.

SPATIAL NONLINEAR ANALYSIS

In the above type of sequential analysis the visual system is oversimplified into an N-channel model, with identical, independent pathways. For the study of the flicker sensitivity to large homogeneous fields this simplification may be justified, but as soon as small fields are considered, the spatial integrative properties of the visual system have to be taken into account. Spatial integration relates to one of the most important features of the visual system. For example there are even special retinal elements, such as horizontal and amacrine cells, whose major task seems the spreading of nervous influences in the plane of the retina. Sequential analysis offers a powerful tool for the study of the location and the characteristics of spatial interactions. We have used this approach to study the spatial interaction in the goldfish retina, which for this purpose is stimulated with a checkerboard pattern. The pattern contains two sets of elements, each of which can be modulated independently (figure 6). Sinewave modulation of one set of squares alone gives a response that (according to the data in figure 2) is similar to a half-wave rectified sinusoid. Counterphase modulation of the other set of squares at the same mean intensity and modulation depth as the first set results, of course, in the same half-wave rectified response but shifted 180° in phase. Simultaneous counterphase stimulation of both sets of checkerboard squares can give one of the two following two responses (figure 6): (a) either a full-wave rectified sinusoid or (b) no spike discharge at all.

This can be understood as follows: if the spatial summation takes place *after* the essential nonlinear element, then the response would consist of a full-wave rectified sinusoid with the same amplitude as the original half-wave rectified response (figure 6a). On the other hand, if spatial summation occurs at a site *preceding* the nonlinear element, then the two sets of input sinusoids counterbalance each other completely and no response results (figure 6b).

Figure 6c gives the actual data for a green-'off' centreprocess. As is evident from this figure, there is no spike discharge when the two sets of squares are modulated simultaneously in counterphase. This holds, of course, only when the strengths of the responses to each set of squares are identical. Since neither the type of pattern nor the size of the pattern elements proved to be of importance, the data demonstrate directly that spatial summation takes place preceding the essential nonlinear element in the goldfish retina. Moreover an algebraic mode of operation governs this interaction, i.e. the interaction is linear (Spekreijse and van den Berg, 1971).

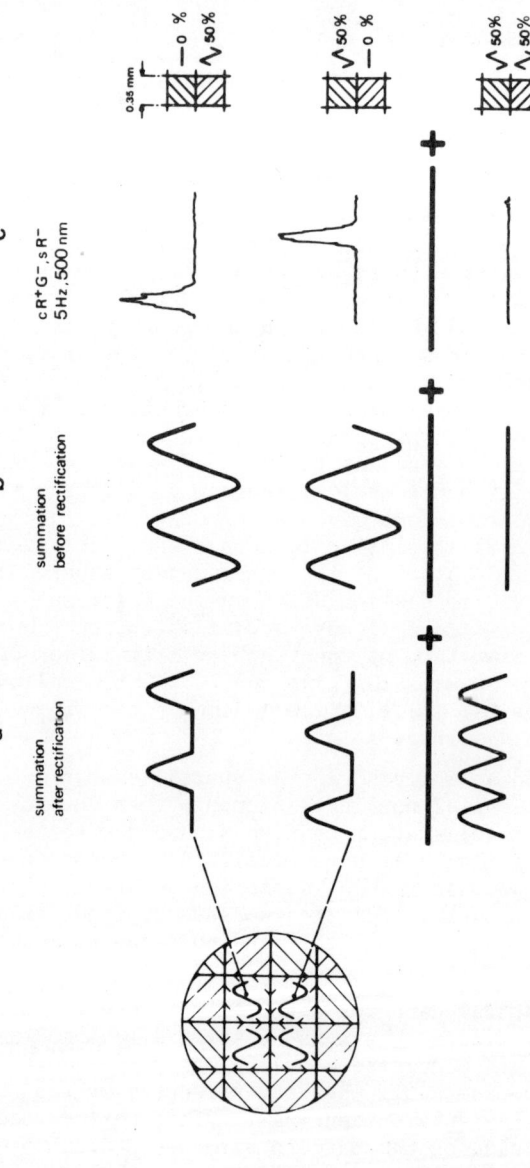

Figure 6 - Schematic representation (columns a and b) of retinal modes of summation between counterphase signals generated by the two sets of counterphase modulated squares of a checkerboard pattern. Column c gives the actual data for a green-off centre process. The top figure is the average spike response to modulation (50%) of one set of squares (0.35 mm width). The other set of squares is not modulated at all but has a steady intensity identical to the mean intensity of the modulated set. Reversing the condition and modulating the other set of squares with the same depth, but in counterphase, results in the mid figure response. Simultaneous counterphase modulation of both sets of squares does not result in a spike discharge at all (bottom figure). The mean intensity of the green stimulus light is approximately 4 µW/cm². The number of summations is 100, the modulation frequency is 5 Hz.

SPATIAL DYNAMIC INTERACTIONS

Figure 1 shows the de Lange curves for man and monkey for three different retinal illuminations. The shapes of these curves are a function of the mean intensity of the flickering light. On the other hand, both van der Tweel (1961) and Kelly (1959) have shown that in man the flicker fusion curves are also a function of the spot size used. This suggests that spatial interactions strongly influence the shapes of the de Lange curves.

Since the diameter of the receptive field centres in the goldfish retina is constant irrespective both of the spectral coding of the central processes and of the presence of peripheral processes (Spekreijse et al., 1972), then it is a straightforward matter to quantify the dependence of the dynamic characteristics of the goldfish ganglion cell responses on intensity and spot size, especially since these diameters, as determined by the area of full summation, extend up to 1 mm in the plane of the retina. In accordance with the checkerboard experiments (figure 6), the dynamic characteristics of the ganglion cells are determined by a simple algebraic summation within a receptive field centre (figure 7).

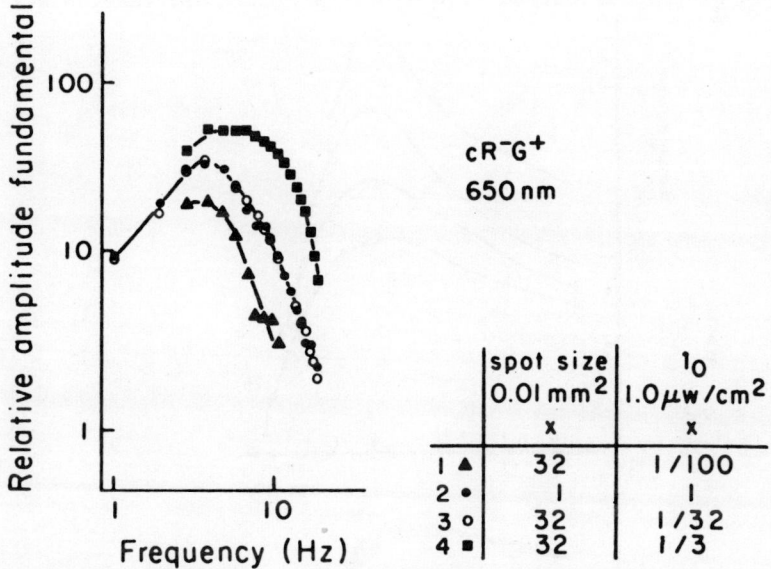

Figure 7 - Amplitude characteristics of the central red off process of a spontaneous ganglion cell are depicted as a function of the luminous flux (power) of a Gaussian noise modulated (σ = 40%) stimulus spot. A constant flux $E = AI_0$, where A is the stimulus area and I_0 the mean stimulus intensity, gives identical curves (2 and 3).

This figure shows that the shape of the amplitude characteristics depends on the luminous flux (power) falling within a receptive field rather than on the intensity of the stimulus spot.

The same amplitude characteristic can be obtained by increasing the stimulated retinal area by a factor of 32 and diminishing the intensity by the same factor or vice versa (curves 2 and 3). This means that firstly all the output signals of the early retinal processes are summed, next the system is 'tuned' - the term Floyd Ratliff (1969) uses for the Limulus eye - according to the absorbed light power. The data demonstrate directly that receptor processes cannot be sole determinants of the shape of the de Lange curves because spatial summation plays such an important rôle.

ORIGIN OF RETINAL NOISE

The dependence of the dynamic characteristics of the ganglion cell responses in goldfish on intensity (Schellart and Spekreijse, 1972) offers also an opportunity to determine the location of retinal noise in the chain of transformations converging in the ganglion cell responses. If the dynamics of the spontaneous spike activity does not depend on the mean level of illumination, then the 'noise' enters at a site after the spatial summation point. The data in figure 8 indicate that this is the case. Although the shape of the dynamic characteristics of the ganglion cell responses changes with illumination, the dynamics of the spontaneous activity

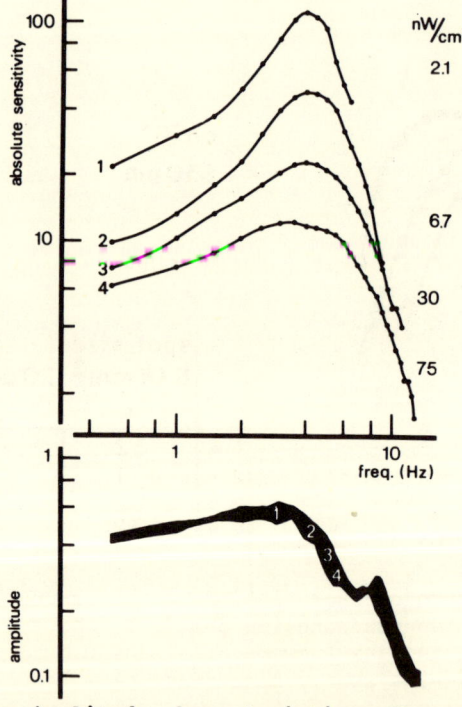

Figure 8 - Amplitude characteristics of a spontaneous ganglion cell as a function of the mean intensity of the stimulus light. Whereas these curves change, the characteristics (bottom half) of the spontaneous activity remain the same irrespective of the level of illumination.

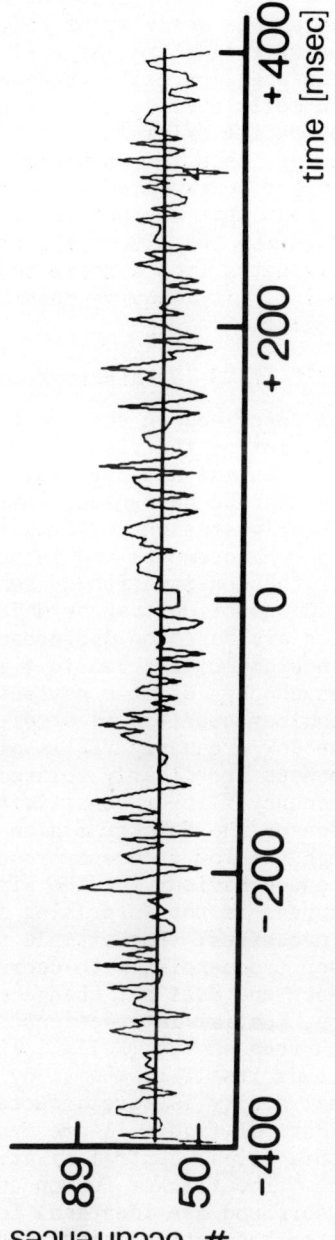

Figure 9 - Cross-intensity function of the spontaneous activity of two neighbouring ganglion cells. The horizontal line represents the theoretical expectation value for uncorrelated activity of the ganglion cells.

remains the same irrespective of the level of illumination. This point can be strengthened by a second argument which concerns the correlation between spontaneous activity of neighbouring ganglion cells. Since the receptive fields are large (1 mm) and located concentrically around the ganglion cell, then the receptive fields of neighbouring ganglion cells overlap each other completely. Therefore, if the retinal noise originates at a stage preceding the spatial summation point, then the spontaneous activity of neighbouring ganglion cells might be expected to be highly correlated. We found experimentally that this was not so (figure 9). This indicates again that in goldfish the stochastic character of the ganglion cell responses originates from a noise-source located after the spatial summation point. It is quite possible that the ganglion cell is a noisy cell!.

APPLICATIONS IN PATHOLOGY

Experiments have been described in the preceding sections in which the nonlinear operation of the visual system is employed to split up the system in sequential and parallel stages. It might at first seem surprising that we have used dynamic characteristics for this purpose since nearly stationary stimuli are observed in everyday vision, although eye movements and in particular saccades may be of importance for the continuation of sensation. Yet sometimes in pathology also distinctions can be made between normal and affected vision which are based on differences specific in high frequency operation. An example is given in figure 10, where the electrophysiology and psychophysics of a patient with the right eye affected with retrobulbar neuritis is studied during 4 subsequent weeks. Although the low frequency VER is almost unaffected, the high frequency responses are clearly related to the return to (about) normal high frequency flicker sensitivity. Abnormality in the high frequency region of the flicker fusion curve is obvious in this patient, although the low frequency responses do not seem to be abnormal. Different behaviour for the high and low frequency tails of the de Lange curves is not surprising since the two seem to depend on different processes. For example the high frequency tail shifts towards lower frequencies with decreasing luminance, although the low frequency end does not change much with luminance (figure 1). Furthermore, spatial interactions seem to operate differently at low and high frequencies (Kelly, 1969). Amblyopia is a visual defect which lends itself to the study of this aspect, since in amblyopia visual acuity is more affected than the luminance sensitivity. The data of figure 11 are from a subject with amblyopia ex anisometropia (0,+4) central fixation and some stereopsis (vis.ac. 1.25;1/6). The flicker fusion curves for homogeneous 3° fields without surround are identical for both eyes (left of figure 11), and counterphase stimulation with 20' checks gives identical curves for frequencies above 20 Hz. However, for low frequencies the sensitivities of the two eyes differ by a factor of 10 (right of figure 11). This finding is in accordance with the general clinical characteristics of amblyopia. At these low frequencies the sensitivity of the amblyopic eye is the same as for

SYSTEM ANALYSIS APPROACH TO THE PROBLEMS OF VISION

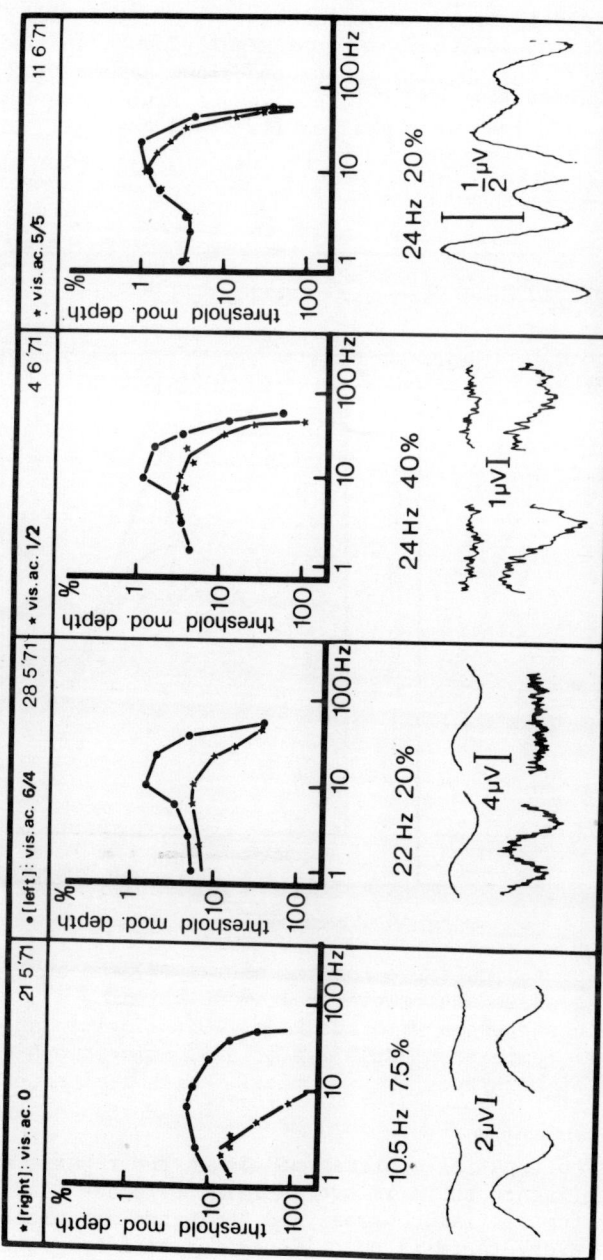

Figure 10 - Psychophysics (top row) and electrophysiology (bottom row) of a patient with a right eye (★) affected with retrobulbar neuritis. With the recovery of visual acuity the high frequency tails of the flicker fusion curves of the right eye become progressively (weekly sessions) more similar to those of the left eye (●). The first picture in the bottom row shows the low frequency (10.5 Hz) occipital response of each eye to sinewave modulated light. From the first session on these responses were similar for both eyes. The other pictures show the high frequency (22-24 Hz) responses. Whereas at the first session no such response could be obtained with the affected eye, at the fourth and last session the two eyes do not differ much. The mean luminance is 5000 asb.

homogeneous fields, although in contrast the sensitivity of the normal eye is enhanced. Spatial contrast models have been proposed to explain this enhanced sensitivity (Kelly, 1971). These models are based on interactions between neighbouring spatial elements. It is tempting to ascribe amblyopia to impairment of such spatial interactions. However, the spatial interactions are assumed to steepen the low frequency fall-off for homogeneous fields, so that impairment should result in a more shallow low frequency tail for the amblyopic eye. This has not been found in practice.

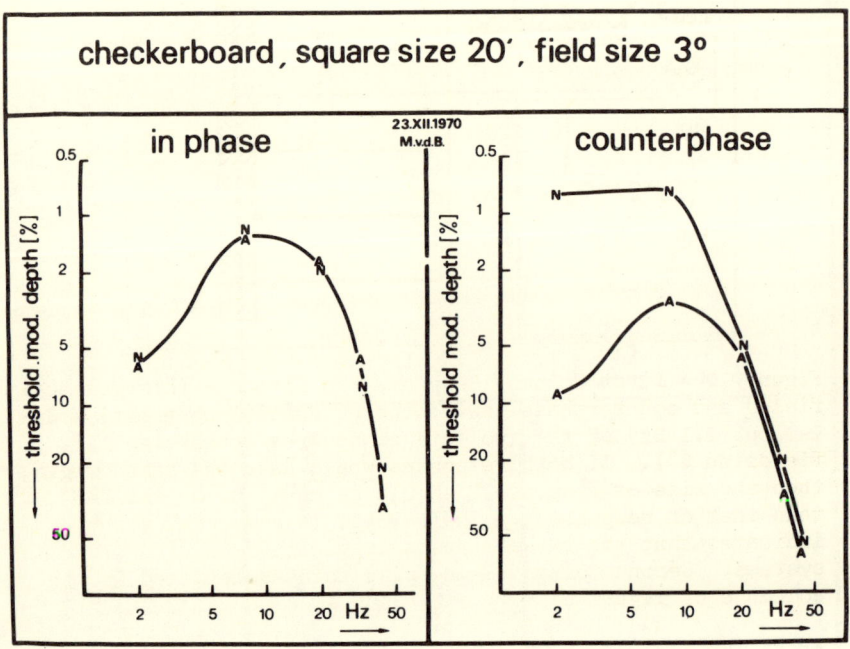

Figure 11 - Flicker fusion curves of the normal (N) and amblyopic (A) eye to in-phase and counterphase modulation of a 3° checkerboard field patterned with checks of 20'. To in-phase stimulation - i.e. luminance modulation of a 3° homogeneous field - the data of both eyes are identical. Mean luminance is 5000 asb.

A common weakness of spatial contrast models is their basis on luminance processing, since there is overwhelming evidence that in the human visual system spatial contrast and luminance are processed separately. However, there is no evidence for similar processing of spatial contrast in the goldfish retina.

In man visual evoked occipital potentials can be recorded that are a function of spatial contrast changes only (figure 12). The left side of figure 12 shows VER's which are obtained with the same checkerboard stimulator that was used for the goldfish experiments described in figure 4.

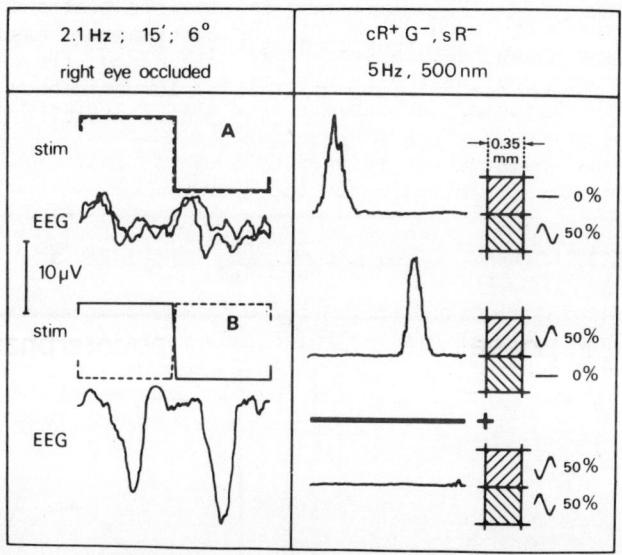

Figure 12 - First Column: Responses to in-phase (homogeneous field) and counterphase (switching of spatial contrast) modulation (2.1 Hz) of the two sets of squares (checksize 15', fieldsize 6°). If both responses would have the same origin, then the size of response B should be equal to or smaller than that of response A. The reverse is the case, which indicates that the two responses originate from different systems. Second Column: Same spike data as depicted in the column c of figure 6.

As in the case of the ganglion cell responses (right side of figure 12) our hypothesis was that no response at all should be produced with counterphase modulation if the checkerboard squares were considerably smaller than the retinal summation fields, since the flicker signals of adjacent checks would cancel before reaching the rectifying stage. Conversely the VER should be similar to that elucidated by homogeneous field stimulation when sufficiently large squares were used. The left side of figure 12 shows that the results for the human VER did not fit our prediction. To our surprise the responses elicited by small checks, modulated in counterphase, were much *larger* (figure B) than the responses to homogeneous field stimulation (figure A). This demonstrates that these two responses originate from different systems, one for luminance and the other one for spatial contrast processing. However, there is still no coherent system analytic approach for the latter type of responses.

CONCLUSION

In this paper I have tried to point out that, although linear system analysis is very convenient, there are situations in which the behaviour of biological systems are not all linear even when 'small' signals are used. I have described an approach to this situation and shown how, in some cases, the system can be split into linear and nonlinear elements and furthermore how these elements can be characterized and arranged into a functional sequence. I have also given examples that not only nonlinearities but also natural visual defects can be used as tools to gain further information about the organization of the system.

ACKNOWLEDGMENTS

I am grateful to Dr. D. Regan for critical reading of the manuscript. This research was supported by a grant (90-6) from the Netherlands Organization for the Advancement of Pure Research (Z.W.O.) and by the Organization for Health Research (T.N.O.), The Hague.

REFERENCES

de Lange, H. Dzn. (1954). Relationship between critical flicker-frequency and a set of low frequency characteristics of the eye, *J. Opt. Soc. Amer.*, **44**, 380-389.

de Lange, H. Dzn: Research into the dynamic nature of the human fovea→cortex systems with intermittent and modulated light; I. (1958). Attenuation characteristics with white and coloured light, *J. Opt. Soc. Amer.*, **48**, 777; II. (1958). Phase shift in brightness and delay in colour perception, *J. Opt. Soc. Amer.*, **48**, 784.

DeVoe, R.D. (1964). Linear electrical flicker responses from the eye of the wolf spider, *Doc. Opthalmol.*, **18**, 128.

Ives, H.E. (1922). Critical frequency relations in scotopic vision, *J. Opt. Soc. Amer. Rev. Sci. Instrum.*, **6**, 254.

Kelly, D.H. (1959). Effects of sharp edges in a flickering field, *J. Opt. Soc. Amer.*, **49**, 730.

Kelly, D.H. (1964). Sine waves and flicker fusion, *Doc. Opthalmol.*, **18**, 16.

Kelly, D.H.: Theory of flicker and transient responses; I. (1971). Uniform fields, *J. Opt. Soc. Amer.*, **61**, 537; II. (1971). Counterphase gratings, *J. Opt. Soc. Amer.*, **61**, 632.

Landis, C. (1953). *An Annotated Bibliography of Flicker Fusion Phenomena*, (Armed Forces - National Research Council, University of Michigan).

Marimont, R.B. (1965). Numerical studies of the Fuortes-Hodgkin *Limulus* model, *J. Physiol.*, **179**, 489.

Ratliff, F., Knight, B.W. and Graham, N. (1969). On tuning and amplification by lateral inhibition, *Proc. Nat. Acad. Sci. U.S.A.*, **62**, 733.

Schellart, N.A.M. and Spekreijse, H. (1972). Dynamic characteristics of retinal ganglion cell responses in goldfish, *J. Gen. Physiol.*, **59**, 1.

Spekreijse, H. (1966). *Analysis of EEG responses in man, evoked by sine wave modulated light*, (Thesis), (Dr. W. Junk, Publr., The Hague).

Spekreijse, H. (1969). Rectification in the goldfish retina. Analysis by sinusoidal and auxiliary stimulation, *Vision Res.*, **9**, 1461.

Spekreijse, H. and Oosting, J. (1970). Linearizing: A method for analysing and synthesizing nonlinear systems, *Kybernetik*, **7**, 23.

Spekreijse, H., Norren, D. van, and Berg, T.J.T.P. van den, (1971). LGN flicker responses in primate and human flicker fusion, *Proc. Nat. Acad. Sci. U.S.A.*, **68**, 2802.

Spekreijse, H. and Berg, T.J.T.P. van den, (1971). Interaction between color and spatial coded processes converging to retinal ganglion cells in goldfish, *J. Physiol.*, **215**, 679.

Spekreijse, H., Wagner, H.G. and Wolbarsht, M.L. (1972). The spectral and spatial coding of ganglion cell responses in goldfish retina, *J. Neurophysiol.*, **35**, 73.

Sperling, G. (1964). Linear theory and the psychophysics of flicker, *Doc. Opthalmol.*, **18**, 3.

Tweel, L.H. van der, (1961). Some problems in vision regarded with respect to linearity and frequency response, *Ann. N.Y. Acad. Sci.*, **89**, 829.

Tweel, L.H. van der, and Spekreijse, H. (1969). Signal transport and rectification in the human evoked response system, *Ann. N.Y. Acad. Sci.*, **156**, 678.

FOOD FOR THOUGHT

I.J. GOOD

The University Professor of Statistics at Virginia Polytechnic Institute and State University, Blacksburg

PBI's

This paper is intended to be an exercise in armchair neurophysiology, a potpourri of partly-baked ideas (pbi's) of possible interest at this brainy conference. If justification is required, F.A. Hayek's remark can be held in mind, that speculation is another name for thinking. *Cogito ergo cogito*. A computer that could speculate would be a computer that could think.

Pbi's can be of various lengths, but should never be very long. To set the tone, let me start with some very short ones.

(1) Could one learn to interpret one's own EEG by listening to it coded in colour and sound (Good, 1967)? This possibility has recently been partially commercialized. (2) Happiness is wide vision. (This can be taken literally or metaphorically). (3) Did immortal men become extinct by Natural Selection (Good, 1967)? That is, were tribes with centenarian chieftains easily defeated in battle? (4) Does the paucity of missing links show that when intelligence reached a certain level its selective advantage suddenly became extremely great? (Good, 1971c). (5) Young children can be trained to apprehend absolute pitch, but the ability apparently atrophies later if not trained early. Is this because absolute pitch was useful a long time ago, when almost the only music was the song of the birds? I don't think birds change key and their twittering might have signalled the approach of wild animals. (Contrast Good, 1968b). (6) The appreciation of chords is probably also "built in" since few natural sounds are pure tones, and vowel sounds are also chords. (7) Why does light span only about an octave? More precisely: why has Natural Selection given us the ability to see only one octave of the electromagnetic spectrum? (8) Do children have good parrot-style memories because they don't yet have enough knowledge (or grammatical skill) to rely very much on higer-level thinking? (9) Is this true of other animals and does it explain imprinting? (10) Neurons in the brain don't regenerate (or divide) because it is better to forget than to remember something that didn't happen (Good, 1967). This pbi applies to acquired long-term memories rather than to the built-in ones. The idea would not apply to lower animals who have little acquired long-term memory, so it is not refuted by some comments made by Dr. Raisman in his paper at this conference. I once dangerously conjectured (Good, 1970a) that the large size of the Golgi apparatus in the cortical cells of humans might be responsible for their failure to regenerate. If this conjecture is correct, the Golgi apparatus

should not be so large relatively in the cortical neurons in the lower animals.

The bakedness of a pbi is sometimes improved after a long delay. For example, consider a communication channel along which pulses are sent, and having various regeneration stations where these pulses are "squared up". The question was raised in 1963 whether it is optimal for these stations to be uniformly spaced, thus explaining the uniform spacing of the nodes of Ranvier (Good 1963; 1967). This question has only recently been tackled (Osteyee and Good, 1972). For a variety of models we found that uniform spacing was optimal except in very noisy channels. Most neurons cannot be very noisy.

Some pbi's are convincing although they merit further development. Consider, for example, the following proof that computers and cybernetics have had an important influence on philosophy.

A great modern philosopher, by definition, is one for whom a volume has been edited by P.A. Schilpp. Therefore Bertrand Russell was a great philosopher. Now Russell claimed (1921) that the following characteristic broadly distinguishes living organisms from dead matter: "The response of an organism to a given stimulus is very often dependent upon the past history of the organism, and not merely upon the stimulus and the *hitherto discoverable* present state of the organism". (Russell's italics). He would hardly have said that thirty years later unless he wanted to argue that electronic computers are alive. (Good, 1970b).

OCKHAM'S LOBOTOMY

Ockham's razor is a well-known principle in the hard sciences. It states that hypotheses should not be multiplied without necessity. A more modern form of the principle is that, of two hypotheses, both of which explain the same set of facts, the simpler one has the larger logical probability. There is also a sharpened and fairly quantitative form of the razor which takes into account the *degrees* to which the hypotheses explain the facts (Good, 1968a) and this might be more appropriate in the present context. At any rate the simpler form of Ockham's razor can be misleading when applied to brain models, and has been called "Ockham's lobotomy" (Good, 1965). The brain has been evolving for thousands of times as long as any human society, but, even in a human society, a really good and economical organizational idea has a fair chance of being adopted in part. Perhaps a form of Ockham's razor adapted to complex "orgs" (organizations or organisms) is that all simple hypotheses that explain some of the main facts have a fair chance of being part of the truth. For simple systems, hypotheses are more likely to be mutually exclusive than for complex systems.

APPARENTLY MUTUALLY EXCLUSIVE THEORIES

Take for example the assembly theory or its elaboration the subassembly theory on the one hand (Hebb, 1949; Milner, 1957; Good, 1962ab, 1965, 1966, 1971b; Kaplan, 1967; John, 1962; Harmon and

Lewis, 1966) and on the other hand the established theory that different parts of the brain have different functions. A brief description of the subassembly theory is given later in this paper. The subassemblies are assumed mostly to be highly localized, but not the assemblies. (Hebb's 'assemblies' are my 'subassemblies'). The theory does not contradict the established fact of localized function; rather it supplements it.

As a related example, there might be a temptation to suppose that the processing of visual information should be either parallel or serial. But both theories *must* be partly true. When looking at a picture the eyes are usually unconsciously moved in a roughly periodic manner, and this suggests a serial model for recognition (Noton and Stark, 1971) yet the effect of the eye movements might very well be to reinforce in a serial manner some ultra-parallel activity in the brain, namely the reverberation of a cell assembly (Good, 1971a). It might be more suggestive to describe the activity in the cerebral cortex as 'serial-parallel', although the expression 'series-parallel' has another specialized technical meaning in circuit theory.

INTROSPECTION

According to some behaviorists, one form of speculation is introspection, which they regard as a no-no. A well-known behaviorist, in conversation with me, wouldn't trust my recall of a prenatal event because he thought it was obviously based on wishful thinking, and he quickly changed the subject. Obviously his reaction was based on behavioral trade-unionism. Each of us was the other's guinea-pig. As the rat said, "I have conditioned the psychologist to give me a pellet of food whenever I press this lever".

Introspection is certainly a powerful technique for planning programs, programs that might eventually tell us much about the mind. A useful non-introspective approach is to ask a chess player, or some other decision maker, to think aloud, and then to analyse a recording of what was said. This approach was used by A.D. De Groot (1946) and it proved some facts about human thinking, such as the importance of "progressive deepening" in problem solving, that is, gradually improved understanding when thinking about a problem several times, with several restarts. Yet the same result, and others, could be obtained, with less conviction but with less effort, by introspection and common observation. Similarly the notion of a decision tree, with the cutting off of variations in quiescent conditions, and with the analysis of forced variations, seemed obvious to some us by introspection (Good, 1948) before Shannon's paper on the subject appeared (1950). (But we might have been influenced by our experience with cryptanalysis, as I think Shannon might have been also). The decision tree can also be applied to medical diagnosis, and will presumably soon be a standard part of a medical education. It applies to most planning and decision problems.

Let's consider another example of introspection. Dr. J.J. Katz visited Blacksburg a few years ago and argued in a lecture that all languages have syntactic features in common, from which he inferred that we must have quite complicated syntactic circuitry (genetically) built in to our speech centres. This opinion, which I believe he shares with Naom Chomsky, was based on the careful study of many examples in many languages. But a baby can think even before it knows a single word. (I know this because I remember an incident in my own experience that proves it; but it is too personal to describe in public). Therefore a baby might very well form the abstraction, at a preconscious level, that one object can operate on or be related to another one. This is the syntactic structure of subject-verb-object. Prelinguistic thought is possible and it must have inherent syntax, but I do not see how we can determine whether it is built in or acquired by experience.

Perhaps prelinguistic reasoning uses the speech centre of the brain. Now, at Oklahoma University, a chimpanzee has been taught nearly a hundred words of the American Sign Language and can form new sentences of the form subject-verb-object. Does a chimpanzee have a cerebral speech centre, perhaps better called a reasoning centre?

The lightning of the neuron and initial probabilities. At the Fourth London Symposium on Information Theory in 1960 Oliver Selfridge said during the unpublished discussion of his joint paper with Marvin Minsky, that he hoped to see the day when a machine could perform genuine intellectual activities. At that exact moment there was a roar of thunder, the only one during the day. Selfridge cast his eyes upwards and sat down amidst moderate chuckling.

The breakdown potential gradient in lightning is about a million volts per meter and the action potential in a neuron is about a tenth of a volt, so we might have correctly guessed that the membrane of an unmielinated neuron is about a tenth of a micron thick. A primitive savage might now infer that the electrical discharges in the atmosphere correspond to a form of thinking by a demiurge. He might have (correctly) predicted that Oliver Selfridge's house would be struck by lightning! If you do not accept the theory of the savage, you must be, like me, a Bayesian, who believes that the initial probabilities of hypothesis, as well as the results of observation, should be taken into account.

PLANARIA, RNA, AND TURKEYS

Since we are all Bayesians, whether we know it or not, we do not readily accept surprising reports of experimental results at their face value. You know the planarian experiments seeming to show that learning could be transferred by feeding planaria with the bodies of the RNA of trained planaria. Physiologists expect most of the RNA to be broken down before it gets into the brain cells and this makes the reported result extra surprising. In terms of Bayesian reasoning, a conventional 5% significance level is nowhere near enough when the initial probability is very low. The initial probability of a theory can be depressed by its complexity and also by background knowledge.

Recently A.M. Schulman (1972) did some analogous experiments with turkeys. Some of the turkeys were imprinted by means of a rotating spiral, and one cc of each of their homogenized brains was then injected intraperitoneally into newly hatched recipient turkeys. (One donor to one recipient). The recipients seemed to become imprinted slightly more quickly than a control group for which the donors had not been exposed to the rotating spirals; and much more quickly than a group that had been injected merely with a saline solution. A conventional significance level was attained in the more interesting part of the experiment. Like the turkey, I am prepared to stick my neck out, and I predict that the result will be found to be due to chance. The more *statistically* significant part of the experiment was not intended to be very interesting since it only shows that protein produces more activity than saline solution, that brain like fish is "good for the brain" or is food for thought.

IS MEMORY STORED IN SINGLE NEURONS OR IN ASSEMBLIES?

If it is true that RNA injected into a neuron can transfer some training to it, then it might be possible to demonstrate this by means of experiments on individual neurons of say a squid of some other animal with thick neurons. If non-specific RNA is just as effective then it must be food for thought, as I predicted just now for the turkey brain. This suggests another question: can we train an individual neuron by means of electrical waveform input? This is an interesting question because the most popular theory is that learning depends mainly on the synapses, more vessicles, closer contacts, bigger neurons, and modified RNA, or possibly even DNA. The last of these proposals is not very Lamarkian if a trained DNA molecule cannot migrate from its original cell.

To say that an input wave-form might lead to the training of a neuron would mean that a repetition of the wave-form would lead more easily to an output pulse along the axon, at least if the original output had been reinforced in some way such as by acetylcholine. Now how could a neuron recognise a repeated pattern? A suggestion made by Peter Fong (1969) is that the wave-forms might cause a coding along the lengths of the RNA molecules by bases projecting form the coils of the helix, and he suggested a fairly specific mechanism for this. We also have to consider whether the RNA strand could then emit specific signals. In principle it might possibly do this by acoustic vibrations, these being perhaps converted into voltages as if in a mercury delay line. It has been speculated in a metaphysical vein that consciousness might correspond to the vibrations of DNA or RNA helices, like the movements of the toy known as Slinky (Good, 1967) and this speculation would accord with the mechanism just mentioned. It is debatable whether it would accord with an idea due to Adrian (1947, p. 92) that "the physical basis of memory is in the nature of a resonance pattern which may be established in local circuits throughout the whole of the cortex". For Adrian presumably had in mind circuits each of which consists of a *number* of neurons, not circuits *within* the neurons.

The expression "resonance pattern" suggests a field theory and inductance/capacity circuits rather than the kind of information-processing that occurs in a digital electronic computer. (Compare Greene, 1962). But "antockhamously", both points of view might well contain a part of the truth about a brain. Beurle (1956) showed theoretically how plane waves could travel in a mass of cells, thus explaining the EEG to some extent, and this work has been developed by others. For example, Griffith (1963, 1965) has shown that, with appropriate choice of parameters in a network, assemblies can reverberate without saturating a complete net. This could presumably also be achieved by means of a feedback mechanism from the reticular or "centrencephalic" system, as proposed by Good (1965, pp. 64-65). Such a feedback mechanism might explain some of the rhythms of the EEG. (The new subject of microsonics might also shed light on the EEG since it deals with surface waves and signal processing (see Vollmer and Gandolfo, 1972)).

Another "field theory" is that of the "encephalohologram", to coin a self-explanatory term. See, for example, Pribram (1966) and van Heerden (1966). It would require some degree of linearity in the propagation of brainwaves, as do the theories of Beurle, Greene, and Griffith.

SEMILINEARITY

Consider the following approximate syllogism: The world has many approximately linear features. The brain has had to adapt to the world. Therefore the brain is also likely *a priori* to have some approximately linear features. Let's elaborate.

Many mechanical systems are approximately linear, so it often happens that positive multiples of a given acoustic spectrum occur in similar circumstances. The ear-brain system must therefore be able to extract invariants in spite of changes of acoustic intensity. Similarly considerable changes in luminosity should not much affect the interpretation of a visual scene. Variations in the size of the pupil do a little of the work, and much light adaptation occurs in the retina (for example, Ratliff, 1961; Dowling, 1972) but brighter scenes still look brighter so it remains necessary to extract invariants with respect to brightness.

In both the acoustic and visual examples, the proportionality constant (for spectral intensities) is *positive*, so we need only *semilinearity*, to coin a term. It is not important that the negative of a photograph should look much the same as the positive, since negatives only occur only artificially.

Semilinearity in the operation of complex nervous networks can be given a reasonable interpretation. We must interpret it in terms of the total frequencies of firing of *pools* or *bundles* of neurons, so as to iron out random effects and to obtain a wide enough dynamic range. The concept that the dynamic range of individual neurons can be extended by treating neurons in bundles was proposed by van Bergeijk (1961) in connection with the spiral arrangement in the auditory nerve. Bundles have the further merit of informational "redundancy".

If a bundle of neurons receives input spike frequencies f_1, f_2, f_3,... at various synapses one might expect its output frequency to be of the form $\max(a_1 f_1 + a_2 f_2 + \ldots, 0)$ where the a's are positive or negative depending on whether the synapses are excitatory or inhibitory, and the absolute values of the a's are the synaptic strengths which depend on the previous history. This assumption is made, for individual units, in the theory of the perceptron: see, for example, Rosenblatt (1962), Papert (1961). (For a recent excellent introduction to perceptrons, see Block (1970). This gives many references and emphasizes that multilayer perceptrons with feedback are important. Compare Good (1962b), p. 125 and Hayek (1952), p. 70). The "max" makes the model only semilinear. Let's assume this is true in the pathways from the output of the peripheral neurons. It is convenient to regard this peripheral output as the *intermediate input* to these pathways. The hypothesized semilinearity refers to the frequency coding used by neurons and bundles of neurons, as is clear from the above "max" formula (but it might also apply to other neural codes). Some support for the hypothesis can be derived from Roll (1955). Semilinearity *throughout* the cortex is not refuted by the fact that our output is not proportional to our input; for the output depends also of course on other internal activity such as memory and set. Thus the hypothesis does not support a crude stimulus-response model.

In principle a semilinear network can do everything that can be done by a linear one fairly simply. For units (bundles of neurons) could occur in pairs, one of each pair having a set of coefficients $(a_1, a_2, \ldots)$ and the other having the coefficients $(-a_1, -a_2, \ldots)$, both units having the same input vector $(f_1, f_2, \ldots)$. The outputs from such a pair of units would contain all the information that could have been derived from a genuinely linear unit with output $a_1 f_1 + a_2 f_2 + \ldots$. For this to be possible it would perhaps be necessary that the microstructure of the brain should be more systematic than is sometimes believed likely. We could imagine it growing layer by layer, with each neuron of one layer giving birth to two in the next, one of the two daughter cells having excitatory "umbilical" connections and the other having inhibitory ones. It would then be possible, for example, that a semilinear network of $2^{n+1} n$ units, arranged in n strata, would be capable of carrying out a mod 2 discrete n-dimensional Fourier or Hadamard transform which gives factorial interactions (see Good, 1958/1960). This might be the basis of a fast Fourier transform that might be incorporated in an encephologram.

Perhaps all the output from a given neuron is excitatory, or all is inhibitory. It can easily be seen that the effect of a model without this constraint could be achieved by at most doubling the number of neurons. Accordingly, for the sake of simpler exposition, this constraint will not be assumed.

Since semilinearity presumably has great survival value, because of its invariant properties (to be described in more detail in a moment), we can make the following guess: *when the intensity of an intermediate input becomes higher than the level at which the semilinearity is approximately true, then the result is usually painful or unpleasant.* Otherwise we would not avoid such situations, and this would lead to great confusions in the interpretation of neural signals; for the breakdown of semilinearity would make it difficult to extract the meaningful invariants of the situation. The theory is that displeasure and pain correspond to situations which it is difficult for us to interpret or to which we can barely adapt. (Panic too might correspond to non-linearity). We have evolved a propensity to avoid such situations, by Natural Selection. The theory does not imply that the lower the intensity of intermediate input the greater the pleasure. There is too much low-intensity intermediate input for it to encourage the curiosity of an animal. As a function of spike frequency, the pleasure plausibly has a graph as in figure 1 under normal circumstances. Inputs of medium intensity are the pleasurable ones; they are informative without being so informative as to overload the communication channels.

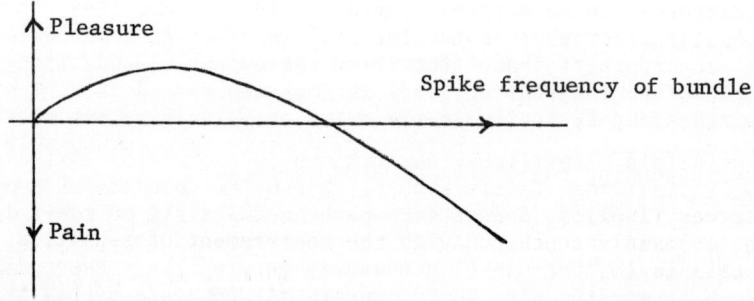

Figure 1 - *A pleasure-pain hypothesis*. We take for granted that there are specialized pathways for the transmission of pain and pleasure information.

This theory suggest that, for a *given* moderate input, a large unit puts out a slow uninteresting spike frequency; a medium-sized unit puts out a moderate and pleasurable spike frequency; and a small units puts out a high and unpleasant spike frequency. Also that the units will tend to grow with use and atrophy with disuse, so that repetition in *learning* circuits (less so in the built-in ones) will tend to decrease displeasure and to change pleasure into monotony. This helps to explain polygamy and the nature of the arts, but the hypnotic effect of local repetition requires separate explanation.

Can this theory explain the facts of harmonious and dissonant chords in music? Any theory (apart from a 'beat' theory such as Helmholtz's, now apparently in disfavor: see Ward 1970, p. 435) that tries to explain why some chords are pleasant and some unpleasant must first explain why the 'same' chord can be identified at different frequencies. A chord depends on the ratios of frequencies so this ratio must be approximately an invariant of perception. Under an assumption of semilinearity of the 'inner' nervous system (that is, excluding the periphery), we are almost forced to assume that logarithms of the acoustic frequencies are 'computed' by the peripheral equipment. This could explain why the inner nervous system is capable of detecting chords, namely by differencing logarithms, and also of apprehending that a tune is much the same when its key is changed.

That the nervous system contains many differencing units is extremely likely once semilinearity is assumed, quite apart from the present application. The assumed differencing units would be expected to be large when they correspond to chords occurring frequently in nature, speech or music, and small in the opposite case. An acoustic frequency ratio of 2, an octave, is too common, is boring, and is here presumed to correspond to large neurons and to small spike frequencies. A ratio of 3/2 is intermediate, and pleasant, a ratio of 9/8 is rare and unpleasant (Ward, 1970, p. 437) and is presumed to correspond to small neurons. Rare chords, i.e. discords, contain more information than common ones, as measured by the logarithms of the reciprocals of their probabilities, and it is important that informative signals should be strongly attracted to our attention. But if they are made less rare by training, as by listening to the music of Stravinsky, or to the noises of a factory, we can grow to tolerate them, presumably after the corresponding small neurons grow larger.

Stevens (1961) is a logarithmophobe and insists on power laws, but he is mainly concerned with the measurement of sensation, and when this is so there is no contradiction with the present discussion. When we study the circumstances in which a subject says one light is twice as bright as another one we are studying his use of language more than his nervous system. Moreover, power laws are often well approximated by logarithmic laws (for example, Uttal, 1972, p. 472, where an earlier reference is given; and, in connection with athletic records, Good, 1971d).

It seems difficult to construct a plausible model for taking fairly accurate logarithms in the inner (presumed semilinear) nervous system: it seems to require too great an accuracy of response. So it is reasonable to suppose that any accurate logarithmic transformations occur peripherally (other than those computed by ordinary arithmetic). But such a transformation is known to relate brightness and spike frequency in the visual cortex of the cat (Jung, 1961, who refers to his joint work with Baumgartner), so our hypothesis would imply that this transformation takes place in the retina.

It might be suggested that it would be useful if the logarithms of distances could be subtracted for the purpose of recognizing shapes. But for this purpose the estimation of angles is sufficient and the magnitudes of angles can be derived by subtraction from knowledge of directions, which knowledge is contained in some cortical neurons of the cat in accordance with the experiments of Hubel and Wiesel. It is certainly difficult to conceive a mechanism by which logarithms of distances could be computed in the retina. But recognition of shape is presumably a 'higher' mental ability than that of a chord, and would be expected to make use of the more complicated circuits of the brain where it is important that semilinearity is not just linearity, and which 'in principle' are capable of any logical operation whatever. These more complicated circuits must be involved in 'thinking' as distinct from the most elementary forms of perception. For example, they must be involved in reading. If you become sleepy when reading, your set for reading dissolves, and your perception sinks to a more elementary form. Instead of seeing words you then see white crooked lines running down the page, between the words. Thus a given visual experience can have two entirely different and unrelated interpretations, when the 'set' of the mind is varied. This may be contrasted with artificial illusions, where the interpretations vary *without* change of set.

ILLUSIONS

In any general discussion of the eye and brain, optical illusions are worth some attention as in Gregory (1966). All animals live in environments that are to some extent specialized and where some phenomena are therefore very rare or virtually non-existent. An economical information-handling device should not be expected to interpret every possible input realistically; in other words it is economical that some inputs lead to optical, auditory, and other sensory illusions. Their existence is thus explicable, and some of them can be explained in more detail.

One of these illusions is provided by the two-hand experiment. With one arm outstretched and the other bent, so that one hand is twice the distance of the other, the two hands look about the same size when they subtend between them a reasonably large angle at the eyes. This is of course to be expected because the situation is of a very common kind where corrections for depth must be made. When we look from one hand to the other, we separately estimate their sizes and so, by long training, the estimates are about equal. If we close one eye we lose the convergence and other information and one hand looks much larger. Likewise, if the angle subtended is small, then the two hands appear to be side by side, and this also leads to large apparent magnification of one hand. Finally, if the angle is small and *also* we close one eye, so that we lose both clues, then the two effects seem to be multiplicative, and one hand look enormous compared with the other. It is as if we had multiplied the two effects together, or perhaps added them in a logarithmic representation. This suggests, though perhaps rather weakly, that there are very rough logarithmic transformations even after information has reached the cortex. It is not difficult to design circuits for taking *very rough* logarithms.

THE SUBASSEMBLY THEORY

I should like to conclude with a few further comments about the subassembly theory without trying to describe it in detail. The main points are that (i) an assembly is suppposed to correspond to a conscious 'unit concept', when it is reverberating, and, while reverberating, it is large enough to prevent (by inhibition) any other assembly from reverberating as a unit. (Note that my terminology differs somewhat from Hebb's). (ii) Assemblies reverberate for only a fraction of a second at a time in most circumstances. (iii) Subassemblies are much smaller, usually reverberate for much longer, and correspond to *preconscious* and *unconscious* thoughts (iv) The next assembly to fire is determined by the subassemblies currently active that have been produced either by the sensory input or by the breaking up of the sequence of assemblies that have recently fired. (v) The brain must be capable of extracting far more kinds of invariants than the simple ones measured before. This can be achieved by a generalized form of 'regeneration' where the word 'regeneration' is here analogous to its use for the squaring up of pulses in binary computers. The notion of assemblies and subassemblies provides a reasonable explanation for such regeneration. Regeneration is a way of bringing an adequate degree of discreteness into the system, and the assemblies and subassemblies serve a similar function in the brain to that served by the words in a language. (vi) Subassemblies sometimes consist of sub-subassemblies and so on, but we often use the word 'subassemblies' for all of these. Assemblies and subassemblies form hierarchies containing many dendriform structures (trees). The recognition of an object depends to a large extent on working upwards in the hierarchy towards an assembly, the lowest level subassemblies corresponding to elementary sensations such as that of a short straight line or angle, or phoneme. The whole recognition process is probabilistic, in other words each activated subassembly or assembly can be regarded as embodying a provisional hypothesis and as temporarily excluding rival hypotheses. A hypothesis made at a high level also implies new hypotheses at a *lower* level, that is the implications go in both directions in the hierarchy, a process called "duality" by Good (1968c). Thus the determination of the next assembly to fire is apt to be a very complex but very fast iterative process (according to the theory), and is not as simple as might have been suggested by heading (iv), although that heading is not contradicted.

What is the relationship of Adrian's 'resonance patterns' to the assembly theory? If the reverberations in the various local circuits were not connected, then the resonance theory, as described by Adrian, would not explain why in general only one concept is in full consciousness at any one time. On the other hand if the local circuits mentioned *are* connected into an integrated whole, then the resonance theory becomes an assembly theory. I infer from this that the assembly theory is a modification of the resonance theory, and is itself modified by the subassembly theory.

I once did a five-second experiment in which the subject was the mathematician A. Nerode. He had trained himself for many decades, from the age of four, to read fast and he was able to read a page of a novel in about five seconds. When he told me of this, he had not yet noticed the motion of his eyes when reading so I asked him to read a page while I watched. Then for the first time he discovered his method, and I was able to confirm it. We found that his eyes moved from left to right a number of times equal to the number of lines on the page but they did not move horizontally across the page. For each line they moved down about six lines in a diagonal movement and then returned so that the page was covered in overlapping diagonal bands six lines wide stepping down one line at a time. He was looking ahead and unconsciously preparing his mind for the next line. Since he had previously been unaware of the method, his observation of 'forthcoming' important words must have been at a subliminal or preconscious level. In terms of the subassembly theory he was feeding in subassemblies which would increase the relevant transition probabilities from one assembly to the next in his understanding of the text. He was making good use of the ultraparallel activity of the brain, an activity of which it is impossible to be entirely conscious because it involves much dynamic activity of subassemblies alone.

When we enter a familiar room in which an article of furniture has been moved, we are often aware of a change before we know what the change is. Can this be explained by the subassembly theory? Since the aggregate of subassemblies is slightly unusual, the probabilities of various unit activities are all somewhat new. Under a behavioral interpretation of 'atmosphere' it follows that the atmosphere of the room will appear slightly different from our memory of it. A more convincing example of an explanation by the subassembly theory is that of the fractionation of stabilized images (Good, 1968c).

THE SUBASSEMBLY THEORY AND THE GESTALT THEORY

On the dust cover and on page 51 of Köhler (1969), he gives an example of a not very complicated diagram seeming to have reasonable unity and which can be apprehended as a whole but which you are very unlikely to have seen before independently (figure 2). Köhler says, "Clearly, therefore, the principles according to which visual objects are established differ from the processes which the empiricist explanation, the explanation of learning, makes one expect". He might have added that he here presents a problem for the subassembly theory, for the various parts of the expression for the square root of 16 are all present, yet the assembly for this, which might well exist already, does not fire.

To answer this implicit objection to the subassembly theory, we note that the low-level subassemblies for the square root of 16 have been mixed up with many other subassemblies of a similar nature. They have been fitted together in a deliberately misleading manner so as to provoke us to think unconsciously or preconsciously of higher-level subassemblies unrelated to the square root of 16.

Thus, in the upwards and downwards traversing of the hierarchy of subassemblies and assemblies, a search (that would find the square root of 16) is required that is much more difficult than normally

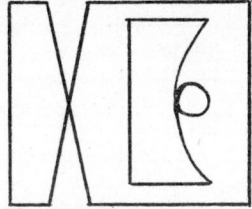

Figure 2 - The square root of 16 vanishes.

occurs in the problem of recognition. There are so many hypotheses competitive to the 'right solution' that even when the right solution is hypothesized it does not seem especially likely to be 'correct' in the sense of having been put there deliberately. (It is easier to see a face in the moon). Indeed a perfectly reasonable hypothesis, on not too deep an analysis, and one which we all adopt if we are not told otherwise, is that the entire pattern was constructed for its own sake. It could be described in about a hundred words so it has a much higher intuitive probability than most of the scenes we see every second of the day, each of which would take thousands of words to describe in detail, and which therefore have intuitive probabilities of less than 10^{-1000}. (The intuitive probability of a *possible* event that has never occurred is not zero, contrary to a naive definition of probability).

ACKNOWLEDGMENTS

This work was supported in part by U.S. Dept. of Health, Education and Welfare Grant No. R01 GM18770-01. Also I wish to thank Mr. Curtis Lee Baker for drawing my attention to some important references.

REFERENCES

1. Adrian, E.D. (1947). *The Physical Background of Perception*, (Oxford).
2. van Bergeijk, W.A. (1961). "Studies with artificial neurons; II: analog of the external spiral innervation of the cochlea", *Kybernetik*, **1**, 102-107.
3. Beurle, R.L. (1956). "Properties of a mass of cells capable of regenerating pulses", *Proc. Roy. Soc.*, **B240**, 55-94.
4. Block, H.D. (1970). "A review of 'Perceptrons: An Introduction to Computational Geometry'", *Information and Control*, **17**, 501-522.
5. Dowling, J.E. (1972). "The site of visual adaptation", in *Sensory Coding*, (ed. Uttal, W.R.), (Little, Brown, Boston), pp. 157-163.
6. Fong, Peter (1969), "Brain memory and ferroelectric recording mechanism of RNA", *Physiol. Chem. and Phys.*, **1**, 24-41.

7. Good, I.J. (1948). A letter to A.M. Turing of 16 September, "If a chess machine analyses forced variations then a suitable definition of a 'forced variation' might be that every move must be considered if it is either a capture or an attack of a piece by one of smaller value".
8. Good, I.J. (1958/60). "The interaction algorithm and practical Fourier analysis", *J. Roy. Statist. Soc., Ser. B*, **20**, 361-372; **22**, 372-375.
9. Good, I.J. (1962a). "The mind-body problem, or could an android feel pain?", in *Theories of the Mind*, (ed. Scher, J.M.), (The Free Press, New York), (Collier MacMillan, London), pp. 490-518.
10. Good, I.J. (1962b). "Botryological speculations", in *The Scientist Speculates*, (eds. Good, I.J. and Maynard Smith, John), Heinemann, London), (Basic Books and Capricorn Books, New York), pp. 120-132.
11. Good, I.J. (1963). "Information Theory: Survey", CRD-IDA Working Paper No. 83, p. 33.
12. Good, I.J. (1965). "Speculations concerning the first ultraintelligent machine", *Advances in Computers*, **6**, 31-88.
13. Good, I.J. (1966). "The function of speculation in science exemplified by the subassembly theory of mind", *Theoria to Theory*, **1**, 28-43.
14. Good, I.J. (1967). "Partly-baked Ideas", *Zenith*, (Hilary Term), pp. 16-17, 19-21.
15. Good, I.J. (1968a). "Corroboration, explanation, evolving probability, simplicity, and a sharpened razor", *Brit. J. Phil. Sci.*, **19**, 123-143.
16. Good, I.J. (1968b). "Olla Podri(d)a", *Mensa J.*, (December), p. 2.
17. Good, I.J. (1968c). "Creativity and duality in perception and recall", in *Pattern Recognition*, (NPL/IEE), pp. 228-237.
18. Good, I.J. (1970a). "Rough and disorderly mass", *Mensa J.*, (May), p.6.
19. Good, I.J. (1970b). "Hotchpot", *Mensa J.* (December), pp. 4-5.
20. Good, I.J. (1971a). Letter in *Scientific American*, **225**, No.4, (October), p. 8, concerning an article "Eye movements and visual perception" (by David Noton and Lawrence Stark).
21. Good, I.J. (1971b). "Human and machine intelligence: comparisons and contrasts", *Impact of Science on Society*, **21**, No. 4, (October), 305-322.
22. Good, I.J. (1971c). "The Baker's Oven, XV", *Mensa J.*, (October), p. 10.
23. Good, I.J. (1971d). "A power law and a logarithmic law in athletics", *The American Statistician*, **25**, (June), 54.
24. Greene, Peter H. (1962). "On looking for neural networks and 'cell assemblies' that underlie behavior: I. A mathematical model", *Bull. Math. Biophys.*, **24**, 247-275.
25. Gregory, R.L. (1966). *Eye and Brain*, (McGraw-Hill).
26. de Groot, A.D. (1946/1965). *Thought and Choice in Chess*, (ed. Baylor, G.W.), (Mouton, The Hague and Paris), (Dutch, 1946; English, 1965).

27. Griffith, J.S. (1963, 1965). "A field theory of neural nets", I and II, *Bull. Math. Biophys.*, **25**, 111-120; **27**, 187-195.
28. Harmon, L.D. and Lewis, E.R. (1966). "Neural modelling", *Physiol. Rev.*, **46**, 513-591.
29. Hayek, F.A. (1952). *The Sensory Order*, (University Press, Chicago).
30. Hebb, D.O. (1949). *The Organization of Behavior*, (Wiley).
31. van Heerden, P.J. (1966). "The basic principles of artificial intelligence", (Polaroid Corporation, Cambridge, Massachusetts), (mimeographed), pp. 113.
32. John, E.R. (1962). "Some speculations on the psychophysiology of mind", in *Theories of Mind*, (ed. Scher, J.M.), (The Free Press, New York; Collier MacMillan, London), pp. 80-121.
33. Jung, Richard (1961). "Neuronal integration in the visual cortex and its significance for visual information", in *Sensory Communication*, (ed. Rosenblith, W.A.), (MIT Press), pp. 627-674, esp. p. 641.
34. Kaplan, Stephen, (1967). "The formation of a percept: an application of a neural net model", (University of Michigan), (mimeographed).
35. Köhler, W. (1969). *The Task of Gestalt Psychology*, (Princeton University Press).
36. Milner, P.M. (1957). "The cell assembly: Mark II", *Psychol. Rev.*, **64**, 242-252.
37. Noton, D. and Stark, L. (1971). "Eye movements and visual perception", *Scientific American*, (June), pp. 34-43.
38. Osteyee, D.B. and Good, I.J. (1972). "Regeneration of a binary signal in a uniform transmission line", (submitted for publication on February 9).
39. Papert, S. (1961). "Some mathematical models of learning", in *Proceedings of the 4th London Symposium on Information Theory*, (Butterworth, London).
40. Pribram, Karl, H. (1966). "Some dimensions of remembering: steps towards a neuropsychological model of memory", in *Macromolecules and Behavior*, (ed. Gaito, J.), (Academic Press), pp. 165-187.
41. Ratliff, F. (1961). "Inhibitory interaction and the detention and enhancement of contours", in *Sensory Communication*, (ed. Rosenblith, W.A.), (MIT Press), pp. 183-203.
42. Roll, W. (1955). "A statistical theory of monosynaptic input-output relations", *J. Cellular Comp. Physiol.*, **46**, 373-411.
43. Rosenblatt, Frank (1952). *Principles of Neorodynamics*, (Washington, D.C., Spartan Books).
44. Russell, Bertrand (1921). *The Analysis of Mind*, (Allen and Unwin, London).
45. Schulman, A.H. (1972). "Transfer of behavior controlled by an imprinted stimulus via brain homogenate injections in turkeys", (to be published).
46. Shannon, C.E. (1950). "Programming a computer for playing chess", *Phil. Mag.*, **41**, 256-275.
47. Stevens, S.S. (1961). "The Psychophysics of Sensory Function", in *Sensory Communication*, (ed. Rosenblith, W.A.), (MIT Press).

48. Uttal, W.R. (1972). "Emerging principles of sensory coding", in *Sensory Coding*, (ed. Uttal, W.R.), (Little, Brown, Boston), pp. 457-481.
49. Vollmer, J. and Gandolfo, D. (1972). "Microsonics", *Science*, **175**, (14 January), 129-133.
50. Ward, W.D. (1970). "Musical Perception", in *Foundations of Modern Auditory Theory*, (ed. Tobias, J.V.), (Academic Press), pp. 405-447.

A LOOK AT BIOLOGICAL AND MACHINE PERCEPTION

R.L. GREGORY

Department of Anatomy, University of Bristol

The study of perception is divided between many established sciences: Physiology, Experimental Psychology and Machine Intelligence; with several others making contributions. But each of the contributing sciences tends to have its own concepts, and ways of considering problems. Each - to use T.S. Kuhn's term - has its own 'paradigm', within which its science is respectable. This can make cooperation difficult, as misunderstandings (and even distrust) can be generated by paradigm differences. This paper is a plea to consider perceptual phenomena from many points of view, and to consider whether a general paradigm for perception might be found. We may say at once that the status of perceptual phenomena is likely to be odd, as science is in general concerned with the object world; but perceptions are not objects, though they are in some sense related to objects. It is this relation between perceptions and objects which is the classical philosophical problem, and it cannot be ignored when we consider perception as a territory for scientific investigation. This territory is essentially odd: its phenomena tend to be illusions - departures from the world - rather than facts of the world. It requires a conceptual somersault to accept illusions as the major facts of a science! But this we must do: and once this decision is taken, we can hardly expect physics (or physiology) to provide the paradigm for perception.

Machine Intelligence and cognitive psychology (though certainly not all perceptual theories) may agree in regarding perceptions as inferences - inferences based on strictly inadequate data. Our reason for seeing perceptions as inferences is that perception is predictive. Perceptual prediction is of two kinds. First: to properties of objects which cannot at that time be sensed directly, or 'monitored'. This applies to hidden parts of objects, to the three-dimensional form of an object given as a plane optical projection, and to non-optical properties such as hardness and mass, which in biological perception are vitally important. The second kind of prediction exhibited by biological perception is prediction to the immediate future. This allows neural conduction and procession time to be cut to zero, so that in skilled performance there is typically zero 'reaction-time'. (This implies that the classical stimulus-response notion, though applicable to reflexes, is not appropriate for perception). Prediction to the future can also allow behaviour to continue appropriately through gaps in the available sensory data. Prediction to the future is vitally important because dangers, rewards, problems and solutions, all lie in the future.

Although it is convenient for experimental purposes to think of perception in stimulus-response terms, the immense contribution of stored data, required for prediction, makes us see perception as largely cognitive. Current sensory data cannot be sufficient for perception or control of behaviour: it must select relevant facts and generalisations from the past, rather than control behaviour directly from present stimuli.

The importance of prediction - which requires stored knowledge makes us see perception in cognitive as well as in physiological terms. Although there must be physiological mechanisms to carry out the cognitive logical processes, of generalising and selecting stored data; the concepts we need for understanding what the physiology is carrying out are not part of physiology. We do not derive a cognitive paradigm from physiology, though every move is made by physiological components. (We find this situation in games, such as chess. The moves are physical moves, of pieces on a board; but we do not understand the game from the moves, without knowing the rules and where success and failure lie). We may suggest that it is just this essential cognitive component of biological perception - which unfortunately is very difficult to investigate - which makes Machine Intelligence potentially important for understanding biological perception. But, again unfortunately, programs adequate for comparable machine perceptual performance do not as yet exist. Judging from biological perception, perceiving machines will not be of intellectual interest, or effective, until they are capable of using sensed data for making these two kinds of predictions: based on stored knowledge of objects. To increase the sensory capacity of machines, to try to avoid this cognitive component, is futile as a solution because there will always be hidden aspects and properties of objects, and the future cannot in principle be monitored. So to produce machines with accurate ranging devices, or other features for reducing the ambiguity of images or other sensory data, is merely to postpone the problem. However ingenious the engineering may be they are conceptually dull and may hide the essential problem by their (limited) success.

When we start to compare the visual perception of animals with present machine perception - by regarding both as giving inferences about external objects from ambiguous sensed data - we strike a paradox. The perceptual performance of quite primitive organisms is greater than the most sophisticated machines designed for scene analysis, or self-guided response to objects. On the other hand even the most advanced brains are weaker at performing logical operations than are simple devices, of cogs or switches. Why is it that machines, such as computers, can perform logical tasks so well where brains fail; and yet cannot begin to compete with biological object-recognition? This may seem strange enough, but if Helmholtz was right (and there is every reason to believe him right) to regard perceptions as conclusions of 'unconscious inference', then we must face a truly odd situation - for if perception involves sophisticated inference why are brains weaker at performing logically than are machines? We might suppose that ability to infer was developed

in brains, at the start of biological perception; but that this
ability was locked away, and is not available for other kinds of
problem solving. Or we might suppose that the processes of perceptual inference are different from what we call logic.

It is clear that the physical characteristics of components
available for seeing machines are very different from those present
in brains. The first are relatively free from drift and noise; but
they are relatively large, and cannot carry so many inputs or outputs. This makes parallel processing convenient for biological
computing, and serial computing more convenient for man-made computers. Can we suppose that these physical differences lead to
the supposed different kinds of inference? If so, biological perception seems to demonstrate powers of *parallel* processing, while
computers demonstrate very different powers of *serial* processing.
In addition, we might argue that the biologically unique power of
human logical problem solving is due (in whole or part) to language,
and special symbolic aids, including: mathematical and logical notations, 'digit' fingers for counting, and the abacus - all helping
us to infer serially.

Can this suggestion be supported? We might start by noting that
in general the more an aid differs from what it aids, the greater
the improvement it can confer. (To take an example: knives, forks
and spoons are so useful, as aids to eating, essentially because
our hands are not like knives, forks or spoons. So, if we know
that Martians eat with such utensils, we could make a shrewd guess
that their 'hands' are not like our knives, or forks, or spoons).
If we accept this as a principle, that: *the greater the difference
between the aid and the aided, the greater the possible improvement,*
then we have some support for the notion that biological non-perceptual problem solving is by *parallel* rather than by serial processing - because it is *serial* aids which are so effective. Although this cannot be claimed as a strong argument, it seems worth
some consideration. Finally, if brains are good at perceptual inferences through adopting *parallel* processing, perhaps it will be
necessary to adopt parallel processing for machine perception.

However this may be, we have now learned, from painful experience,
that machine perception is extremely difficult to achieve. This implies that we do not understand biological perception adequately to
design corresponding machines; but perhaps we can learn some useful
things from living systems, including ourselves, clearly capable of
perception. Continuing our emphasis on the cognitive component of
biological perception, we will assume that the details of the physiology are less important in this context than the kinds of inference, from stored and sensory data, than are the cognitive strategies by which objects, and the future, are inferred. But of course
perceptual inference is not infallible. There are errors, and these
may occur systematically in certain situations. Much as the logician may use logical paradoxes for revealing the nature of logic,
so cognitive psychology can use perceptual phenomena for revealing
perceptual assumptions and inference procedures. This is, however,
to assume that at least some perceptual phenomena are due to

misplaced strategies of inference rather than to *physiological malfunction*. Such visual phenomena as after-images, we may safely attribute to the physiology of the system, because the pattern of intense stimulation of the retina transfers to (is superimposed on) any other pattern. Other visual phenomena are specific to the pattern or to its probable significance in terms of the object world. These phenomena we may attribute to inference strategies rather than to the mechanism carrying out the strategy.

It seems useful, if we regard perceptions as the results of inference, to call perceptions *hypotheses*. This draws attention to their similarity, on this view, with hypotheses in science. In both cases slender data serve to make decisions appropriate through inference to situations which cannot be monitored directly, and which may lie in the future. A detailed comparison of perceptions as hypotheses in this sense could be rewarding. Meanwhile, we are in a position to describe *perceptual phenomena* as 'inappropriate hypotheses'. By asking why inappropriateness is generated, we may learn something of the inference procedures (and sometimes the physiology) of perception. As an example, we shall consider some new visual phenomena in these terms. These phenomena are not distortions, but are perceptually created visual features. If they are generated by misplaced inference, we may call them: 'Cognitive Creations'. This loaded term will be used; but they will be considered in terms of alternative paradigms.

COGNITIVE CREATIONS

It is possible to devise simple line figures which evoke illusory contours and create large areas of enhanced or diminished brightness. Unlike the well-known brightness contrast effects, these illusory contours can occur in regions far removed from regions of physical intensity difference; and they can be orientated at any angle to physical present contours. Figure 1 is the figure described by Kanizsa. An illusory triangle is observed whose apices are determined by the blank sectors of the three discs. The 'created' object appears to have sharp contours, which bound a large region of enhanced brightness.

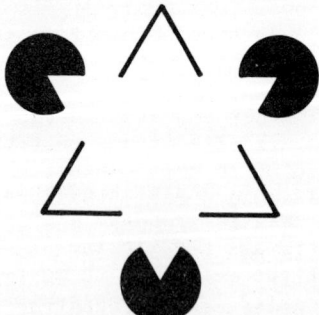

Figure 1 - Illusory triangle with apices in the blank sectors of the discs.

BIOLOGICAL AND MACHINE PERCEPTION

We may discover what features are necessary for producing these creations by removing parts of this figure. Figures 2,3,4 show such a sequence. Three dots spaced as the apices of an equilateral triangle (figure 2) give no created contours, although they are readily seen as indicating a triangle. The broken triangle (figure 3) does not evoke the figure (except perhaps slightly after the effect has been observed in figure 1): but combining the equilaterally spaced dots with the broken triangle (figure 4) does evoke the illusory object, though less markedly than with the sectored discs of figure 1. We can discount eye movements as important for these

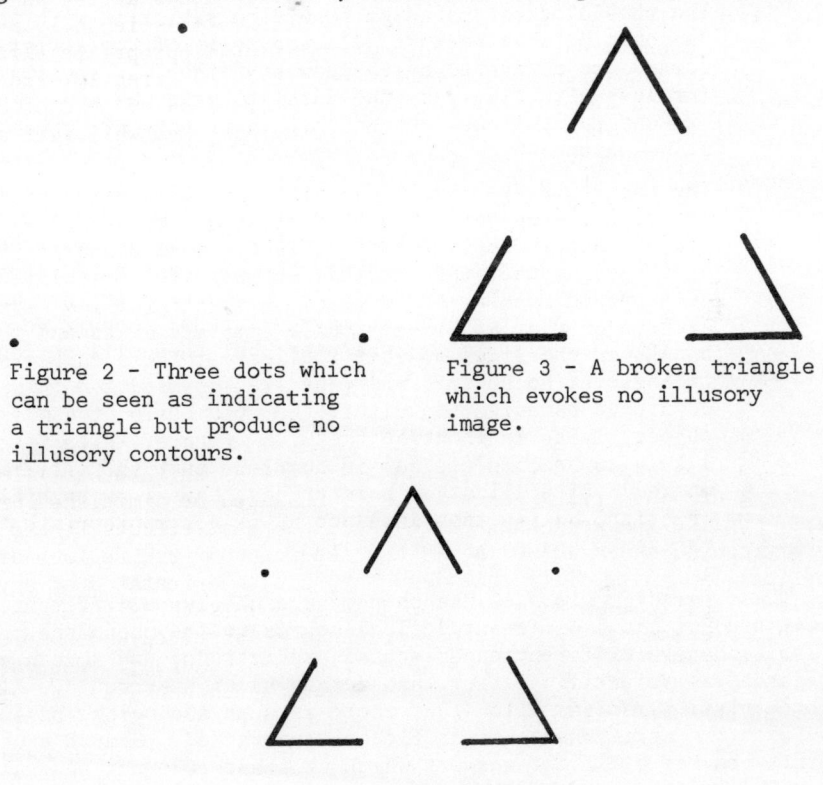

Figure 2 - Three dots which can be seen as indicating a triangle but produce no illusory contours.

Figure 3 - A broken triangle which evokes no illusory image.

Figure 4 - A combination of figures 2 and 3 which does evoke an illusory triangle.

effects, for if the retinal image is stabilised, (as by viewing the figures as after-images, produced with an intense electronic flash) then the effects are seen in the after-images, fixed to and moving precisely with the retina, with movement of the eyes. (When the initial positive after-image changes to a negative after-image, the whiter-than-white created area changes to a corresponding blacker-than-black area, just as when the figures are changed from negative to positive by optical means and viewed normally).

These effects have particular theoretical interest, for they might be explained in terms of at least three very different perceptual paradigms. They might, with at least initial plausibility, be described in terms of: (1) gestalt, (2) physiological, or, (3) cognitive-hypotheses paradigms.

(1) The gestalt paradigm, is satisfied by supposing that the 'created' shapes are 'good figures', having high 'closure' and so on: as accepted by Kanizsa (1955), for the first figure.

(2) The physiological paradigm, would be satisfied with the supposition that feature detector cells of the striate cortex are activated by the edges of the disc sectors, (or less effectively by the dots) to give the appearance of continuous lines, though only their ends are given by stimulation.

(3) The cognitive-hypothesis paradigm, in which perceptions are regarded as going beyond available data, to give 'object hypotheses', (Gregory, 1970) would be satisfied by supposing that the created features are 'postulated', as supposed masking objects, to 'account' for the blank sectors of what are likely to be complete discs and the breaks in the lines of what is likely to be a complete triangle. The sectors and gaps are supposed, on this cognitive paradigm, to elicit the hypothesis of a masking object, lying in front of the given figure, which is likely to be complete but if complete must be partially masked. Like all other perceptions, this is a cognitive creation; but in this instance it is not appropriate to the facts and so is an illusion.

These paradigm views of the phenomena each give a different logical account and a different logical status to the phenomena. They also each have different experimental predictions, and so can be regarded as scientific rather than metaphysical statements. All three rival paradigms allow that there is a physiological basis; so each can ask: "Where is the fiction generated?" Simple experiments provide clear cut answers which at least rule out several possibilities.

By adopting the technique devised in 1899, by Witasek, of sharing parts of the figures between the two eyes with a stereoscope, it is easy to show that the effect is not retinal in origin, but must be after the level of binocular fusion. This follows because the effect holds when the sectored discs are viewed with one eye and the interrupted line triangle with the other eye, when they are stereoscopically fused. By changing the angles of the disc sectors, so that they no longer meet by straight line interpolation, we find that the effect still occurs. The created form is now changed, to give interpolation with a *curved fictional contour*. This may be seen in figure 5. This new effect seems to increase the plausibility of the cognitive fiction notion - for it seems unlikely that 'curved edge' detectors would be selected by the mis-aligned sectors: and it seems that these concave curved (and other) figures which are created, are not especially 'good' figures in the gestalt sense.

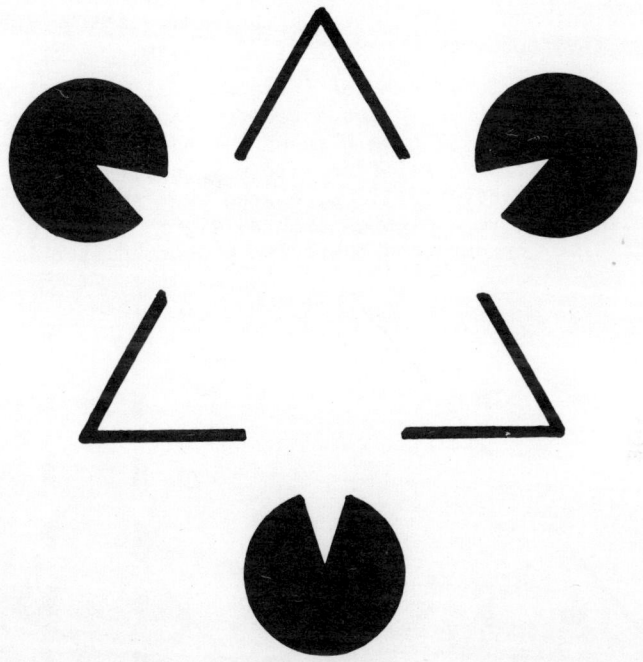

Figure 5 - Illusory triangle with curved contours.

The black line on white background figures give a homogeneous whiter-than-white fictional region. The corresponding negative white line on black background gives a blacker-than-black region. The illusory intensity difference can be measured with a reference light spot, as in a matching photometer. The measured brightness is about 10 per cent. Both the black and the white illusory triangles are reported as by our subjects as appearing somewhat in front of the rest of the figure. We have measured this objectively, by matching a stereoscopically viewed marker light spot to the apparent distance of the physical and created parts of the figures. This is compatible only with the cognitive paradigm.

Not only contours, but large homogeneous areas of different brightness are created - but could such areas of different brightness be created by the line detectors of the physiological paradigm? Consider figure 3. We have lines with gaps; but there is no observed difference in brightness between the inside and the outside of this triangle - and no contours between the gaps. So why should there be contours, and a brightness difference, with the created triangle? The lack of contours in the gaps of figure 3, and the absence of enhanced brightness show that aligned features are not sufficient for producing these effects. What seems to be needed is a high probability of an over-lying object which if it existed would give gaps by masking. This, however, would require processes of a logical sophistication beyond those believed to occur at the striate region; and concepts beyond those of classical physiology - the cognitive concepts of our third paradigm.

We find that at least some of the classical distortion illusions can be generated by these created contours and created regions of different brightness. Figure 6 shows a kind of Poggendorf figure, in which the usual parallel lines are physically absent, but are generated by four sectored discs, placed well away from the interrupted oblique figure. Figures such as figure 7 also evoke apparently cognitive contours and they also produce distortion illusions.

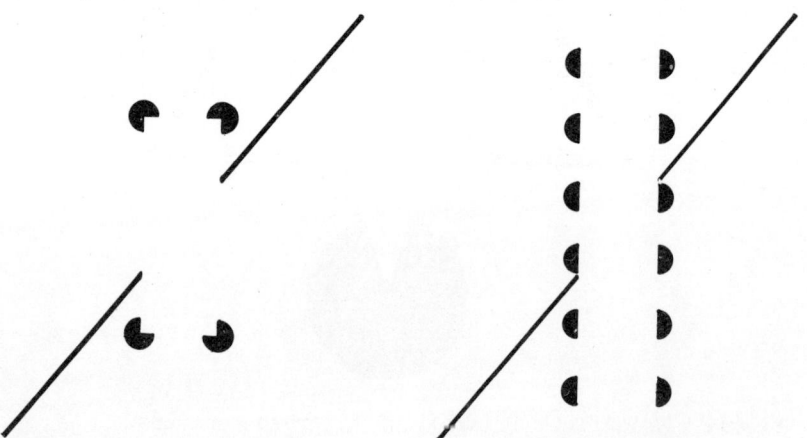

Figure 6 - Poggendorf figure generated from 'cognitive contours'.

Figure 7 - A second Poggendorf figure generated from illusory contours.

This seems significant, for how could these distortions be generated by physiological processes, signalling borders, if these borders are not signalled directly by sensory patterns but are, rather, called up from store as fictional hypotheses? It would seem that these effects are not due to physiological interaction effects, such as lateral inhibition, but they are compatible with the notion (Gregory, 1965,1970) that distortions can occur as a result of scaling being set inappropriately, to the surrounding objects, or line figures, by following usually predictive assumptions which do not apply to the given objects of line figures. (this happens especially when perspective features occur on flat picture planes). On this view, it is not the physiology which generates the errors: it is the strategy which leads to error, though of course the strategy is carried out by physiological events. If we do not understand the strategy we will not understand the phenomena, even though we may understand the physiology in every detail. If this view is approximately correct, we have an example where simply taking over paradigms of physics or physiology may be unhelpful, or seriously misleading. This remains true though we are not violating any physical or physiological principle with our cognitive paradigm.

The phenomena of perception deserve consideration though they may appear trivial. There is nothing new in this: some of physics' most dramatic successes came from questioning, and using as tools, trivial-looking phenomena which may have been children's toy things. Studying how pith balls, suspended on silk threads, are affected by rubbed amber; and how lode stones, floating freely, point to the only fixed star in the sky, lead to new ways of seeing - to new paradigms of the physical object world. Perhaps only phenomena (and not philosophy) have the power to suggest new paradigms: to break down old barriers which prevent us seeing how we see.